THIRD EDITION

Medical Terminology
in a **Flash!**

A Multiple Learning Styles Approach

THIRD EDITION

Medical Terminology
in a **Flash!**

A Multiple Learning Styles Approach

Lisa Finnegan, PTA, ACCE
Physical Therapy Educator
Academic Coordinator of Clinical Education
College of Southern Nevada
Las Vegas, Nevada

Sharon Eagle, RN, MSN

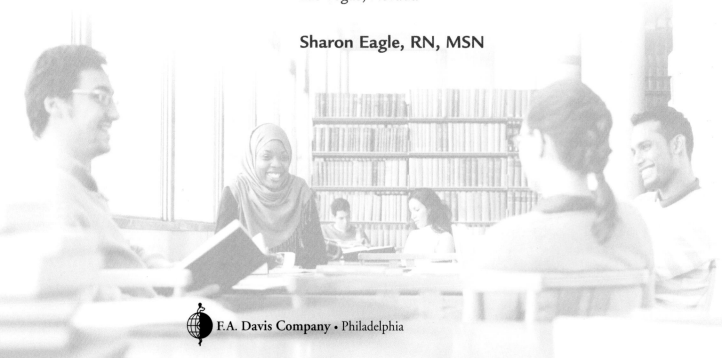

F.A. Davis Company • Philadelphia

F. A. Davis Company
1915 Arch Street
Philadelphia, PA 19103
www.fadavis.com

Copyright © 2016 by F. A. Davis Company

Printed in the United States of America

Last digit indicates print number: 10 9 8 7 6 5 4

Publisher: Quincy McDonald
Director of Content Development: George W. Lang
Developmental Editors: Joanna E. Cain and Pamela Speh
Art and Design Manager: Carolyn O'Brien

As new scientific information becomes available through basic and clinical research, recommended treatments and drug therapies undergo changes. The author(s) and publisher have done everything possible to make this book accurate, up to date, and in accord with accepted standards at the time of publication. The author(s), editors, and publisher are not responsible for errors or omissions or for consequences from application of the book, and make no warranty, expressed or implied, in regard to the contents of the book. Any practice described in this book should be applied by the reader in accordance with professional standards of care used in regard to the unique circumstances that may apply in each situation. The reader is advised always to check product information (package inserts) for changes and new information regarding dose and contraindications before administering any drug. Caution is especially urged when using new or infrequently ordered drugs.

ISBN 978-0-8036-4368-0

DEDICATION

For Tommy, Ryan, Jason, and Grandma Wolf

"Pantophobia. Not the fear of pants, though, if that's what you're thinking. It's the fear of everything. Including pants, I suppose, in that case."

The Doctor, *Doctor Who*

"There must exist certain words, in a certain specific order, that can explain all of this."

Walter White, *Breaking Bad*

PREFACE

Medical Terminology in a FLASH! 3rd edition was created for students of all ages, with all types of learning styles. Visual, auditory, verbal, and hands-on learners are supported through textbook and online resources.

For Instructors:

The third edition has been reorganized to facilitate use in all types of classrooms. The **new structure** allows instructors of traditional, online, flipped, and self-study courses to effortlessly use all or part of each chapter and utilize the book across multiple semesters if they choose. The addition of the **Medical Language Lab** will be especially appealing to instructors who would like to include an online component to their course. ***Davis Plus*** (http://davisplus. fadavis.com) continues to be the instructor's one-stop shop for important instructor resources. These resources include:

- ExamView Pro Electronic Test Bank
- PowerPoint Presentations for each chapter
- Image Resource (including all images from the book in jpeg format)
- Instructor's Manual (with additional teaching tips and activities)
- Teaching Guide (extensive teaching resource which offers lecture guidance, suggested homework assignments, and in-class activities for every lecture in a traditional one-term course)
- LMS Resource Kits (provides all of the resources on the DavisPlus site for *Medical Terminology in a Flash! 3e* in convenient-to-upload packets for the most popular learning management systems)

Updates to this edition include **Flash Cards** for every suffix, prefix, combining form, abbreviation, and pathology term in the book. New **Boxes** and improved **Flashpoint** features offer more information on certain topics as well as where to find additional information online. The **Learning Style Tips** feature has been improved by adding ideas to engage multiple learning styles in a single activity and by offering suggestions on how technology can be used to boost learning. The **Structure and Function** section of each chapter has been enhanced by supplying new exercises to strengthen the students' knowledge of key terms and definitions. Many of the exercises throughout the book are written by the author, and all of the answer keys are now located only in the Instructor's Guide to ensure that students are dedicating enough time to their assignments. There are **more abbreviations** in this edition, some of which will appeal to those in rehabilitation professions. The new **Pharmacology** section in each chapter is a great introduction to medications that will benefit those students who will soon be taking pharmacology courses.

New! The Medical Language Lab

The Medical Language Lab is an interactive, online experience for mastering the language of medicine. The MLL uses proven language methodology to give students the practice needed to become a fluent medical language speaker. Step by step, it guides students from basic through advanced levels of proficiency to become confident medical language speakers while also providing instructors administrative capabilities to create, customize, and manage classes and gradebooks.

Each lesson in the *Medical Language Lab* enables students to develop skills to listen critically for important terms, respond to others using medical terminology, and generate their own terminology-rich writing style and speech. By following the activities in each lesson, students graduate from simple memorization to becoming stronger users of the medical language.

For Students:

Medical Terminology in a FLASH! includes many features to facilitate your success in this course.

In the Textbook

- **Nearly 200 flash cards** including all suffixes and prefixes. Hundreds more are online on *Davis Plus (http://davisplus.fadavis.com).* The *IN A FLASH* icon will appear throughout each chapter to remind you to use your flash cards before moving on to the next section. See *Flash Card Game*s on page xxi for new ways to use your cards.
- **A workbook format** supports your learning by encouraging you to write directly in the book. The act of writing actively engages your brain in a way that reading alone cannot. Perforations allow you to remove as many pages as you'd like. You are able to tear out a few pages and carry them with you instead of carrying the whole book. This can be especially helpful when you are experiencing "wasted" moments in your day such as waiting in a line. If you have a few pages in your bag, you are able to have a quick study session!
- **Learning style tips** throughout the book help you learn and retain new information through activities that use your visual, auditory, verbal, and kinesthetic (hands-on) senses. Look for the learning style tip icons that represent the four learning styles Learning Style Tip. They will help you choose the activities that may be best for you.
- **Flashpoints and boxes** provide more information on certain topics within each chapter.
- **Clearly marked sections in each chapter** enable you to quickly and easily find specific assignments or information on which you need to focus. This is especially helpful if you are a self-study, online, or flipped classroom student. Chapters 1 and 2 help you to discover your learning style preferences and provide the suffix and prefix word parts

necessary for using medical terminology. Each chapter that follows includes a section on:

- **Structure and Function** with key medical terms and full-color anatomical illustrations of the body systems. Body parts are labeled, and combining forms are listed. This information is reinforced at the end of the section in matching and labeling exercises.
- **Combining Forms and Abbreviations** that pertain to each body system with color-coded tables. You will notice that **prefixes** are coded **green**, **suffixes** are coded **blue, combining forms** (word root + a vowel) are coded **teal**, **abbreviations** are coded **orange**, and **pathology terms** are coded **purple.** This color coding directly corresponds with the color-coded flash cards in the textbook. When you go to *DavisPlus* to print out more flash cards, consider using colored paper or markings that correspond to the color of the table.
- **Pathologies, Procedures, and Pharmacology** that pertain to each body system. You will find more than 300 medications described by their generic name, brand name, therapeutic classification, and common use. In addition, you will gain some insight into how the medications act on the body.
- **Exercises that correspond to each section** for courses that do not cover the entire chapter or that divide the material into multiple semesters. You can easily find the exercises that pertain only to the sections you studied.
- **End-of-chapter exercises** provide even more practice on everything you learned in the chapter.

Online at Davis Plus

Go to **http://davisplus.fadavis.com/** for free access to several more student resources including:

- Hundreds more printable flash cards!
- Practice quizzes for every chapter!

Online at Medical Language Lab

Go to **http://www.medicallanguagelab.com** and register using the access code provided in new copies of *Medical Terminology in a FLASH! 3e.* Your free access includes:

- Interactive eBook version of the entire text.
- Lecture videos covering every chapter in the text
- Audio tutorials and pronunciation guides
- Critical listening exercises
- Response exercises
- Term generation exercises; both spoken and written
- Word building exercises
- Labeling exercises
- Crosswords, and more!

The Flash Cards

Flash cards that correspond to all of the tables are provided for you. The back of this book contains all of the flash cards for chapters 2 and 3 as well as all of the combining form cards for chapter 4. All of the combining form cards for chapters 5 through 14 are online, ready for you to print out. You will also find cards for the abbreviation and pathology tables from every chapter online. Many of the flash cards contain visual cues, while others have an area for you to draw your own visual cue, which has meaning for you.

Be sure to practice with the flash cards after you complete each related section of the book. Take them with you when you exercise or go on road trips. Additionally, each day select a few cards to take with you in your purse or pocket, so that they are on hand during otherwise "wasted" moments such as when you're stuck waiting in a line.

- If you review five to 10 different flash cards several times each day, you can easily memorize 35 to 70 new terms each week without using your "official" study time. Over 10 weeks, that adds up to 350 to 700 new terms! Repetition is the key to memorization; flash cards make repetition easy.
- With color-coded flash cards, you will not only memorize the meanings of the word parts but will also memorize whether the word parts are suffixes, prefixes, combining forms, or pathology terms, without even making a conscious effort!
- The flash cards have terms with the same or similar meanings grouped together. Therefore, you will easily memorize two, three, or more terms in the same time it would normally take to memorize just one.

Flash Cards Games

Partner Flash/Two Players
Need one set of any number of flash cards. This is a good exercise to use when your partner is a friend or family member who is not learning medical terminology.

Give selected cards to your partner to shuffle. The partner will flash each card in front of you, one at a time. You will agree on a preset amount of time (5 seconds or less) to name the correct meaning, or correct term, depending upon which side is being flashed. Run through the cards until you can name each of them within the designated time limit. If you make a pile of cards for those you answered correctly and a pile for those you answered incorrectly, you will know which terms you need to practice a bit more.

Single Player Flash
Need one set of any number of flash cards.

Run through your cards alone, while racing against the clock. Challenge a classmate with the same set of cards to see who can complete the cards correctly, in the shortest amount of time.

Single Player Video Flash
Need one set of any number of flash cards and a video recording device.

Shuffle your cards. One at a time, show a term on your card to your video recorder. Hold it there for 3 to 5 seconds before you flip your card, showing the meaning. As you watch your completed recording, the hold time will allow you to guess the meaning of the term before you see the correct answer. Make another recording where you start by showing the meaning and then need to guess the term.

Single Player Audio Flash
Need one set of any number of flash cards and an audio recording device.

Shuffle your cards. One at a time, read a term aloud into your audio recorder. Pause quietly for 3 to 5 seconds and then flip your card and read the meaning aloud. As you listen to your completed recording, the quiet pause will allow you to guess the meaning of the term before you hear the correct answer. Make another recording where you start by reading the meaning aloud and then need to guess the term.

Systems Game/One or More Players

Need the same set of systems flash cards for each player and a blank piece of paper with the name of each system written on top.

Start by playing with cards from two systems such as the integumentary system and the nervous system. Slowly add cards from more systems to make your game more challenging.

Players use their own cards and their own papers. The papers with the system names are laid out in front of each player in whatever order they choose. Shuffle the cards and, when ready, begin matching cards to the system they belong to by laying them down on the correct sheet of paper. The first player to correctly match all of his or her cards to the correct system is the winner. This game can also be played alone while racing against the clock.

Speed/Two Players

Need two sets of the same flash cards. Be sure to label your cards with an identifying mark or color so that your cards can be returned to you at the end of the game.

Players shuffle their cards, face each other and, when ready, begin laying down cards (each in a separate pile) at the same time. When players happen to lay down identical cards, the first one to correctly say the term and name the correct definition takes the matching cards from both piles and puts them aside. Matches will be infrequent at the beginning but will occur more and more frequently as cards are eliminated from play. The game continues until all cards are out of play. The winner is the one who collects the most pairs.

Score Four/Three or More Players

Need one set of the same cards per player. Be sure to label your cards with an identifying mark or color so that your cards can be returned to you at the end of the game.

Each player contributes a set of the same cards related to one or more body systems. All cards are shuffled together, and four are dealt to each player. Remaining cards are placed in a "draw" pile in the center of the table. The object of the game is to collect all four cards of a term. Because the cards have identifying data on both sides, the players will have to hold the cards so that no one else can see them. Players take turns asking other players for cards with a specific term. For example, the first player already has two cards with the term "gastr/o" and wants to collect the other two. On her turn, she would name another player and ask for all cards with the term "gastr/o" and would also pronounce the correct translation "stomach." The other player must hand over all cards with that term. If the other player does not have that card, then the first player must draw a card from the draw pile. Once a player has collected all four cards, that player should lay them on the table and state the term and the correct translation aloud. If the player forgets these steps when laying down the cards, another player may claim the cards by stating the magic words "Score Four!" and must then pronounce the term and identify the correct translation. If the player is unable to name the correct translation (without looking), the original player keeps control of the cards. The winner of the game is the one with the most four-card matches when all cards have been played.

REVIEWERS

Dr. Ana T. Alvarez-Calonge, MLT, RMA, BMO, AHI, DHSc
Program Director/Clinical Coordinator
Southeastern College
Miami Lakes, FL

Ann Hardison Black, MSN, RN
Practical Nursing Faculty
Montgomery Community College
Troy, NC

Cynthia R. Callahan, MEd, MLS(ASCP)CM
Program Director
Stanly Community College
Locust, NC

Cindy J. Drenning, MSN, CRNP
Assistant Professor
Saint Francis University
Loretto, PA

Bobbie Drodwell, RN, BSN, MSN
Nursing Instructor
ATS Institute of Technology
Chicago, IL

April Imes, RMA
Medical Assistant Instructor
Southeastern Institute
Charlotte, NC

Terri L. Kines, RN
Adjunct Instructor
Horry Georgetown Technical College
Myrtle Beach, SC

Kimberly Martin, BSN, MEd, PHN, RN
Director of Nursing
Stanbridge College
Irvine, CA

Rita Mattson, CST
Instructor/Program Director
Erwin Technical Center
Tampa, FL

Shannon B. Morris, CPC
Advanced Medical Coding Instructor
Catawba Valley Community College
Hickory, NC

Stephen J. Nardozzi, EMT-P, BA, Graduate Certificate EMS Planning
Assistant Professor and Chair
Westchester Community College
Valhalla, NY

Bradley W. Sage, MEd, LAT, ATC
Lecturer, Coordinator of Clinical Education
Mercyhurst University
Erie, PA

La Tanya Young Thomas, BSN, MMSc, MPH, RN, PA-C
Program Chair
Atlanta Technical College
Atlanta, GA

Rajinder Virk, BEd (Candidate), RCT(A), MLT
Professor, Program Coordinator
Mohawk-McMaster Institute for Applied Health Sciences
Hamilton, Ontario, Canada

ACKNOWLEDGMENTS

I believe that everything happens for a reason. In some cases, it takes many years before you even realize you have been on a journey. I would like to express my gratitude to everyone involved in the series of events that led to this moment. I think it may have begun with my instructors in the CSN Physical Therapist Assistant Program, Joann Gutschick and Dr. Joe Cracraft. Thank you for changing my life twice. I was thrilled to return to the PTA program as an instructor and am so happy to be doing for others what you did for me. I continue to learn from you and am honored to be your colleague and friend. Thank you to Dr. Mark Guadagnoli at the University of Nevada Las Vegas. I just happened to pick your class from a list of possibilities. Because of you and your teaching style, I developed an interest in brain-based learning, and I changed my teaching methods. Many of those changes became learning activities that are represented throughout this book. Often, when a student compliments me or I have a really great day in the classroom, I smile and think to myself, "I learned that from Dr. G." Thank you to all of my students in the Physical Therapist Assistant Program who challenge me to be a better teacher every semester. Special thanks to the class of 2013 for suggesting I write a book about the learning activities I created for them. When my sales rep from F. A. Davis stopped by one day, I decided to take their advice. Thank you to Greg Middleton at F. A. Davis for listening to my sales pitch and for remembering me at exactly the right moment. Because of you, I met Quincy.

Thank you to Quincy McDonald at F. A. Davis for choosing me for this project. It has truly been a pleasure working with you and your whole team. It was very easy to do my best work for a group of people who treated me with kindness and professionalism every step of the way. Thank you to Sharon Eagle for allowing me to join in your vision for student success. I also want to express an enormous amount of gratitude to Joanna Cain and Pamela Speh of Auctorial Pursuits, Inc. for your guidance, organization, encouragement, and kindness. Thank you Gayle Crist for ensuring that I used the right words at the right time. Finally, thank you to all of the reviewers. Your input and advice facilitated some great improvements. When I entered the PTA Program 15 years ago, I had no idea that I was beginning this journey. Thank you so much to everybody who supported me and who helped me reach this destination.

TABLE OF CONTENTS

LEARNING STYLES

1

Chapter Outline

Overview

Learning style theory suggests that individuals learn information in different ways according to their unique abilities and traits. Therefore, while all humans are similar, the ways in which you best perceive, understand, and remember information may be somewhat different from the ways other people learn.

In truth, all people possess a combination of styles. You may be especially strong in one style and less so in others. You may be strong in two or three areas or may be equally strong in all areas. As you learn about the styles described in this chapter, you may begin to recognize your preferences and will then be able to modify your study activities accordingly. Try using multiple learning styles as you study rather than choosing one in particular. This will help you make the most of your valuable time, enhance your learning, and support you in doing your very best in future classes.

Sensory Learning Styles

Experts have identified numerous learning styles and have given them various names. Some are described in an abstract and complex manner, while others are relatively simple and easy to grasp. For ease of understanding, this book uses the learning styles associated with your senses. You use your senses to see and hear information. You use touch and manipulation or your sense of taste or smell. You may find it useful to think aloud as you discuss new information with someone else. Because the senses are so often involved in the acquisition of new information, many learning styles are named accordingly: visual, auditory, verbal, and kinesthetic (hands-on or tactile).

Visual Learning

Most people have a preference for visual learning. To most accurately and quickly grasp new information, these types of learners need to see the information represented visually. The more complex the data, the more this is true. Visual learners especially like data that are colorful and visually striking. Within the classroom, they prefer instructors who use written outlines and many visual aids. During exams, they may recall information by "seeing" it in their mind's eye, whether it is an actual picture or diagram or a fragment of written text. Visual information can be presented in many ways. Examples include:

Written words	Flowcharts
Diagrams	Time lines
Shapes	Maps
Patterns	Handouts
Colors	Posters
Symbols	Flash cards
Illustrations	PowerPoint presentations
Graphs	Internet data
Photos	Videos
Tables	Live demonstrations

Study Strategies for Visual Learning

Try using any study or memory technique that aids you in visually seeing and recalling information. You may find *mnemonics* (memory aids) especially helpful for remembering lists or sequenced pieces of information. Generally speaking, the more creative, whimsical, funny, or absurd they are, the better you will remember them. There are many different types of mnemonics. Some examples follow.

- Children use the well-known alphabet song, a *musical* mnemonic, to learn their ABCs.
- Students in anatomy classes use one of several mnemonic variations to remember the 12 cranial nerves (olfactory, optic, oculomotor, trochlear, trigeminal, abducens, facial, acoustic, glossopharyngeal, vagus, spinal accessory, and hypoglossal). One example is "On old Olympus' tower tops, a Finn and German viewed some hops." Note that the first letter of each word is the same as the first letter of each cranial nerve's name.
- When spelling, most people use this *rhyming* mnemonic to remember where to place the *I* and *E* in a word: "I before E, except after C."

Another form of commonly used mnemonics is the *acronym*. An acronym is an abbreviation created by using the first letters or word parts in names or phrases. Examples of acronyms include:

LASER—**L**ight **a**mplification by **s**timulated **e**mission of **r**adiation
INTERPOL—**Inter**national Criminal **Pol**ice Organization
FAQ—**F**requently **a**sked **q**uestions
PIN—**P**ersonal **i**dentification **n**umber
OLD CART—**O**nset, **l**ocation, **d**uration, **c**haracter, **a**ggravating factors, **r**elieving factors, **t**reatments

The seven warning signs of cancer can be remembered in the acronym CAUTION:

Change in bowel or bladder habits
A sore throat that does not heal
Unusual bleeding or discharge
Thickening or a lump in the breast or other area

Indigestion or difficulty swallowing
Obvious change in a mole or wart
Nagging cough or hoarseness

And finally, the warning signs of malignant melanoma are shown by the acronym ABCD:

Asymmetry—One half of the mole does not match the other half.
Border—The edges of the mole are irregular or blurred.
Color—The color varies throughout, including tan, brown, black, blue, red, or white.
Diameter—The mole is larger than 6 millimeters.

Auditory Learning

Many people have a preference for auditory (or aural) learning. In order to most accurately and quickly grasp new information, these people need to hear it spoken. The more complex the data, the more this is true. The most common example of auditory information sharing is a classroom lecture; however, there are other ways to hear information. Examples include audiotapes, videotapes, computer tutorials (with audio content), and oral discussions.

Study Strategies for Auditory Learning

Try using any study or memory technique that allows you to hear information. It can be the spoken word, data set to music, a recording of a lecture, or any other auditory format. Recordings can be valuable study tools because you can listen to them during times when you normally cannot study, such as while driving, exercising, or performing household chores. Auditory learners are usually verbal learners as well. If this is true for you, then you may learn best when you have the chance for a verbal exchange. This allows you to speak to and listen to others. For this reason, you may sometimes prefer studying with a partner or in a study group. You can also use your verbal and auditory styles together by making a recording of your own voice. Speak into the recorder as if you were "teaching" the information to another person. Like the visual learner, you may find mnemonics helpful, especially if they include rhymes or are catchy and fun to say aloud.

Verbal Learning

It is sometimes said that some people must think (first) in order to speak. For those who prefer verbal learning, the reverse may be true: They feel compelled to speak in order to think. What this means is that speaking aloud helps them process information and think things through. This is especially true when the information is complex or the situation feels stressful.

Verbal learning can include both the spoken and written word. Note that when reading aloud, the spoken word is also heard, and the written word is also seen. This is an example of how three learning styles are used simultaneously. You may feel that you are verbal learner, but if you read aloud, you are actually using auditory and visual styles as well.

Study Strategies for Verbal Learning

Try using study or memory techniques that allow you to speak aloud in order to recite data or explain concepts. Like auditory learners, you may find mnemonics helpful, especially if they are fun to say or include rhyming. You may also find writing to be very helpful. Writing down important data, such as outlines and summaries, in a form that is meaningful for you and then reciting those things aloud helps you remember the content. You may benefit from studying with a partner or in a study group. This provides ample opportunity for discussion. It is helpful to explain challenging concepts or "teach" your study partners about a given topic. For example, the members of your study group may decide to teach one another about the four major joint types in the body: hinge, ball-and-socket, pivot, and gliding. Each person describes the appearance and function of a type of joint and gives an example. One person may compare a hinge joint, like those found in the knee and elbow, to a door hinge. While doing so, the student describes how it moves back and forth like a door that swings open and shut. The next person may compare a pivot joint, such as the one in the neck, to a chair that turns back and forth in a 180-degree half-circle. Other students may then go on to teach about their assigned joints and give examples. This type of exercise may also involve visual and kinesthetic learning as the members of the group demonstrate what they are verbalizing. To maximize the value of this exercise for verbal learners, you can add a requirement that all members of the group must verbally repeat key information or phrases after the "teacher."

Kinesthetic Learning

Most people have some kinesthetic (tactile) aspects to perceiving, understanding and remembering information. People who are strong kinesthetic learners use their bodies as they learn. They like to touch and manipulate objects. This is especially important when learning physical skills. Kinesthetic learners are often also using their visual, verbal, and auditory learning styles at the same time. Examples of physical learning include:

- Demonstrations
- Simulations
- Practicing a skill

Study Strategies for Kinesthetic Learning

Try using study or memory techniques that allow you to move your body or touch objects. For example, if you are learning the bones of the body, touch that bone on your own body or combine it with the visual learning style and point to it on a partner or on a model of a skeleton. Add the verbal and auditory learning styles by saying the name of the bone aloud as you touch it. When learning skills or procedures, your best strategy is to actually get your hands on the needed supplies and practice the procedure. Consider again the study group in which you and your friends are each describing major types of body joints. In addition to verbally describing the joints and giving examples, add a requirement that each person must somehow act out or physically mimic the joint movement—something like a charades game with talking allowed. The person describing the hinge joint now must physically get up and find a door to open and shut while describing its function. Better yet, the person might play the part of the door by moving the body back and forth. The next person compares a pivot joint, such as the one in the neck, with a chair that turns back and forth in a 180-degree half-circle. While describing this, the individual literally turns the head back and forth and then turns the chair back and forth in a 180-degree circle. After each person performs a physical demonstration, other members of the group must perform the same movement. This gives everyone full kinesthetic value from the activity in addition to verbal, auditory, and visual benefits.

When actual physical practice of a skill is not possible, visualization is a great alternative. It gives you the chance to "practice" skills in your mind and even move your body, arms, and hands as you would when performing the actual skill. When the content is theoretical, you still benefit from physical movement. Play learning games, use flash cards, complete activities included in your textbook or online, and interact with a study partner or group.

Social Preferences

In addition to sensory preferences, you may also have a social inclination for learning. If you notice that interacting with others helps you to grasp and understand information, you may benefit from a social learning environment. On the other hand, you may feel that you do your best when working alone without the distraction of others, in a solitary learning environment. Don't limit yourself to one or the other. Learning can be enhanced by studying in both environments.

Social Learning

Many people learn effectively when they are able to interact with other people. They enjoy group *synergy* (the enhanced action of two or more agents working together cooperatively) and are able to think things through with the verbal exchange that occurs during a lively discussion. Examples of social learning include:

- Discussions about specific topics
- Question-and-answer sessions
- Group projects
- Group games
- Role-playing
- Peer assessments

Study Strategies for Social Learning

If you prefer social learning, you may find that you feel restless and have difficulty staying focused when you try to study alone. You need to seek out opportunities to study with one or more additional people. If there isn't a study group available, consider starting one. Your study group will be most effective if you set and adhere to some ground rules that provide structure. Here are some suggestions:

- Identify a group leader—preferably someone with some knowledge or experience in the subject being studied.
- Have the group complete specified readings or assignments prior to each meeting.
- Have the group members agree to stay on task so the group doesn't deteriorate into a social group or complaint session.
- Set and follow time limits.
- Encourage all members to contribute.

Solitary Learning

Many people learn effectively when they are able to study alone without distraction from others. Solitary learners can participate in group study sessions by using technology. Discussion boards, social media, and online collaboration tools allow solitary learners to provide input or focus on the information they feel is most relevant while still studying alone.

Study Strategies for Solitary Learning

If you prefer solitary learning, you may feel frustrated when trying to study with a partner or a group. You may feel like they are wasting your time and believe you would do better by yourself. You focus and concentrate best when alone. You may be a self-starter who doesn't need anyone else to prompt you or provide structure.

There are many ways that solitary learners study. They may read the textbook, review and revise notes, make and listen to audio recordings, create and use flash cards, complete online activities, use digital "apps," watch videos, or practice a skill. For these learners, the important thing is that they do it alone.

Global Versus Analytical Preferences

In addition to the sensory and social styles described above, most people tend to initially grasp information either as a whole, looking at the "big picture," or in a more sequential fashion in which the individual parts are studied first to comprehend the whole. If you are in the first group, you have a preference for global learning. If you are in the second group, you prefer analytical learning.

Global Learning

Global learners, sometimes called *holistic* learners, generally see the big picture first and later pay more attention to details. For example, when studying the human body, global learners first see the body as a whole, complete organism. With that picture in mind, they are then able to begin studying the parts. This is true even when studying individual body systems, such as the cardiovascular system. Global learners first grasp the big picture of the entire system as it circulates blood throughout the body. With further study and thought, they appreciate how the system delivers oxygen and nutrients and eliminates waste through a complex network of vessels including veins, arteries, and capillaries.

Study Strategies for Global Learning

If you prefer global learning, you may process information best using your visual and auditory abilities. When you find studying details to be tedious and boring, try to find other, more creative and fun ways to learn the same material. For example, you may prefer drawing your own colorful diagrams or may enjoy using audiovisual tutorials or other activities that are often available online or in digital "apps."

Use your strengths. It's likely that you are flexible and a multitasker. Don't be afraid to mix it up a bit to make your study efforts more lively and enjoyable. You are good at seeing the overall picture and recognizing relationships; therefore, begin each study session by identifying the relationship between what you are currently studying and your future career ambitions.

Beware of your tendency to overlook details. You can compensate with strategies that help you identify and remember details of significance. While reading, make note of terms, concepts, or sections that you skipped over or did not understand. You can do this by highlighting these areas in a specific color or by writing notes in the margins. Once you've completed your initial read, force yourself to return to each of these areas and investigate them further. When deciding how much time and energy to devote to each one, ask yourself the following questions:

- Is there a learning objective in the syllabus that pertains to this content?
- Might this content impact my understanding of the whole?
- How likely is the instructor to include a test question on this content?
- How relevant is this content to the remainder of this class, to future classes, or to my future career?

Analytical Learning

Analytical learners, sometimes called *logical, linear, sequential,* or *mathematical* learners, generally need to see the parts before fully comprehending the whole. Analytical learners readily identify patterns and like to group data into categories for further study. They may create and follow agendas, make lists with items ranked by priority, and approach problem-solving in a logical, methodical manner.

Some of the same qualities that are your strengths can, at times, become a source of frustration. For example, you may get stuck in "analysis paralysis" as you study details. This can stall forward movement and impair decision-making. To you, facts are only facts when they are indisputably accurate and supported by reliable data. In turn, other people may become frustrated by your need to gather more data and process information in detail (often verbally). In most cases, they really don't want to hear all of your logic and rationale and instead wish you would just get to the point.

Study Strategies for Analytical Learning

If you prefer analytical learning, you may process information verbally, which means you sometimes talk to yourself and think aloud. You may also have a visual dimension to your preferred learning style that lends itself so well to grouping information into categories and drawing connections.

Use a variety of styles to maximize learning, but take care not to get stuck in analysis paralysis or sidetracked with insignificant detail. Put your organizational talent to work to make your study efforts productive: Make an agenda or create a list of topics to be studied. Prioritize topics to ensure that you address the most important things first. This is your "Need to Know" list. Set and follow time limits, but don't overanalyze your plan. It is most important to get busy studying. Rather than getting sidetracked with interesting (but low-priority) items, make another list of topics as you go along titled "Nice to Know." Come back to this list later if—and only if—time permits. Use your gift for identifying patterns by noting patterns within the material you are studying. This can be useful when you prepare for exams, because test questions often focus on features that are similar and those that are different. For example, a myocardial infarction (MI) and angina both cause chest pain. In both cases, the pain is caused by inadequate blood supply to the heart. These are two important and similar features when comparing these disorders—chest pain and lack of oxygen. On the other hand, an MI causes actual death of heart muscle tissue, while angina does not. This is an important difference.

To make the most of some study strategies, you must give yourself permission to be illogical or even silly. If a technically "inaccurate" mnemonic or silly song will help you remember something, then why not use it? Your global-learner classmates can help you with this if you will let them.

It's likely that you are a good reflective thinker and are able to evaluate your own performance. However, this can also become a flaw, because you are probably a perfectionist and may be too hard on yourself. You must learn to let the small stuff go, not let other people bug you, and give yourself permission to be less than perfect. If other students distract or annoy you with their behaviors or chosen study tactics, try to ignore them. You may need to physically separate yourself from them to do so. You need to do your "analytical thing" and allow them to do their "global thing." You will both achieve the same goals in different ways. The exception is when you must work with others as part of a group assignment. This can be challenging for students of different styles, but this mirrors real life. In fact, this is the main reason instructors assign group work: It gives you the opportunity to practice communication and teamwork skills. In this case, it will help if everyone on the team begins by sharing information about their individual styles, including strengths, flaws, and needs. Group roles and tasks can be divided according to each person's style and strengths.

Identifying Your Style

In reading through this chapter, you probably recognized yourself in more than one of the styles described. Try using multiple learning styles instead of selecting one in particular. Think of your brain as a busy city. Is there only one way to reach your destination or are there multiple routes to choose from? If you limit yourself to only one method of learning, you are creating only one pathway to retrieve the information you stored in your memory. Using multiple learning styles will enable you to create multiple pathways and improve your chances of reaching your destination with ease! Soon, you'll begin to understand yourself better and will recognize your preferences for learning. This will help you to identify study strategies that will be most effective for you and will allow you to make the most of limited study time.

Learning Styles and Medical Terminology

Any course in medical terminology requires students to learn and remember a huge amount of information. As you learn various terms and their meanings, you must find a way to commit this knowledge to memory. In other words, you must *memorize* large amounts of data. There is no way around it; you are learning a foreign language, and to become fluent in this language, you must develop a large, accurate vocabulary and must know how to use it.

So how does learning style theory apply to learning medical terminology? By having a clear understanding of your style preferences, you will be able to use your strengths and abilities to their fullest. Knowing what *not* to do becomes as important as knowing what to *do*. Because learning and remembering memorized data are key to this course, understanding how memory works will help you to accomplish this.

Memory

Human memory is the process by which people store, retain, and retrieve information (Fig. 1-1). Perceiving, processing, and storing information are complex processes that involve many parts of your brain. It is beyond the scope of this

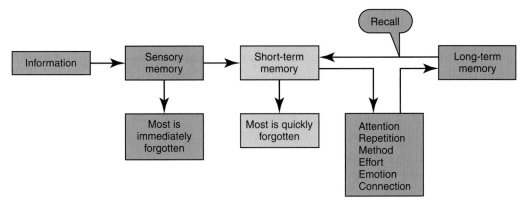

FIGURE 1-1 **Memory.**

book to describe the process in detail. However, a few key points are worth mentioning.

Sensory memory involves the first brief impression during which your brain registers patterns, sounds, smells, or other sensory data. You then almost immediately forget it, although you do store some data for later retrieval.

Perception and storage of information requires a complex combination of electrical and chemical functions within the nervous tissue of your brain, usually in your *short-term memory.* This allows you to retrieve the information for a very short span of time, usually several seconds to several minutes. In general, most people are able to retrieve four to seven items of information from short-term memory. This capability increases if the data are clustered into groups; this is known as *chunking.* For example, you may have noticed that it is easier to remember a string of numbers, such as a telephone number, if you chunk the numbers, such as in 233-467-9012 rather than 2334679012.

Memorization is a method that allows you to recall data through a process known as rote learning. It can be an effective strategy for you if you use it in the right way. It has been shown that most people's ability to retain memorized information is enhanced if they rehearse the data intermittently over an extended period of time rather than using a last-minute cram-and-forget method. In other words, cramming may or may not get you through the next exam, but it certainly will not support your long-term success in future classes or your future career. To get important memorized data into your *long-term memory,* you must do more than cram. Long-term memory is capable of storing an infinite amount of data for an indefinite period of time, perhaps for a lifetime. However, getting the information you wish to remember into your long-term memory is sometimes challenging. A number of factors are required, among them healthy functioning of several parts of the brain and a sufficient quantity and quality of sleep. Other factors important to long-term memory retention include:

- Attention (the extent to which you consciously attend to and focus on the data)
- Repetition (rehearsal of the data over and over)
- Information processing methods (strategies used to analyze and remember data; examples include chunking or other means of organizing data and using creative tricks such as mnemonics and acronyms)

- Study effort (the time and energy you devote; the greater your effort, the better your recall)
- Emotional relationship (relating the information being studied to strong emotions or significant events)
- Connection (relating new information to a prior experience or previously learned information)

Some activities hamper your ability to store and recall information in both your short-term and long-term memory banks. Examples include:

- Interference (stimuli that hamper your ability to attend to information as you learn)
- Cramming (extensive memorization of a large amount of data over a short period of time; cramming results in very poor recall and may displace other data in short-term memory)

Some general measures can help you in this process. General self-care activities that enhance memory include healthy nutrition; stress-reduction activities; regular exercise; socialization activities; and regular, good-quality sleep.

Plan for Success

To ensure your success in this course, you must take a bit of time now to do a self-assessment. It won't take long, and the information you gather will pay off big time. Completing the chapter activities below will guide you in this process. Once you've identified your preferences for learning, then you will be able to get the most from this book. You will notice specific *Learning Style Tips* scattered throughout all chapters (Fig. 1-2). The four styles you have learned about are labeled with icons that allow you to quickly find those that may be most relevant to you. However, it would be to your benefit to read them all; your style is probably a blend of the various styles, and you may want to consider trying all of the tips to find the ones that fit you best.

Learning Style Tips

Special tips for visual, auditory, verbal, and kinesthetic learners are placed throughout this book. You can identify each type by the icons shown below.

 Tip for visual learners

 Tip for verbal learners

 Tip for auditory learners

 Tip for kinesthetic learners

FIGURE 1-2 **Learning style tips.**

Chapter Activities

1. Investigate websites that provide free self-assessment tests such as those listed below. Take two or three different tests and compare your results. Describe what you learned about your strengths and what may be your preferred learning style(s). Be prepared to discuss your answers with your classmates.
   - http://vark-learn.com/the-vark-questionnaire
   - http://www.edutopia.org/multiple-intelligences-assessment

2. Briefly describe some study strategies that were suggested and that you are willing to try.

3. Create a plan that you believe will help you to be most effective in this course. Include approximate study times and techniques, and note which will be solitary and which will be social in nature.

4. Identify the activities you plan to employ to transfer as much medical terminology data as possible into your long-term memory.

As you continue through this book, you will find study tips included in every chapter. These tips suggest study techniques for all learning styles. Keep an open mind as you move forward and be willing to try any strategies that you believe may be helpful. Make notes as you do so about what did and did not work well and anything you might do differently next time. By the end of this course, you will have developed a good working knowledge of medical terminology. You will also have learned more about yourself and your learning preferences than you know now. Both of these things will serve you extremely well in your future classes and career.

Practice Exercises

Matching

Match the following terms with the correct description. Each answer is used once.

Exercise 1

1. _____ Visual

    a. Prefers to study alone

2. _____ Auditory

    b. Needs to see data with the eyes

3. _____ Verbal

    c. Needs to speak in order to think

4. _____ Kinesthetic

    d. Needs to hear the spoken word

5. _____ Social

    e. Enjoys group synergy and lively discussions

6. _____ Solitary

    f. Needs to touch and manipulate things

True or False

Decide whether the following statements are true or false.

Exercise 2

1. True   False   Most people have only one predominant learning style.

2. True   False   For visual learners, the more complex the data, the more important it is for them to see it.

3. True   False   Written text is an example of visual data.

4. True   False   Most auditory learners are also solitary learners.

5. True   False   Kelly enjoys meditation and traveling alone. She is a solitary learner.

Multiple Choice

Select the one best answer to the following multiple-choice questions.

Exercise 3

1. Colors, tables, and live demonstrations all appeal to which type of learners?

    a. Visual

    b. Auditory

    c. Kinesthetic

    d. Verbal

2. Visual learners are most likely to make which of the following statements?

   a. "That sounds like an experience I had."

   b. "This doesn't feel right to me."

   c. "I see what you mean."

   d. "Let's cooperate on this project."

3. Which of the following is the **best** example of an auditory way to get information?

   a. Reviewing flash cards

   b. Watching a PowerPoint presentation

   c. Listening to a lecture

   d. Asking a question

4. Jonathon loves music and is always humming, whistling, or singing something. In a recent conversation, he told his friend, "I hear you loud and clear." Jonathon is most likely:

   a. A visual learner   c. An auditory learner

   b. A social learner   d. A kinesthetic learner

5. Brian fidgets in the classroom and struggles to get through lectures, yet when he is in the laboratory, he does very well and enjoys learning. His dominant learning style is most likely:

   a. Auditory   c. Kinesthetic

   b. Solitary   d. Verbal

6. Which of the following is an example of an acronym?

   a. "I before E except after C"

   b. FAQ - frequently asked questions

   c. The alphabet (ABCs) song

   d. "On old Olympus' tower tops, a Finn and German viewed some hops."

7. All of the following statements are true regarding analytical learners **except:**

   a. They are sometimes called holistic learners.

   b. They like to take a methodical approach to studying.

   c. They readily identify patterns and like to group data into categories for further study.

   d. They create and follow agendas and make lists with items ranked by priority.

8. Which type of learner would benefit in a study group that is taking turns describing information aloud while performing a physical demonstration?

   a.   kinesthetic only

   b.   verbal only

   c.   visual only

   d.   kinesthetic, verbal, visual and auditory

9. Which of the following statements is **not** true about using a multiple learning styles approach?

   a.   It will help you to identify study strategies that will be most effective for you and will allow you to make the most of limited study time.

   b.   It is too difficult and is not recommended.

   c.   It creates multiple pathways in the brain for retrieving information from your memory.

   d.   It will help you to recognize your preferences for learning.

10. Which of the following statements about memory is true?

   a.   Sensory memory involves the first brief impression during which the brain registers sensory data such as patterns, sounds, or smells.

   b.   Short-term memory allows you to retrieve data in a very short span of time, usually several seconds to several minutes.

   c.   Chunking is a technique that increases the number of items one can recall.

   d.   All of the statements are true.

True or False

Decide whether the following statements are true or false.

Exercise 4

1. True   False   Many learning styles are named according to the special senses.

2. True   False   Few people are strong visual learners.

3. True   False   Verbal learners need to listen as others speak.

4. True   False   *Auditory* and *aural* have similar meanings.

5. True   False   Kinesthetic learners like to touch and manipulate objects.

Multiple Choice

Select the one best answer to the following multiple-choice questions.

Exercise 5

1. Diagrams, shapes, and patterns are examples of which type of data?

    a. kinesthetic

    b. visual

    c. solitary

    d. verbal

2. Using flash cards with a partner benefits which type of learner?

    a. visual learners only

    b. auditory learners only

    c. social learners only

    d. verbal learners only

    e. visual, auditory, social and verbal learners

3. Which of the following statements is **not** true regarding solitary learners?

    a. They can use all learning styles when studying.

    b. They can participate in group study sessions.

    c. They can focus and concentrate best when alone.

    d. All of the statements are true

4. Which of the following techniques may **not** appeal to visual learners?

    a. musical mnemonics

    b. acronyms

    c. group discussion

    d. rhyming mnemonics

5. Oral discussions appeal to students with which learning style?

    a. verbal only

    b. auditory only

    c. social only

    d. verbal, auditory and social

6. Which of the following statements are true regarding global learners?

   a.   They are sometimes called sequential learners.

   b.   They like to analyze details.

   c.   They may overlook details.

   d.   They approach problem-solving in a very logical manner.

7. All of the following words of advice are specifically appropriate for global learners **except:**

   a.   You are flexible, so don't be afraid to mix it up a bit and make your study efforts more lively and enjoyable.

   b.   Begin each study session by identifying the relationship between what you are currently studying and your future career ambitions.

   c.   Beware of your tendency to get stuck in analysis paralysis.

   d.   While reading, make note of terms or concepts that you skipped over and later take time to look them up.

8. All of the following words of advice are appropriate for students working on a group project **except:**

   a.   Do not put global and analytical learners in the same group.

   b.   Divide tasks according to learning style preferences and strengths.

   c.   Practice communication and teamwork skills because this mirrors real life.

   d.   Share information with each other about strengths, flaws and needs.

9. All of the following words of advice are specifically appropriate for analytical learners **except:**

   a.   Prioritize items of importance for studying.

   b.   Identify patterns within the material you are studying.

   c.   Give yourself permission to be illogical or even silly.

   d.   All of these are appropriate words of advice for analytical learners.

10. Which of the following statements about memory is true?

   a.   Most data move easily from short-term to long-term memory.

   b.   Emotions affect whether some information is stored in long-term memory.

   c.   Cramming is an effective method of transmitting data into long-term memory.

   d.   All of these statements are true.

MEDICAL WORD ELEMENTS

2

Chapter Outline

Word Parts

Most medical words derive from Greek or Latin and therefore may look and sound odd to you. However, once you have taken the time to learn the meanings of the word parts, you will be able to understand most of the medical terms you encounter, regardless of how big or complex they appear. There are three types of word parts that you need to know: (1) suffixes, (2) prefixes, and (3) combining forms (created by joining a *word root* to a *combining vowel*). You will use these word parts in a three-step process to find the meanings of medical terms. You also need to know the abbreviations and pathology terms that are used in health care; however, the three-step deciphering process often does not work with these terms.

Flashpoint
Word Root (WR) +
Combining Vowel (CV) =
Combined Form (CF)

Suffixes

A **suffix** is a word part that comes at the end of the medical term. If the suffix *-meter* (instrument used to measure) is added to the combining form therm/o, the result is the creation of the word therm/o/**meter,** an instrument used to measure heat.

Prefixes

A **prefix** is a word part that comes at the beginning of the medical term. For example, again consider the word root therm. If it is joined with the prefix *hypo-* (beneath or below) and the suffix -ia (condition), then a new word is created: *hypo*/therm/ia, a condition of low heat. As you may already know, this term is used in reference to a condition of low body temperature.

Combining Forms

The **combining form** is created by joining a **word root** with a **combining vowel**. A word root (WR) is the main stem, or primary meaning, of the word. An example using a nonmedical term is the word *walking*. The main stem or root of this word is *walk*. A combining vowel (CV) is used to make the medical term easier to pronounce. You could say that it makes medical terms more user-friendly for the tongue. A combining vowel is not always necessary. When it is needed, in nearly all cases the combining vowel is an *o,* although there are a few exceptions.

The combining vowel has no impact on the meaning of the term; it is placed between word parts to link them together. For example, consider the root *therm,* which means *heat.* If this word root is combined with the combining vowel *o,* the result is the combining form *therm/o.* Combining vowels are typically used to link word parts together regardless of whether the following part is a suffix or another combining form.

When to Use a Combining Vowel

To determine the need for a combining vowel, notice whether the following word part begins with a consonant or a vowel. If it begins with a consonant, as in the word *therm/o/meter,* then a combining vowel (often *o*) is usually needed. However, if the next word part begins with a vowel *(a, e, i, o, u),* then a combining vowel is usually not needed. This is because the vowel at the beginning of the next word part serves as the combining vowel. For example, when the root *arthr,* which means *joint,* is combined with the suffix *-itis,* which means *inflammation,* no combining vowel is needed. The *i* in *-itis* serves as the combining vowel. The new term *arthr/itis* is created, which means *inflammation of a joint.* This term may already be familiar to you.

The terms we have been using are diagrammed below so that you can clearly see how the word parts fit together, as well as when and why combining vowels are used.

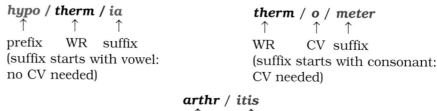

hypo / **therm** / ia
↑   ↑   ↑
prefix   WR   suffix
(suffix starts with vowel: no CV needed)

therm / o / meter
↑   ↑   ↑
WR   CV   suffix
(suffix starts with consonant: CV needed)

arthr / itis
↑   ↑
WR   suffix
(suffix starts with vowel: no CV needed)

Three Simple Steps

There are just three simple steps to follow as you begin deciphering medical terms:

1. Translate the *last* word part first.
2. Translate the *first* word part next.
3. Translate *following* word parts in order.

It's that simple. Here's an example: Consider the term *esophagogastroduodenoscopy.* This term is quite a mouthful and may seem rather intimidating.

However, we will follow the three simple steps described above, and you will see how easy it can be to decipher this word's meaning. You may find it helpful to put slashes between the word parts: esophag/o/gastr/o/duoden/o/scopy. After practicing these steps a few times, you won't need to do this anymore.

Step 1
-Scopy is a **suffix** that means visual examination.
Step 2
Esophag/o is a **combining form** that means esophagus.
Step 3
Gastr/o is a **combining form** that means stomach.
Duoden/o is a **combining form** that means duodenum, which is the first part of the small intestine.

Now put it all together. The final translation of esophagogastroduodenoscopy: visual examination of the esophagus, stomach, and duodenum, also known as an upper endoscopy.

  ## Learning Style Tip

Reading the terms aloud helps verbal and auditory learners. If you are a verbal learner, you need to say them. If you are an auditory learner, you need to hear them, even if it is in your own voice.

Flashpoint
It may help you to remember the order in which to complete these steps if you consider the order in which you write your name on most legal forms: last, first, middle.

Abbreviations

Abbreviations save time and simplify the speaking, reading, and writing of medical terms. They are used extensively in health care because there are so many terms that are lengthy and difficult to pronounce. *EGD* is the abbreviation for the large term you just learned, *esophagogastroduodenoscopy.* Many abbreviations are **acronyms**, abbreviations formed by using the first letter of each word. An example of this type of abbreviation is *CAD,* which stands for *coronary artery disease.* Some abbreviations do not even contain letters found in the medical term. For example, *c̄* is the abbreviation for the word *with.* **Symbols** are also used to save time and space when **documenting**, or writing in the patient's chart, and in written communication with other medical professionals. An example of a symbol is ↑, which means *upward* or *increase.* As you continue through this book, you will notice that each chapter contains a table of abbreviations that pertain to the body system you are studying. See Table 2-14 on page 40 for abbreviations and symbols that do not pertain to a particular body system but do have an important role in documentation and written communication with other medical professionals.

It is very important that you use only abbreviations that are commonly recognized and have been approved by the facility in which you work. Making up your own abbreviations or using ones not recognized by your facility can lead to communication errors and can potentially jeopardize patient well-being. For example, some people may interpret the abbreviation *hs* to mean *half strength* while others interpret it as *at bedtime.* The Joint Commission (formerly the Joint Commission on Accreditation of Healthcare Organizations or JCAHO) has developed a "Do Not Use" list of abbreviations to help ensure patient safety.

Flashpoint
The Joint Commission provides accreditation and certification to more than 20,000 health-care organizations in the United States. Their standards and initiatives have been developed to ensure the highest quality and safety in patient care. For more information, go to www.jointcommission.org

Pathology Terms

Pathology terms are used extensively in health care; they refer to diseases and disorders of all body systems. An example is ***multiple sclerosis,*** a chronic disease in which nerves lose the ability to transmit messages to the muscles. Students sometimes struggle with these terms because the three-step deciphering process that you just learned often does not work with these terms. Learning and remembering pathology terms requires study and memorization. However, this book includes some helpful tips to assist you with this process. Many of the pathology terms have pictures that accompany the definition and the terms are included in the learning exercises in each chapter. There are also flash cards for the pathology terms from each chapter on the Davis*Plus* website.

Closer Look

Let's take a closer look at the concepts mentioned previously.

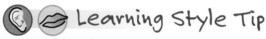 Learning Style Tip

Study with a partner so you can take turns quizzing each other. Verbalizing terms and definitions helps verbal learners; listening to each other helps auditory learners.

Suffixes

Flashpoint
Suffixes always change the meaning of the term.

Suffixes are word parts that appear at the ends of words and modify the meaning in some way. Consider the combining form ***appendic/o,*** which means *appendix.* If the suffix ***-itis*** *(inflammation)* is added, the term *appendic/itis* is created. As you may already know, this term means *inflammation of the appendix.*

This chapter introduces you to a large number of suffixes. They have been grouped according to several general categories. Note that the suffixes are usually arranged in alphabetical order; however, where there are two or more suffixes with the same or similar meanings, they are grouped together. This will make them easier for you to learn. Don't worry about word building yet. Just focus on learning and memorizing these suffixes. To help you with this process, study the suffix tables using the following steps:

1. Read the suffix in the first column.
2. Practice pronouncing the suffix correctly by using the guide in the second column.
3. Read the meaning aloud in the third column.
4. Write the suffix in the fourth column as you again pronounce it aloud.

Table 2-1 shows suffixes that indicate medical specialty, and Table 2-2 contains suffixes that indicate surgeries, procedures, or treatments. Note that these suffixes will be reviewed again throughout the following chapters.

TABLE 2-1
SUFFIXES THAT INDICATE MEDICAL SPECIALTY

Suffix	Pronunciation Guide	Meaning	Write the Suffix
-iatrics, -iatry	ī-ă-trĭks, ī-ă-trē	field of medicine	
-iatrist, -ician, -ist	ī-ă-trĭst, ĭ-shŭn, ĭst	specialist	
-logist, -ologist	lō-jĭst, ŏl-ō-jĭst	specialist in the study of	
-logy, -ology	lō-jē, ŏl-ō-jē	study of	

TABLE 2-2
SUFFIXES THAT INDICATE SURGERIES, PROCEDURES, OR TREATMENTS

Suffix	Pronunciation Guide	Meaning	Write the Suffix
-centesis	sĕn-tē-sĭs	surgical puncture	
-cidal, -cide	sī-dăl, sīd	destroying, killing	
-desis	dē-sĭs	surgical fixation of bone or joint, binding, tying together	
-dilation	dī-lā-shŭn	widening, stretching, expanding	
-ectomy	ĕk-tō-mē	excision, surgical removal	
-graphy	gră-fē	process of recording	
-metry	mĕ-trē	measurement	
-pexy	pĕk-sē	surgical fixation	
-plasty	plăs-tē	surgical repair	
-rrhaphy	ră-fē	suture, suturing	
-scopy	skō-pē	visual examination	
-therapy	thĕr-ă-pē	treatment	
-tomy	tō-mē	cutting into, incision	
-tripsy	trĭp-sē	crushing	

Practice Exercises

Fill in the Blanks

Choose the term that matches the description. Each term may be used more than once.

Exercise 1

Suffix   Prefix   Combining form
Word root   Combining vowel   Abbreviations

Pathology terms	Acronyms	Symbols
Documenting		

1. _____ Used to make the medical term easier to pronounce

2. _____ Unrecognized and unapproved use of these may jeopardize patient well-being

3. _____ A word part that comes at the end of the medical term

4. _____ Writing in the patient's chart

5. _____ Created by joining a word root with a combining vowel

6. _____ Letters used to save time and simplify the speaking, reading, and writing of medical terms

7. _____ Abbreviations formed by using the first letter of each word

8. _____ Does **not** include a prefix, suffix, or combining vowel

9. _____ Is **not** used if the next word part begins with a vowel

10. _____ A word part that comes at the beginning of the medical term

11. _____ The main stem, or primary meaning, of the word

12. _____ Nonletters used to save time and space in documentation and communication with other health-care professionals

13. _____ Refer to diseases and disorders of all body systems

14. _____ When deciphering medical terms, translate this word part first

15. _____ The three-step deciphering process often does not work with these

Fill in the Blanks

Fill in the blanks using suffixes from Tables 2-1 and 2-2.

Exercise 2

1. Suffixes that mean *field of medicine* are _____ and

    _____ .

2. Suffixes that mean *specialist in the study of* are _____ and

    _____ .

3. The suffix that means *surgical repair* is _____ .

4. Suffixes that mean *destroying* or *killing* are _____ and

    _____ .

5. The suffix that means *process of recording* is _____ .

6. The suffixes *-logy* and *-ology* mean _____ .

7. The suffix *-desis* means _____ .

8. The suffix *-ectomy* means _____ .

9. The suffix *-metry* means _____ .

10. The suffix *-scopy* means _____ .

True or False

Decide whether the following statements are true or false.

Exercise 3

1. True False   The suffix *-graphy* means *measurement.*

2. True False   The suffix *-dilation* means *widening, stretching,* or
                    expanding.

3. True False   The suffix *-plasty* means *surgical repair.*

4. True False   The suffix *-therapy* means *treatment.*

5. True False   The suffix *-ician* means *technician.*

6. True False   The suffix *-pexy* means *pain.*

7. True False   The suffix *-rrhaphy* means *suture* or *suturing.*

8. True   False   The suffix -tomy means *cutting into* or *incision.*

9. True   False   The suffix -tripsy means *treatment.*

10. True   False   The suffix -centesis means *centimeter.*

The SOAP Note

When documenting information in a patient's chart, or medical record, medical professionals often use the SOAP note format. Information is categorized as subjective and objective data followed by an assessment of the data and a plan for future care.

***Subjective* (S:)** data include what the patient said. This section includes the patient's chief complaint as well as statements regarding any changes in their condition since their last visit. It is not observable or measurable information. Statements in this section often begin with, "Patient states," "Patient reports," or "Patient complains of." Here are some examples of subjective information:

S: Patient complains of pain at right lateral ankle and notes she is unable to put any weight on right foot.
S: Patient reports pain and swelling in right ankle is improving.
S: Patient states pain in her right ankle is "much better."

In contrast, ***objective* (O:)** data include information that can be observed, measured, or quantified in some way. Examples of objective information are a patient's temperature, blood pressure, or pain level. If the patient has a wound, the location, size, depth, and amount of drainage would be entered into the objective portion of the SOAP note. The objective section also includes all treatments provided by the medical professional. In addition, anything the patient did during the visit, such as exercises, is considered objective data. Here are some examples of objective information:

O: Pain at right ankle 8/10. Noted redness, heat, and swelling. Instructed patient in RICE protocol.
O: Volumetric measurement right ankle 600 mL
O: Patient walked on treadmill for 30 minutes with an increase in speed to 2.5 and a 10% incline.

The ***assessment* (A:)** section of the SOAP note is where the medical professional synthesizes the subjective and objective information. This section can include expectations, or treatment goals, as well as how the patient is reacting to the current treatment and whether he or she is or is not making progress toward the treatment goals. In one of the previous examples, a patient complained of pain at the right ankle and inability to walk on the right foot. In the observation portion of the SOAP note, the medical professional wrote the signs of inflammation that were observed and the instructions given to the patient to help relieve the pain and swelling. In the assessment portion of this SOAP note, the medical professional may write an expectation for "decreased pain and swelling within 1 week." On subsequent visits, assessment statements may include, "right ankle swelling has decreased since last visit" and "patient able to tolerate increased speed and incline on treadmill with no complaints of increased ankle pain."

The ***plan* (P:)** section of the SOAP note is where you write what you will *do* to help the patient make progress toward the treatment goals. This part includes statements about continuing with the current treatment or making changes to the treatment. It also includes recommendations for consultation or collaboration with other medical professionals. "Continue as per plan of care" and "will contact orthotist regarding ankle brace adjustment" are examples of statements that belong in the plan section of the SOAP note. Most facilities provide guidelines regarding the specific information they want included in the medial record as well as how they want it documented.

Suffixes That Indicate Sensation, Feeling, Action, or Movement

Table 2-3 includes suffixes that indicate sensory experience, sensation, or subjective feeling. Table 2-4 includes suffixes that indicate action or movement.

Flashpoint

An easy way to remember the difference between subjective and objective is that *subjective* data are based on what the patient *said*. *Objective* data are based on what you *observed* or measured.

TABLE 2-3
SUFFIXES THAT INDICATE SENSORY EXPERIENCE, SENSATION, OR SUBJECTIVE FEELING

Suffix	Pronunciation Guide	Meaning	Write the Suffix
-acusia, -acusis, -cusis	ă-koo-zē-ă, ă-koo-sĭs, koo-sĭs	hearing	
-algesia, -algesic, -algia, -dynia	ăl-jē-zē-ă, ăl-jē-zĭk, ăl-jē-ă, dĭ-nē-ă	pain	
-dipsia	dĭp-sē-ă	thirst	
-esthesia	ĕs-thē-zē-ă	sensation	
-opia, -opsia, -opsis, -opsy	ō-pē-ă, ŏp-sē-ă, ŏp-sĭs, ŏp-sē	vision, view of	
-osmia	ŏz-mē-ă	smell, odor	
-phobia	fō-bē-ă	fear	
-phoria	fō-rē-ă	feeling	

TABLE 2-4
SUFFIXES THAT INDICATE ACTION OR MOVEMENT

Suffix	Pronunciation Guide	Meaning	Write the Suffix
-clasis, -clast	klăs-ĭs, klăst	to break	
-ectasis	ĕk-tă-sĭs	dilation, expansion	
-emesis	ĕm-ĕ-sĭs	vomiting	
-gen, -genesis, -genic, -genous	jĕn, jĕn-ĕ-sĭs, jĕn-ĭk, jĕn-ŭs	creating, producing	
-kinesia, -kinesis	kĭ-nē-zē-ă, kĭ-nē-sĭs	movement	
-lysis	lĭ-sĭs	destruction	
-pause, -stasis	pawz, stă-sĭs	cessation, stopping	
-phage, -phagia	fāj, fā-jē-ă	eating, swallowing	
-phasia	fā-zē-ă	speech	
-rrhage, -rrhagia	rĭj, ră-jē-ă	bursting forth	
-rrhea	rē-ă	flow, discharge	
-rrhexis	rĕk-sĭs	rupture	
-spasm	spă-zŭm	sudden involuntary contraction	
-uresis	ū-rē-sĭs	urination	

Some refer to conscious actions and individual tasks, such as speech (-*phasia*) and movement (-*kinesia*). Others indicate unconscious action within the body, such as a sudden involuntary contraction (-*spasm*). Note that many of these suffixes will be reviewed again in the chapters that follow.

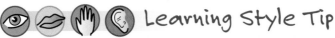 Learning Style Tip

Kinesthetic learners need to move. So imagine you are playing charades—or gather a group to actually play the game—and challenge yourself to act out each of the terms as you study them.

Practice Exercises

Fill in the Blanks

Fill in the blanks below using suffixes from Tables 2-3 and 2-4.

Exercise 4

1. Suffixes that mean *hearing* are _____, _____, and _____.

2. Suffixes that mean *vision* or *view of* are _____, _____, _____, and _____.

3. The suffix that means *feeling* is _____.

4. The suffix that means *smell* or *odor* is _____.

5. Suffixes that mean *creating* or *producing* are _____, _____, _____, and _____.

6. Suffixes that mean *bursting forth* are _____ and _____.

7. Suffixes that mean *eating* or *swallowing* are _____ and _____.

8. The suffix that means *vomiting* is _____.

9. The suffix that means *destruction* is _____.

10. The suffix that means *rupture* is _____.

True or False

Decide whether the following statements are true or false.

Exercise 5

1. True   False   The suffixes *-acusia*, *-acusis*, and *-cusis* mean *pain*.

2. True   False   The suffix *-dipsia* means *feeling*.

3. True   False   The suffixes *-opia*, *-opsia*, *-opsis*, and *-opsy* mean *vision* or *view of*.

4. True   False   The suffix *-osmia* means *sound*.

5. True   False   The suffix *-esthesia* means *sensation*.

6. True   False   The suffixes *-algesia*, *-algesic*, *-algia*, and *-dynia* mean *pain*.

7. True   False   The suffix *-phobia* means *fear*.

8. True   False   The suffixes *-clast* and *-clasis* mean *cessation*.

9. True   False   The suffix *-pause* means *relaxation*.

10. True   False   The suffix *-phasia* means *eating* or *swallowing*.

Suffixes That Indicate Diseases, Disorders, or Conditions

Many suffixes in the medical language indicate diseases, disorders, or conditions; these are listed in Table 2-5. Some terms, such as *-derma (skin)*, *-emia (a condition of the blood)*, and *-thorax (chest)*, provide specific clues about the body part involved. Other terms, such as *-constriction (narrowing)*, *-edema (swelling)*, and *-itis (inflammation)*, provide clues about the nature of the disease or disorder. Note that many of these suffixes will be reviewed again throughout the chapters that follow.

Flashpoint
Many suffixes provide clues about the nature or location of the disorder.

TABLE 2-5
SUFFIXES THAT INDICATE DISEASES, DISORDERS, OR CONDITIONS

Suffix	Pronunciation Guide	Meaning	Write the Suffix
-cele	sēl	hernia	
-constriction	kŏn-strĭk-shŭn	narrowing	
-cytosis	sī-tō-sĭs	a condition of cells	
-derma	dĕr-mă	skin	
-edema	ĕ-dē-mă	swelling	
-emia	ē-mē-ă	a condition of the blood	
-gravida	gră-vĭ-dă	pregnant woman	
-ia, -ism	ē-ă, ĭz-ŭm	condition	

Continued

TABLE 2-5

SUFFIXES THAT INDICATE DISEASES, DISORDERS, OR CONDITIONS—cont'd

Suffix	Pronunciation Guide	Meaning	Write the Suffix
-iasis	ī-ă-sĭs	pathological condition or state	
-itis	ī-tĭs	inflammation	
-lepsy, -leptic	lĕp-sē, lĕp-tĭk	seizure	
-lith	lĭth	stone	
-malacia	mă-lā-sē-ă	softening	
-megaly	mĕg-ă-lē	enlargement	
-necrosis	nĕ-krō-sĭs	tissue death	
-oid	oyd	resembling	
-oma	ō-mă	tumor	
-osis	ō-sĭs	abnormal condition	
-oxia	ŏk-sē-ă	oxygen	
-paresis	pă-rē-sĭs	slight or partial paralysis	
-partum, -tocia	părt-ŭm, tō-sē-ă	childbirth, labor	
-pathy	pă-thē	disease	
-penia	PĒ-nē-ă	deficiency	
-pepsia	pĕp-sē-ă	digestion	
-phonia	fō-nē-ă	voice	
-plasia, -plasm	plā-zē-ă, plăz-ŭm	formation, growth	
-plastic	plăs-tĭk	pertaining to formation or growth	
-plegia	plē-jē-ă	paralysis	
-plegic	plē-jĭk	pertaining to paralysis	
-pnea	nē-ă	breathing	
-pneic	nē-ĭk	pertaining to breathing	
-ptosis	tō-sĭs	drooping, prolapse	
-salpinx	săl-pĭnks	uterine (fallopian) tube	
-sclerosis	sklĕ-rō-sĭs	hardening	
-static	stă-tĭk	not in motion, at rest	
-stenosis	stĕ-nō-sĭs	narrowing, stricture	
-thorax	thōr-ăks	chest	
-trophy	trō-fē	nourishment, growth	
-uria	ū-rē-ă	urine	

Practice Exercises

Fill in the Blanks

Fill in the blanks below using suffixes from Table 2-5.

Exercise 6

1. The suffix that means *pregnant woman* is _____.

2. The suffix that means *stone* is _____.

3. Suffixes that mean *seizure* are _____ and _____.

4. The suffix that means *hernia* is _____.

5. The suffix that means *softening* is _____.

6. The suffix that means *voice* is _____.

7. The suffix that means *not in motion* or *at rest* is _____.

8. The suffix that means *narrowing* or *stricture* is _____.

9. The suffix that means *tumor* is _____.

10. The suffix that means *resembling* is _____.

True or False

Decide whether the following statements are true or false.

Exercise 7

1. True   False   The suffix *-lith* means *little*.

2. True   False   The suffixes *-ia* and *-ism* mean *condition*.

3. True   False   The suffix *-derma* means *down*.

4. True   False   The suffix *-megaly* means *motion*.

5. True   False   The suffix *-necrosis* means *tissue death*.

6. True   False   The suffixes *-partum* and *-tocia* mean *person*.

7. True   False   The suffix *-osis* means *oxygen*.

8. True   False   The suffix *-trophy* means *nourishment* or *growth*.

9. True   False   The suffix *-thorax* means *chest*.

10. True   False   The suffix *-rrhea* means *flow or discharge*.

Other Suffixes

There are literally thousands of medical instruments used for countless procedures and treatments. Many are categorized according to their general purpose. Cutting instruments go by various names, many ending with the suffix *-tome*. Recording instruments also have many different names; however, many of them end with the suffix *-graph*. Many instruments used for measurement end with the suffix *-meter,* and many of those used for viewing various parts of the body end with the suffix *-scope*. These terms are listed in Table 2-6. Another group of commonly used suffixes all mean *pertaining to* (Table 2-7). Still other suffixes not easily categorized are listed in Table 2-8. Table 2-9 lists the rules for changing the endings of some terms from the singular to the plural form.

Flashpoint

The suffixes of many instrument names provide clues about their purpose or function.

TABLE 2-6
SUFFIXES THAT INDICATE INSTRUMENTS

Suffix	Pronunciation Guide	Meaning	Write the Suffix
-graph	grăf	recording instrument	
-meter	mĕ-tĕr	measuring instrument	
-scope	skōp	viewing instrument	
-tome	tōm	cutting instrument	

TABLE 2-7
SUFFIXES THAT MEAN "PERTAINING TO"

Suffix	Pronunciation Guide	Meaning	Write the Suffix
-ac, -al, -ar, -ary, -eal,	ăk, ăl, ăr, ār-ē, ē-ăl, ē-ăl,	pertaining to	
-ial, -ic, -ical, -ory, -ous,	ĭk, ĭ-kăl, ō-rē, ŭs, tĭk, tŭs		
-tic*, -tous*			

*-tic, a variation of -ic, is sometimes used; -tous, a variation of -ous, is sometimes used.

TABLE 2-8
OTHER SUFFIXES

Suffix	Pronunciation Guide	Meaning	Write the Suffix
-cyte, -cytic	sīt, sīt-ĭk	cell	
-gram	grăm	record	
-ole, -ule	ōl, ūl	small	
-prandial	prăn-dē-ăl	meal	
-stomy	stō-mē	mouthlike opening	

TABLE 2-9

PLURAL ENDINGS

Singular Form	Plural Form	Rule	Singular Example	Plural Example
-a	-ae	retain -a and add -e	vertebra	vertebrae
-ax	-aces	drop -x and add -ces	thorax	thoraces
-is	-es	drop -is and add -es	diagnosis	diagnoses
-ix, -ex	-ices	drop -ix or -ex and add -ices	appendix	appendices
-um	-a	drop -um and add -a	diverticulum	diverticula
-us	-i	drop -us and add -i	thrombus	thrombi
-y	-ies	drop -y and add -ies	ovary	ovaries

Practice Exercises

Fill in the Blanks

Fill in the blanks below using Tables 2-6 through 2-9.

Exercise 8

1. The suffix that means *recording instrument* is _____.

2. The suffix that means *cutting instrument* is _____.

3. The suffix that means *measuring instrument* is _____.

4. The suffix that means *viewing instrument* is _____.

5. Suffixes that mean *cell* are _____ and

   _____.

6. The suffix that means *meal* is _____.

7. Suffixes that mean *small* are _____ and

   _____.

8. The suffix that means *mouthlike opening* is _____.

9. The suffix that means *deficiency* is _____.

10. The suffix that means *record* is _____.

True or False

Decide whether the following statements are true or false.

Exercise 9

1. True False   The suffixes *-al, -ial, -tic,* and *-tous* mean *pertaining to.*

2. True False   The suffixes *-ole* and *-ule* mean *pertaining to.*

3. True False   The suffixes *-cyte* and *-cytic* mean *small.*

4. True False   The plural form of the word *appendix* is *appendixes.*

5. True False   The plural form of the word *diagnosis* is *diagnoses.*

6. True False   The suffixes *-ac, -ar, -ory,* and *-ous* mean *pertaining to.*

7. True False   The plural form of the word *thrombus* is *thrombuses.*

8. True False   The suffixes *-y, -um,* and *-ex* mean *pertaining to.*

9. True False   The suffixes *-ary, -ical, -ic,* and *-eal* mean *pertaining to.*

10. True False   The plural form of the word *diverticulum* is *diverticula.*

IN A FLASH!
Remove the Suffix Flash Cards from the back of this book and run through them at least three times before you continue.

Prefixes

Prefixes are always located at the beginnings of words, and they always modify the meaning of the word in some way. As an example, let's take another look at the word *hypothermia.* The prefix **hypo-** means *beneath* or *below.* Therefore, this term indicates *a condition of heat that is below normal.* A common cause of hypothermia is exposure to cold weather without adequate clothing.

Now let's see what happens when we change the prefix to **hyper-,** which means *excessive* or *above.* The newly created word, *hyperthermia,* means *a condition of excessive heat.* This term refers to high body temperature. As you can see, changing the prefix can drastically change the meaning of the term. Hyperthermia might refer to a fever caused by an illness such as the flu. Another example of hyperthermia is heatstroke, a life-threatening condition caused when a person becomes too hot and dehydrated. This typically occurs when a person is exposed to a hot, humid environment and does not use adequate cooling measures.

This chapter introduces you to a large number of prefixes. They have been grouped according to several general categories. Table 2-10 includes prefixes

Flashpoint
Prefixes always change the meaning of the term.

TABLE 2-10
PREFIXES THAT INDICATE SIZE, QUANTITY, OR NUMBER

Prefix	Pronunciation Guide	Meaning	Write the Prefix
a-, an-, in-	ā, ăn, ĭn	without, not, absence of	
ambi-	ăm-bē	both, both sides, around, about	
bi-	bī	two	
di-	dī	twice, two, double	
hemi-, semi-	hĕm-ē, sĕm-ē	half	
iso-	ī-sō	same, equal	
macro-	mă-krō	large	
micro-	mī-krō	small	
mono-, uni-	mŏ-nō, ū-nĭ	one, single	
multi-	mŭl-tē	many	
poly-	pŏ-lē	much	
oligo-	ō-lĭ-gō	deficiency	
pan-	păn	all	
quadri-, tetra-	kwŏ-drĭ, tĕ-tră	four	
tri-	trī	three	

that indicate size, quantity, or number. In some cases, the term is quite specific. For example, the prefix *tri-* means *three,* and the prefixes *quadri-* and *tetra-* mean *four.* In other cases, the terms are less specific and refer to general amounts. Examples are the terms *multi-,* which means *many,* and *poly-,* which means *much.* Other terms such as *a-* and *an-* indicate the absence of something. The term *anuria,* for example, indicates *absence of urine,* and the term *anacusia* indicates *absence of hearing.* To begin familiarizing yourself with these prefixes, read through the following tables and answer the questions in the practice exercises that follow them. Note that the prefixes are generally arranged in alphabetical order; however, where there are two or more terms with the same or very similar meanings, they are grouped together. This will make them easier for you to learn. Don't worry about word building yet. Just focus on learning and memorizing these prefixes. To help you with this process, study these tables using the following steps:

1. Read the prefix in the first column.
2. Practice pronouncing the prefix correctly by using the guide in the second column.
3. Read the meaning aloud in the third column.
4. Write the prefix in the fourth column as you again pronounce it aloud.

Note that most of these prefixes will be reviewed again throughout the chapters.

Learning Style Tip

Make a recording of your voice saying the terms and their definitions. Record a term and then pause for a count of three before you record the definition. As you listen to the recording, the pause will allow you to try to say the correct definition aloud before you hear it. This is a great self-quiz too!

Practice Exercises

Fill in the Blanks

Fill in the blanks below using prefixes from Table 2-10.

Exercise 10

1. Prefixes that mean *one* are _____ and _____.

2. The prefix that means *deficiency* is _____.

3. The prefix that means *small* is _____.

4. Prefixes that mean *without, not,* or *absence of* are _____, _____, and _____.

5. Prefixes that mean *four* are _____ and _____.

6. Prefixes that mean *half* are _____ and _____.

7. The prefix that means *both* or *both sides* is _____.

8. The prefix that means *large* is _____.

9. The prefix that means *much* is _____.

10. The prefix that means *same* or *equal* is _____.

True or False

Decide whether the following statements are true or false.

Exercise 11

1. True   False   The prefix *ambi-* means *half.*

2. True   False   The prefix *macro-* means *small.*

3. True   False   The prefix *iso-* means *same* or *equal.*

4. True   False   The prefix *pan-* means *none* or *zero.*

5. True   False   The prefix *tri-* means *three.*

6. True   False   The prefixes *bi-* and *di-* mean *three.*

7. True   False   The prefix *micro-* means *small.*

8. True   False   The prefixes *quadri-* and *tetra-* mean *two.*

9. True   False   The prefix *multi-* means *many.*

10. True   False   The prefixes *semi-* and *hemi-* mean *half.*

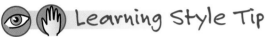 Learning Style Tip

Use the flash cards every day. They were created especially for you! Read both sides, and be sure to note the visual cues on most of them.

Prefixes That Indicate Location, Direction, or Timing

The prefixes in Table 2-11 indicate location, direction, or timing. For example, the prefix *epi-* in *epigastric* indicates a physical location *above* the stomach. The prefix *circum-* in *circumoral* indicates a physical location *around* the mouth. The

TABLE 2-11
PREFIXES THAT INDICATE LOCATION, DIRECTION, OR TIMING

Prefix	Pronunciation Guide	Meaning	Write the Prefix
ab-	āb	away from	
ad-	ād	toward	
anti-	ăn-tē	against	
brady-	bră-dē	slow	
con-	kŏn	together, with	
contra-	kŏn-tră	against, opposite	
circum-	sĕr-kŭm	around	
dia-, trans-	dī-ă, trănz	through, across	
ec-, ecto-	ĕk, ĕk-tō	out, outside	
en-, end-, endo-, in-, intra-	ĕn, ĕnd, ĕn-dō, ĭn, ĭn-tră	in, within, inner	
epi-	ĕ-pĭ	above, upon	
eso-	ĕs-ō	inward	
ex-, exo-, extra-	ĕks, ĕk-sō, ĕk-stră	away from, outside, external	
hyper-, super-, supra-	hī-pĕr, soo-pĕr, soo-pră	excessive, above	
hypo-, infra-, sub-	hī-pō, ĭn-fră, sŭb	below, beneath	

Continued

TABLE 2-11

PREFIXES THAT INDICATE LOCATION, DIRECTION, OR TIMING—cont'd

Prefix	Pronunciation Guide	Meaning	Write the Prefix
inter-	ĭn-tĕr	between	
para-, peri-	pă-ră, pĕr-ĭ	beside, near	
post-	pōst	after, following	
pre-	prē	before	
pro-	prō	before, forward	
re-, retro-	rē, rĕ-trō	behind, back	
tachy-	tăk-ē	rapid	
ultra-	ŭl-tră	beyond	

prefixes *brady-* and *tachy-* are commonly used to indicate timing or speed. *Bradykinesia* indicates *slow movement,* and *tachycardia* indicates *rapid heartbeat.* Other terms may indicate direction. For example, the prefix *ab-* in *abduction* indicates movement *away from* the body and the prefix *ad-* in *adduction* indicates movement *toward* the body.

Practice Exercises

Fill in the Blanks

Fill in the blanks below using prefixes from Table 2-11.

Exercise 12

1. The prefix that means *beyond* is _____.

2. The prefix that means *away from* is _____.

3. Prefixes that mean *across* or *through* are _____ and _____.

4. Prefixes than mean *in, within,* or *inner* are _____, _____, _____, _____, and _____.

5. The prefix that means *toward* is _____.

6. The prefix that means *slow* is _____.

7. The prefix that means *above* or *upon* is _____.

8. Prefixes that mean *out* or *outside* are _____ and

   _____.

9. Prefixes than mean *away from*, *outside*, or *external* are

   _____, _____, and

   _____.

10. The prefix that means *around* is _____.

True or False

Decide whether the following statements are true or false.

Exercise 13

1. True   False   The prefix *anti-* means *against*.

2. True   False   The prefix *tachy-* means *rapid*.

3. True   False   The prefixes *re-* and *retro-* mean *behind* or *back*.

4. True   False   The prefix *epi-* means *below*.

5. True   False   The prefix *con-* means *together* or *with*.

6. True   False   The prefix *contra-* means *against* or *opposite*.

7. True   False   The prefix *eso-* means *outward*.

8. True   False   The prefixes *hyper-*, *super-*, and *supra-* mean *excessive* or *above*.

9. True   False   The prefixes *para-* and *peri-* mean *beside* or *near*.

10. True   False   The prefix *pro-* means *between*.

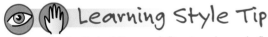 Learning Style Tip

Physically holding and flipping through flash cards (while reading them, of course) helps kinesthetic and visual learners learn and remember.

Other Prefixes

Table 2-12 includes prefixes that indicate a variety of other meanings.

TABLE 2-12

OTHER PREFIXES

Prefix	Pronunciation Guide	Meaning	Write the Prefix
auto-	aw-tō	self	
dys-	dĭs	bad, painful, difficult	
eu-	ū	good, normal	
mal-	măl	bad, inadequate	
neo-	nē-ō	new	
tox-	tŏks	poison, toxin	

Practice Exercises

Fill in the Blanks

Fill in the blanks below using prefixes from Table 2-12.

Exercise 14

1. The prefix that means *poison* is _____.

2. The prefix that means *good* or *normal* is _____.

3. The prefix that means *new* is _____.

4. The prefix than means *bad, painful,* or *difficult* is _____.

5. The prefix that means *self* is _____.

True or False

Decide whether the following statements are true or false.

Exercise 15

1. True   False   The prefix *mal-* means *against.*

2. True   False   The prefix *neo-* means *new.*

3. True   False   The prefix *tox-* means *try.*

4. True   False   The prefix *auto-* means *car.*

5. True   False   The prefix *dys-* means *self.*

IN A FLASH!
Remove the Prefix Flash Cards from the back of this book and run through them at least three times before you continue.

Pronunciation

It often takes a considerable amount of practice before the pronunciation of medical terms comes easily and naturally. It will help if you develop good habits right from the start. Carefully review the pronunciation guidelines in Table 2-13. These guidelines will help you learn correct pronunciation.

Abbreviations and Symbols

Table 2-14 contains abbreviations and symbols regarding information and instructions. They do not pertain to a particular body system but do play an important role in documentation and written communication with other health-care providers. While some of the abbreviations are on "Do Not Use" lists, you need to know all of them as you will still occasionally see them in written documentation. Make sure the abbreviations you use are approved by your facility and, if you see an abbreviation that should not have been used, be sure to clarify the meaning with the person who wrote it.

TABLE 2-13
PRONUNCIATION GUIDE

Letters	Guidelines	Examples
ae and oe	pronounce only the *e*	pleurae (PLOO-rē)
-es	when located at the end of a word, may be pronounced as a separate syllable	nares (NĀR-ēz)
g and c	pronounce as *j* and *s* before *e, i,* and *y*	generic (jě-NĔR-ĭk) gelatin (JĔL-ă-tĭn) cycle (SĪ-kĭl) cytology (sī-TŎ-lō-jē)
g and c	pronounce as *g* and *k* before other letters	gait (gāt) gastric (GĂS-trĭk) caffeine (kă-FĒN) calcium (KĂL-sē-ŭm)
-i	when located at the end of a word, generally indicates a plural; pronounce as *ī* or *ē*	alveoli (ăl-VĒ-ō-lī) bronchi (BRŎNG-kī)
pn-	pronounce only the *n*	pneumonia (nū-MŌ-nē-ă) pneumatic (nū-MĂT-ĭk)
ps-	pronounce only the *s*	psoriasis (sō-RĪ-ă-sĭs) psychology (sī-KŎL-ō-jē)

TABLE 2-14

ABBREVIATIONS AND SYMBOLS

A&O	alert and oriented	pc	after meals
ā	before	PE	physical examination
ac	before meals	per	by / through
ad lib.	as desired, at discretion	PLOF	prior level of function
ADLs	activities of daily living	p.o.	by mouth
AMA	against medical advice	post-op	after surgery (operation)
B/S	bedside	pre-op	before surgery (operation)
bid	twice a day	prn	as needed
BRP	bathroom privileges	Pt. or pt.	patient
c̄	with	PTA	prior to admission
c/o	complains of	q	every
CC or C/C	chief complaint	qd	every day, once daily
cont.	continue	qid	four times a day
D/C or d/c	discharge, discontinue	qh	every hour
DNR	do not resuscitate	q2h	every two hours
DOB	date of birth	qod	every other day
Dx	diagnosis	re:	regarding, concerning
ELOS	estimated length of stay	R/O or r/o	rule out
EOB	edge of bed	ROS	review of systems
eval.	evaluate, evaluation	Rx	prescription, intervention plan
FH	family history	s̄	without
h or hr.	hour	S/P or s/p	status post
H&P	history and physical	sig	directions for use, give as follows, let it be labeled
h/o	history of	S:	Subjective
		O:	Objective
		A:	Assessment
		P:	Plan
HOB	head of bed	stat.	immediate(ly)
ht.	height	STG	short-term goal
Hx	history	Sx	symptoms
LOS	length of stay	tid	three times a day
LTG	long-term goal	tiw	three times a week
Meds	medications	TO or t.o.	telephone order
Noc	night, at night	tol	tolerate, tolerated, tolerance
NPO or npo	nothing by mouth	Tx	treatment, traction

TABLE 2-14

ABBREVIATIONS AND SYMBOLS—cont'd

OOB	out of bed	VO or v.o.	verbal order
OTC	over the counter	y/o or y.o.	year old
p̄	after	wt.	weight
Symbols			
~ or ≈	approximately	/	per
Δ	change	1°	primary
↓	down, downward, decreased, diminished	→	to, progressing toward, approaching
♀	female	2°	secondary, secondary to
♂	male	↔	to and from
Ø	no, none	↑	up, upward, increased
#	number (#5) or pounds (5# wt.)		
✕	number of times (✕5, 5✕) or minutes (✕5 min)		

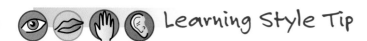 Learning Style Tip

Use a set of handheld white boards/dry-erase boards for a game show–type study session. Each person, or team, gets a board on which to write the answers. One person calls out a term or definition to decipher. The first team to hold up the board with the correct answer gets a point. The first team to get 10 points wins.

IN A FLASH!

Go to the Davis*Plus* website to print out the Abbreviations and Symbols Flash Cards and run through them at least three times before you continue.

End-of-Chapter Practice Exercises

Deciphering Terms

Occasionally, you will find a word made up of only a prefix and a suffix. Some examples are listed below. Write the correct meaning of these medical terms.

Exercise 16

1. toxic _____

2. autograph _____

3. polyphobia _____

4. anesthesia _____

5. atrophy _____

6. multigravida _____

7. tetraplegia _____

8. hyperemesis _____

9. postprandial _____

10. dyspnea _____

11. bilateral _____

12. hypoxia _____

13. euphoria _____

14. anacusis _____

15. anosmia _____

16. hemiplegia _____

17. polyuria _____

18. bradykinesia _____

19. postpartum _____

20. neoplasm _____

Deciphering Terms

Write the correct abbreviations or symbols for these medical terms.

Exercise 17

1. date of birth _____

2. nothing by mouth _____

3. patient _____

4. history of _____

5. every _____

6. before _____

7. do not resuscitate _____

8. change _____

9. as needed _____

10. without _____

11. by/through _____

12. primary _____

13. symptoms _____

14. after _____

15. rule out _____

16. secondary to _____

17. female _____

18. with _____

19. year old _____

20. male _____

Multiple Choice

Select the one best answer to the following multiple-choice questions.

Exercise 18

1. Which of the following prefixes is matched with the correct definition?

   a. *ambi-*:   against

   b. *an-*:   with

   c. *pan-*:   without

   d. *bi-*:   two

2. The prefixes *hemi-* and *semi-* mean:

   a. both, both sides

   b. twice, two, double

   c. half

   d. whole

3. Which of the following prefixes is matched with the correct definition?
   a. *infra-*:   above
   b. *pro-*:   beyond
   c. *re-*:   behind, back
   d. *ultra-*:   after

4. Which of the following prefixes means *bad* or *inadequate*?
   a. *mal-*
   b. *eu-*
   c. *tox-*
   d. *auto-*

5. The prefix *auto-* means:
   a. new
   b. poison
   c. self
   d. none of these

6. The suffix *-pexy* means:
   a. widening, stretching, expanding
   b. surgical fixation
   c. surgical puncture
   d. measurement

7. Which of the following suffixes is matched with the correct definition?
   a. *-phoria*:   fear
   b. *-phobia*:   feeling
   c. *-dynia*:   pain
   d. *-algia*:   sound

8. Which of the following suffixes is matched with the correct definition?
   a. *-edema*:   eating
   b. *-lith*:   loosening
   c. *-malacia*:   softening
   d. *-megaly*:   measurement

9. Which of the following suffixes is matched with the correct definition?

    a. *-paresis*:   pregnancy

    b. *-partum*:   partial

    c. *-plegia*:   pain

    d. *-pnea*:   breathing

10. All of the following suffixes mean *pertaining to* **except:**

    a. *-ar*

    b. *-ory*

    c. *-itis*

    d. *-tic*

11. All of the following prefixes mean *without, not,* or *absence of* **except:**

    a. *an-*

    b. *in-*

    c. *uni-*

    d. *a-*

12. Which of the following prefixes means *all?*

    a. *pan-*

    b. *ambi-*

    c. *multi-*

    d. *micro-*

13. The prefix *di-* means:

    a. diagonal

    b. diagram

    c. dilate

    d. none of these

14. The prefixes *a-, an-,* and *in-* all mean:

    a. both, double

    b. without, not, of

    c. many, much

    d. none of these

15. Which of the following prefixes is matched with the correct definition?

    a. *mono-:*   one, single

    b. *multi-:*   twice

    c. *a-:*   with

    d. *hemi-:*   whole

16. Which of the following prefixes is matched with the correct definition?

    a. *neo-:*   new

    b. *eu-:*   good, normal

    c. *dys-:*   bad, painful

    d. all of these

17. Which of the following prefixes means *bad, painful,* or *difficult?*

    a. *tox-*

    b. *eu-*

    c. *dys-*

    d. *neo-*

18. The prefix *neo-* means:

    a. self

    b. bad

    c. new

    d. none of these

19. The suffix *-ician* means:

    a. field of medicine

    b. study of

    c. specialist

    d. physician

20. Which of the following suffixes is matched with the correct definition?

    a. *-lysis:*   flow, discharge

    b. *-cele:*   pregnant woman

    c. *-kinesia:*   movement

    d. *-uresis:*   eating, swallowing

21. Which of the following suffixes is matched with the correct definition?

    a. *-ology*: study of

    b. *-opsy*: vision, view of

    c. *-cidal*: destroying, killing

    d. all of these

22. Which of the following suffixes is matched with the correct definition?

    a. *-iasis*: illusion

    b. *-necrosis*: tissue death

    c. *-oma*: hernia

    d. *-oxia*: air

23. All of the following suffixes mean *pain* **except:**

    a. *-algesic*

    b. *-dynia*

    c. *-phobia*

    d. *-algia*

24. Which of the following terms has been correctly changed to the plural form?

    a. thorax: thoraces

    b. diagnosis: diagnoses

    c. diverticulum: diverticula

    d. all of these

25. Which of the following prefixes means *in, within,* or *inner?*

    a. *endo-*

    b. *contra-*

    c. *super-*

    d. *trans-*

3

LEVELS OF ORGANIZATION

Chapter Outline

Structure and Function

The human body is arranged in a complex yet orderly fashion (Fig. 3-1). Therefore, a systematic approach to studying it is helpful. Chemistry courses typically study the human body at the atomic and molecular levels. Some biology courses, such as cellular biology, study the body at the cellular level. Other courses, such as anatomy and physiology and medical terminology, generally study the body at the organ and organ-system levels. This will be our approach.

Cell Level

Cells are the structural units that form all body tissues. Their functions are consistent with the functions of the tissues they comprise. Their walls are composed of a membrane made up of lipids (fats), proteins, and other components that selectively allow certain substances, such as nutrients, to enter and other substances, such as wastes, to leave. Within the cell is a gelatinous substance called cytoplasm. It surrounds a variety of tiny structures called organelles that are important to cellular function. The largest of these is the nucleus. Contained within the nucleus is deoxyribonucleic acid (DNA), which is the genetic material that makes up the blueprint for your body. It includes information that determines your gender, skin, hair and eye colors, and numerous other features.

Tissue Level

Tissue is composed of a group of similar cells that perform a specific function. The types of tissue are epithelial, connective, nervous, and muscle.

Flashpoint

Each cell contains organelles that perform a specific function. Some of the major organelles found in human cells behave like an online shopping service that takes your order, packages the items, and delivers them to your home. Ribosomes process genetic instructions. The Golgi apparatus packages the molecules. The endoplasmic reticulum transports the molecules to their destination, and the mitochondria provide the energy, or fuel, for the transportation.

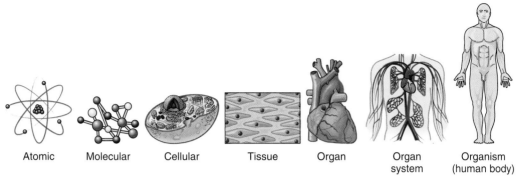

Atomic   Molecular   Cellular   Tissue   Organ   Organ system   Organism (human body)

FIGURE 3-1 Levels of organization.

Epithelial tissue forms the epidermis (top layer of the skin) and surface layer of the membranes. It may be composed of a single layer (simple) or of several layers (stratified). It is also classified according to the cell shape: squamous (flat), cuboidal (cube shaped), or columnar (cylindrical) (Fig. 3-2). Epithelial tissue has many functions, including protection, absorption, and secretion.

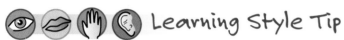 Learning Style Tip

Sketch simple drawings of the three cellular shapes with colorful markers and then label them. Speak aloud as you do this. Kinesthetic learners will remember this even better if they make models of cells out of clay.

Simple Squamous Cells
Simple squamous cells are flat in shape.

Simple Cuboidal Cells
Simple cuboidal cells are cube shaped.

Simple Columnar Cells
Simple columnar cells are cylindrical in shape.

Connective Tissue
Connective tissue is composed of cells that are able to form tissues of various consistencies. These tissues act to connect and support other body tissues. The

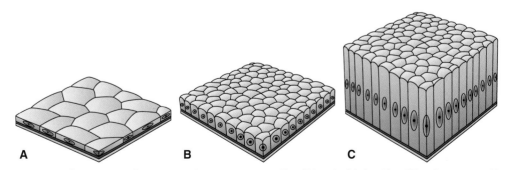

FIGURE 3-2 Common cell shapes: (A) squamous cells, (B) cuboidal cells, (C) columnar cells.

Flashpoint

Muscle tissue has a normal resting length when there is no stimulus or force applied to it. It is the only tissue in the body with these four characteristics:
1. *Irritability:* The ability to respond to a stimulus
2. *Contractility:* The ability to shorten, or contract, when it receives a stimulus
3. *Extensibility:* The ability to stretch, or lengthen, when a force is applied
4. *Elasticity:* The ability to return to its normal resting length when the shortening stimulus or stretching force is removed

various types of connective tissue include cartilage, adipose (fat), bone, and even blood.

Nervous Tissue

Nervous tissue is composed of cells called neurons, which function to transmit nerve impulses by the release of chemicals called neurotransmitters. Nervous tissue comprises the brain, spinal cord, and nerves for the entire body.

Muscle Tissue

Muscle tissue is composed of cells called contractile fibers. As each muscle cell contracts or relaxes, it shortens or lengthens. Consequently, the muscle also shortens or lengthens. Muscles help you move your body, make your heart beat, help many of your internal organs function, and maintain your blood pressure.

Organ and Organ-System Level

Organs are structures made up of two or more types of tissue that perform specialized functions. For example, the heart is composed of cardiac muscle tissue, various types of membranes, and special nervous tissue. Many organs and related structures function together as organ systems to accomplish a specific purpose. For example, the heart acts as a pump; along with a complex network of arteries, veins, and capillaries, it comprises the cardiovascular system. This system circulates blood throughout your body for your entire lifetime. There are many other organ systems as well. You will learn about each of these as you read this book.

Directional Terms and Anatomical Position

Accurate communication is critically important in the world of health care. To ensure that this occurs, all health-care workers must speak the language of medical terminology in a clear and efficient manner. You will begin learning this language by learning directional terms. The use of these terms will enable you to accurately communicate descriptive data about your patient to other members of the health-care team, both verbally and in writing.

Flashpoint

If the patient is in the anatomical position and turns the palms inward, with the thumbs facing forward, they have changed from the anatomical position to the fundamental position.

References to the human body are always made as if the patient is standing in the **anatomical position** (Fig. 3-3). This applies regardless of the actual position of the patient. In the anatomical position, the patient is standing upright, with arms at the side and palms facing forward. The patient's legs are straight, and the toes are pointing forward. The midline is an imaginary line that runs from the head to the feet and through the umbilicus and divides the body into right and left halves. The **midline** is often used as a point of reference. In general, the **axial** portion of the body includes the head, neck, and trunk. The **appendicular** portion of the body includes the arms, or upper extremities, and the legs, or lower extremities.

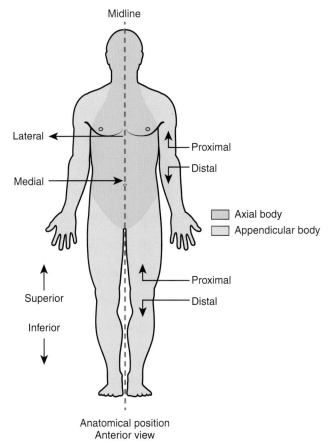

FIGURE 3-3 Directional terms and anatomical position.

Body Planes and Movements

Body planes are imaginary slices or cuts through the body that divide it vertically or horizontally (Fig. 3-4). They are used as points of reference. To visualize
this, imagine a person standing in an upright position. Now imagine dissecting
this person into two pieces with imaginary vertical and horizontal planes. The
sagittal plane runs vertically from front to back and divides the body into right
and left halves. The **frontal** plane (also known as the *coronal* plane) runs vertically from left to right and divides the body into front and back portions. The
transverse plane (also known as the *horizontal* plane) is horizontal and divides
the body into upper and lower portions.

Most movements of the body occur in these planes (Fig. 3-5). When the
motion of the body, or body part, is in an anterior or posterior direction, it is
moving in the sagittal plane. These motions include *flexion* and *extension*.
When motion occurs in a medial or lateral direction, it is moving in the frontal
plane. These motions include *abduction* and *adduction, radial* and *ulnar deviation,* and *eversion* and *inversion*. When motion occurs in a horizontal direction

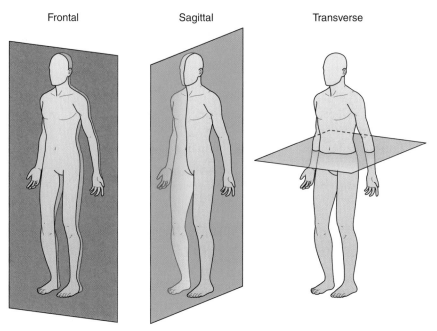

FIGURE 3-4 Body planes.

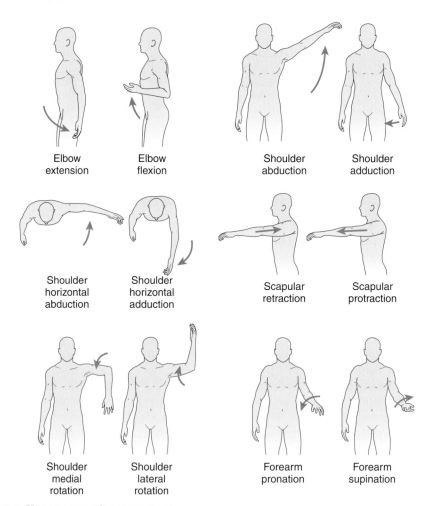

FIGURE 3-5 Upper extremity movements.

or produces a rotation of the body part, it is moving in the transverse plane. These motions include *medial and lateral rotation*, *pronation* and *supination*, and *horizontal adduction and abduction*.

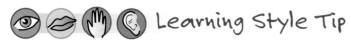 Learning Style Tip

Study with several classmates or enlist the help of family or friends. Identify one person as your patient. Write directional terms on pieces of tape and take turns placing them on the appropriate parts of the patient's body. For the midline, use one long piece of tape; for the planes, pretend to slice the patient into sections. Ask your patient to perform the body movements that occur in each plane. Speak aloud throughout the activity to achieve the full verbal and auditory benefit.

Body Cavities, Regions, and Quadrants

The body is divided into a dorsal cavity and a ventral cavity (Fig. 3-6). The **dorsal cavity** is located on the posterior or back part of the body. It is further divided into the **cranial cavity,** which contains the brain, and the **vertebral cavity,** which contains the spinal column. The **ventral cavity,** located on the anterior or front side of the body, consists of the thoracic and abdominopelvic

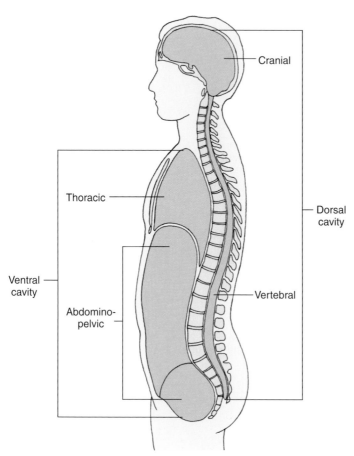

FIGURE 3-6 **Body cavities.**

cavities. The **thoracic cavity** contains the lungs, heart, great vessels, trachea, and thymus. The abdominopelvic cavity is one large cavity, but an imaginary line is sometimes drawn to create a boundary between the abdominal and pelvic cavities. The **abdominal cavity** contains the stomach, pancreas, liver, gallbladder, and large and small intestines. The kidneys lie at the back of the abdomen in an area called the **retroperitoneal space,** just lateral to (to the side of) the spinal column. The **pelvic cavity** contains the sigmoid colon, rectum, bladder, and—in females—the uterus, fallopian tubes, and ovaries.

Two systems are commonly used to visually divide the abdominopelvic cavity for communication and documentation purposes. The nine-region system divides the cavity into nine approximately equal sections. The four-quadrant system divides it into four equal sections, which intersect at the umbilicus (Fig. 3-7). The midline is an imaginary parallel line that runs through the umbilicus and divides the body into right and left halves.

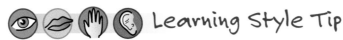 Learning Style Tip

Like the previous Learning Style Tip, you can do this activity with classmates, family, or friends. Identify two people to serve as the patients. Use strips of tape to divide one patient's abdomen into quadrants and the other patient's abdomen into regions. Next, add pieces of tape with the correct names to label each quadrant or region.

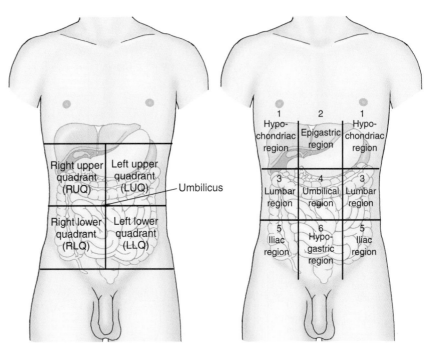

FIGURE 3-7 Abdominal quadrants and regions.

Structure and Function Practice Exercises

Fill in the Blanks

Choose the term that matches the description.

Exercise 1

Cells	Organs	Dorsal cavity
Tissue	Anatomical position	Cranial cavity
Epithelial tissue	Midline	Vertebral cavity
Simple squamous	Axial body	Ventral cavity
Simple cuboidal	Appendicular body	Thoracic cavity
Simple columnar	Body planes	Abdominal cavity
Connective tissue	Sagittal	Retroperitoneal space
Nervous tissue	Frontal	Pelvic cavity
Muscle tissue	Transverse	

1. _____ An imaginary line that runs from the head to the feet and divides the body into right and left halves

2. _____ Cells that are cylindrical in shape

3. _____ The plane that divides the body into upper and lower portions

4. _____ Two or more types of tissue that perform specialized functions

5. _____ The structural units that form all body tissues

6. _____ The cavity that contains the lungs, heart, great vessels, trachea, and thymus

7. _____ The plane that divides the body into front and back portions

8. _____ A group of similar cells that perform a specific function

9. _____ Points of reference which are imaginary slices or cuts through the body that divide it vertically or horizontally

10. _____ The cavity that contains the spinal column

11. _____ Acts to connect and support other body tissues

12. _____ The cavity that contains the stomach, pancreas, liver, gallbladder, and large and small intestines

13. _____ The head, neck, and trunk portion of the body

14. _____ Forms the top layer of skin

15. _____ The cavity that contains the sigmoid colon, rectum, and bladder, and, in females, contains the uterus, fallopian tubes, and ovaries

16. _____ Standing upright with the toes and the palms facing forward

17. _____ The cavity that is located on the anterior or front side of the body

18. _____ Cells that are flat in shape

19. _____ The arms and legs of the body

20. _____ The cavity that contains the brain

21. _____ Comprises the brain, spinal cord, and nerves for the entire body

22. _____ The space at the back of the abdomen just lateral to the spinal column

23. _____ Composed of cells called contractile fibers

24. _____ The cavity that is located on the posterior or back part of the body

25. _____ The plane that divides the body into right and left halves

26. _____ Cells that are cube shaped

Fill in the Blanks

Write the body plane in which each motion occurs. Choose sagittal, frontal, or transverse.

Exercise 2

1. Horizontal adduction _____

2. Adduction _____

3. Inversion _____

4. Pronation _____

5. Radial deviation _____

6. Horizontal abduction _____

7. Abduction _____

8. Eversion _____

9. Medial rotation _____

10. Flexion _____

11. Supination _____

12. Ulnar deviation _____

13. Extension _____

14. Lateral rotation _____

Fill in the Blanks

Label Figure 3-8 with the correct names of the body cavities.

Exercise 3

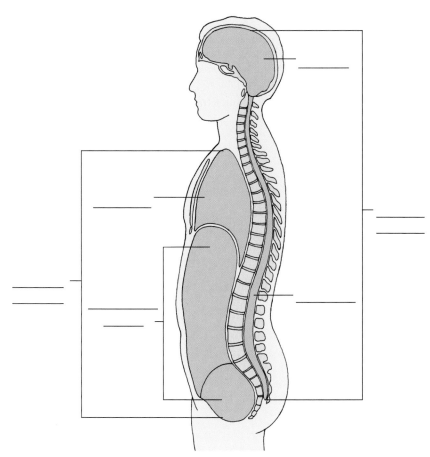

FIGURE 3-8 **Body cavities with blanks.**

Fill in the Blanks

Label Figure 3-9 with the correct names of the abdominal quadrants and regions.

Exercise 4

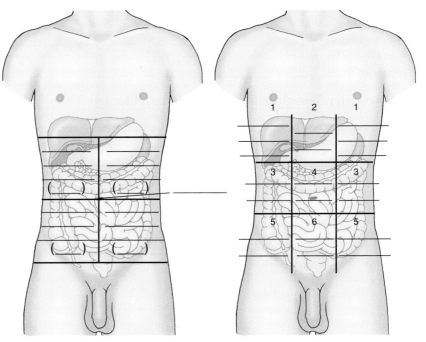

FIGURE 3-9 Abdominal quadrants and regions with blanks.

Locating Body Parts Using Directional Terms

Place the following letters at the specified locations on Figure 3-10.

Exercise 5

1. Place the letter A just superior to the right elbow on the anterior surface of the arm.

2. Place the letter B on the anterior, superior surface of the head.

3. Place the letter C on the distal portion of the left arm on the anterior surface, just proximal to the wrist.

4. Place the letter D slightly inferior to the umbilicus.

5. Place the letter E just inferior to the right knee.

6. Place the letter F on the anterior chest wall, lateral to the sternum (center) on the left.

7. Place the letter G lateral to the umbilicus on the right.

8. Place the letter H proximal to the left knee.

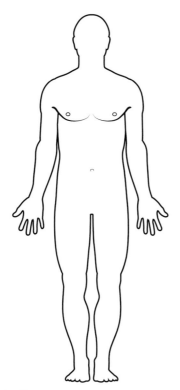

FIGURE 3-10 **Human body illustration.**

Fill in the Blanks

Label Figure 3-11 with the correct names of the body movements.

Exercise 6

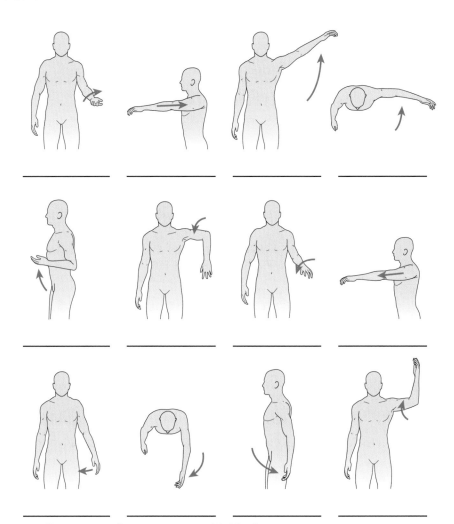

_____   _____   _____   _____

_____   _____   _____   _____

_____   _____   _____   _____

FIGURE 3-11 Upper extremity movements with blanks.

Combining Forms and Abbreviations

Combining Forms

Table 3-1 includes commonly used directional terms and provides a list of anatomical orientations.

IN A FLASH!
Remove the Chapter 3 Combining Forms Flash Cards from the back of this book, and run through them at least three times before you continue.

TABLE 3-1

DIRECTIONAL TERMS AND ANATOMICAL ORIENTATIONS

Term	Combining Form	Meaning	Term	Combining Form	Meaning
abduction		movement toward the side, away from the body	adduction		movement toward the side, toward the body
anterior	anter/o	toward or near the front; ventral	posterior	poster/o	toward or near the back; dorsal
base		the lower or supporting part of any structure	apex		the pointed tip of a conical structure
bilateral		both sides	unilateral		one side
contralateral		the opposite side	ipsilateral		the same side
deep		further into the body	superficial		nearer to the surface of the body
eversion		movement of the ankle causing the bottom of the foot to face toward the side or laterally	inversion		movement of the ankle causing the bottom of the foot to face toward the midline or medially
flexion		movement toward the front or anterior (exception at the knee joint)	extension		movement toward the back or posterior (exception at the knee joint)
horizontal adduction		movement of the arm toward the midline, or anterior, when at shoulder level	horizontal abduction		movement of the arm away from midline, or posterior, when at shoulder level

Continued

TABLE 3-1

DIRECTIONAL TERMS AND ANATOMICAL ORIENTATIONS—cont'd

Term	Combining Form	Meaning	Term	Combining Form	Meaning
medial	medi/o	toward the midline; nearer to the middle	lateral	later/o	away from the midline; toward the side
medial rotation		rotation movement of the shoulder or hip toward the midline; internal rotation	lateral rotation		rotation movement of the shoulder or hip away from the midline; external rotation
pronation		rotation movement of the forearm to palm down; palm facing posterior	supination		rotation movement of the forearm to palm up; palm facing anterior
protraction		movement of the scapula away from the spinal column; scapular abduction	retraction		movement of the scapula toward the spinal column; scapular adduction
proximal	proxim/o	nearer to the axial body	distal	dist/o	further from the axial body
radial deviation		movement of the wrist toward the radius or away from the body; wrist abduction	ulnar deviation		movement of the wrist toward the ulna or toward the body; wrist adduction
superior	super/o	toward or nearer to the head; cranial	inferior	infer/o	toward or nearer to the feet: caudal
supine		lying horizontally facing upward	prone		lying horizontally facing downward
ventral	ventr/o	front; anterior	dorsal	dors/o	back; posterior

Abbreviations

Table 3-2 lists some of the most common abbreviations related to body organization and directional terms as well as others often used in medical documentation.

IN A FLASH!

Go to the Davis*Plus* website to print out all of the Chapter 3 Abbreviations Flash Cards, and run through them at least three times before you continue.

TABLE 3-2
ABBREVIATIONS

abd	abduction	add	adduction
ant	anterior	post	posterior
AP	anteroposterior	PA	posteroanterior
flex	flexion	ext	extension
L	left	R	right
lat	lateral	med	medial
LE	lower extremity; leg	UE	upper extremity; arm
LLQ	left lower quadrant	LUQ	left upper quadrant
RLQ	right lower quadrant	RUQ	right upper quadrant

Combining Forms and Abbreviations Practice Exercises

Multiple Choice

Select the one best answer to the following multiple-choice questions.

Exercise 7

1. What term describes the position of the elbow relative to the wrist?

   a. anterior

   b. distal

   c. lateral

   d. proximal

2. What term describes the position of the mouth relative to the nose?

   a. medial

   b. distal

   c. superior

   d. inferior

3. What term describes the position of the toes relative to the ankle?

   a. superior

   b. medial

   c. distal

   d. anterior

4. Movement toward the front or anterior direction is known as:

   a. inversion

   b. abduction

   c. extension

   d. flexion

5. Movement toward the side or lateral direction is known as:

   a. adduction

   b. abduction

   c. frontal

   d. transverse

6. Where is the right lung relative to the heart?

    a. lateral

    b. anterior

    c. proximal

    d. ventral

7. Where is the heart relative to the rib cage?

    a. proximal

    b. superficial

    c. midline

    d. deep

8. Movement of the forearm causing the palm to face anteriorly is known as:

    a. flexion

    b. supination

    c. medial rotation

    d. eversion

9. Movement of the wrist in the lateral direction is known as:

    a. radial deviation

    b. ulnar deviation

    c. adduction

    d. inversion

10. What term describes the position of the great toe relative to the other four toes on the same foot?

    a. lateral

    b. medial

    c. proximal

    d. distal

Fill in the Blanks

Fill in the blanks below.

Exercise 8

1. The abbreviation *lat* stands for _____.

2. The pointed tip of the heart is the _____.

3. The abbreviation *UE* stands for _____.

4. A person who is lying down and facing upward is in the
   _____ position.

5. The abbreviation *RLQ* stands for _____.

6. Pain located near the body surface is said to be _____.

7. The abbreviation *PA* stands for _____.

8. A person who is lying facedown is in the _____ position.

9. The abbreviation *LUQ* stands for _____.

10. The bottom of the right lung may be described as the
    _____.

Pharmacology

In each of the chapters that follow, a list of common medications that pertain to that particular organ system is provided. Each of these organ systems may also require the use of antibiotic, anti-inflammatory, pain, or cancer medications that are listed in Table 3-3 of this chapter.

TABLE 3-3

PHARMACOLOGY

Therapeutic Classification	Generic Name	Brand Name	Common Use
		Antibiotics	
Aminoglycoside	neomycin	Neo-Fradin, Mycifradin	Inhibit protein synthesis
	streptomycin		
	tobramycin	Nebcin	
Cephalosporin	cephalexin	Biocef, Keflex	Prevent bacteria cell wall formation
Fluoroquinolone	ciprofloxacin	Cipro	Prevent growth of bacteria
	levofloxacin	Levaquin	
Macrolide	azithromycin	Zithromax	Inhibit protein synthesis
	erythromycin	E-Mycin, Pediazole	
Penicillin	amoxicillin	Amoxil	Prevent bacteria cell wall formation
	ampicillin	Omnipen, Principen	
Tetracycline	tetracycline	Panmycin, Sumycin	Inhibit protein synthesis
	doxycycline	Microdox, Periostat, Vibramycin	

TABLE 3-3

PHARMACOLOGY—cont'd

Therapeutic Classification	Generic Name	Brand Name	Common Use
		Pain and Anti-inflammatory Medications	
Analgesic and antipyretic	acetaminophen	Tylenol	Relieve minor aches and pains, reduce fever
Corticosteroid	dexamethasone	Decadron	Reduce inflammation, suppress the immune system
	hydrocortisone	Cortaid, Preparation H	
	methylprednisolone	Medrol, Solu-Medrol	
	prednisolone	Prelone	
	prednisone	Deltasone	
Nonsteroidal anti-inflammatory (NSAID)	aspirin	Bayer, Bufferin, Ecotrin	Reduce inflammation, pain, and fever
	celecoxib	Celebrex	
	diclofenac	Voltaren	
	ibuprofen	Motrin	
	indomethacin	Indocin	
	ketoprofen	Orudis	
	ketorolac	Toradol	
	nabumetone	Relafen	
	naproxen	Aleve, Naprosyn	
	oxaprozin	Daypro	
	piroxicam	Feldene	
	sulindac	Clinoril	
Opioid/Narcotic analgesic	codeine		Relieve moderate to severe pain
	fentanyl	Actiq, Duragesic, Fentora	
	hydrocodone	Lorcet, Lortab, Norco, Vicodin	
	hydromorphone	Dilaudid, Exalgo	
	meperidine	Demerol	
	methadone	Dolophine, Methadose	
	morphine	Avinza, Kadian, MS Contin, Oramorph SR	
	oxycodone	Oxycontin, Oxyfast, Percocet, Roxicodone	
	oxymorphone	Opana	

Continued

TABLE 3-3

PHARMACOLOGY—cont'd

Therapeutic Classification	Generic Name	Brand Name *Cancer Medications*	Common Use
Alkylating agents	bendamustine	Treanda	Direct damage to DNA to prevent the cancer cell from reproducing
	chlorambucil	Leukeran	
	cyclophosphamide	Cytoxan	
	ifosfamide	Ifex	
	lomustine	CeeNU	
	mechlorethamine	Mustargen	
	melphalan	Alkeran	
	streptozotocin	Zanosar	
Antimetabolites	capecitabine	Xeloda	Interfere with DNA and RNA through substitution of the building blocks
	cladribine	Leustatin	
	clofarabine	Clolar	
	cytarabine	Cytosar	
	fludarabine	Fludara	
	gemcitabine	Gemzar	
	hydroxyurea	Hydrea	
	methotrexate		
	pemetrexed	Alimta	
	pentostatin	Nipent	
Antitumor antibiotics	bleomycin	Blenoxane	Interfere with enzymes involved in DNA replication
	daunorubicin		
	doxorubicin	Adriamycin	
	epirubicin	Ellence	
	idarubicin	Idamycin	
	mitomycin-c	Mutamycin	
Differentiating agents	arsenic trioxide	Arsenox	Force cancer cells to mature into normal cells
	bexarotene	Targretin	
	tretinoin	Atralin	
Immunotherapy	alemtuzumab	Campath	Stimulate the immune system to recognize and attack cancer cells
	interferon-alfa	Intron A, Roferon-A	
	lenalidomide	Revlimid	
	rituximab	Rituxan	
	thalidomide	Thalomid	

TABLE 3-3			
PHARMACOLOGY—cont'd			
Therapeutic Classification	**Generic Name**	**Brand Name**	**Common Use**
Mitotic inhibitors	docetaxel	Taxotere	Stop mitosis or inhibit enzymes from making proteins needed for cell reproduction
	estramustine	Emcyt	
	ixabepilone	Ixempra	
	paclitaxel	Taxol	
	vinblastine	Velban	
	vincristine	Oncovin	
	vinorelbine	Navelbine	
Targeted therapies	bortezomib	Velcade	Attack specific cancer cells
	gefitinib	Iressa	
	imatinib	Gleevec	
	sunitinib	Sutent	

End-of-Chapter Practice Exercises

Multiple Choice

Select the one best answer to the following multiple-choice questions.

Exercise 9

1. Levels of organization of the human body from smallest to largest are:

    a. molecular, tissue, atomic, cellular, organ, organ system, human body

    b. atomic, molecular, cellular, tissue, organ, organ system, human body

    c. tissue, cellular, atomic, molecular, organ, organ system, human body

    d. none of these

2. All of the following are types of tissues in the human body **except:**

    a. staphylococci

    b. connective

    c. nervous

    d. muscle

3. Which of the following statements is true?

   a. the arrangement of the human body is simple.

   b. chemistry courses typically study the body at the cellular level.

   c. cellular biology courses study the body at the chemical level.

   d. medical terminology generally studies the body at the organ and organ-system levels.

4. Which of the following statements is true regarding cells?

   a. They are composed of body tissues.

   b. Their walls protect them by not allowing any substances to enter or leave.

   c. The fluid within cells is called plasma.

   d. The genetic blueprint of the body is contained within the cell nucleus.

5. Which of the following statements is true?

   a. Squamous cells are cube shaped.

   b. Cuboidal cells are cylindrical in shape.

   c. Columnar cells are cube shaped.

   d. None of these

Matching

Choose the correct letter to match the term with the meaning.

Exercise 10

1. _____ Rotation movement of the shoulder or hip toward the midline; internal rotation

2. _____ Movement toward the side, toward the body

3. _____ Movement of the wrist toward the ulna or toward the body; wrist adduction

4. _____ The same side

5. _____ Toward or near the back; dorsal

6. _____ Away from the midline; toward the side

7. _____ Further from the axial body

8. _____ Movement toward the side, away from the body

9. _____ Nearer to the surface of the body

a. horizontal adduction

b. medial

c. proximal

d. abduction

e. medial rotation

f. pronation

g. adduction

h. flexion

i. superior

10. _____ Toward or nearer to the feet: caudal

    j. deep

11. _____ Movement toward the back or posterior

    k. lateral

12. _____ Movement toward the front or anterior

    l. distal

13. _____ Toward the midline; nearer to the middle

    m. ulnar deviation

14. _____ Movement of the scapula toward the spinal column; scapular adduction

    n. eversion

15. _____ Further into the body

    o. inferior

16. _____ Toward or nearer to the head; cranial

    p. posterior

17. _____ Movement of the arm toward the midline, or anterior, when at shoulder level

    q. superficial

18. _____ Rotation movement of the forearm to palm down; palm facing posterior

    r. ipsilateral

19. _____ Nearer to the axial body

    s. extension

20. _____ Movement of the ankle causing the bottom of the foot to face toward the side or laterally

    t. retraction

Fill in the Blanks

Fill in the blanks below.

Exercise 11

1. The abbreviation _ant_ stands for _____.

2. The abbreviation _lat_ stands for _____.

3. The abbreviation _R_ stands for _____.

4. The abbreviation _abd_ stands for _____.

5. The abbreviation _post_ stands for _____.

6. The abbreviation _ext_ stands for _____.

7. The abbreviation _med_ stands for _____.

8. The abbreviation _add_ stands for _____.

9. The abbreviation _flex_ stands for _____.

10. The abbreviation _L_ stands for _____.

Fill in the Blanks

Using Table 3-3, write the therapeutic classification of the medication next to each generic or brand name.

Exercise 12

1. fentanyl _____

2. interferon alfa _____

3. Motrin _____

4. methotrexate _____

5. Cortaid _____

6. Cytoxan _____

7. naproxen _____

8. Zithromax _____

9. Lortab _____

10. Oncovin _____

11. Percocet _____

12. daunorubicin _____

13. amoxicillin _____

14. Levaquin _____

15. prednisone _____

16. ifosfamide _____

17. Celebrex _____

18. paclitaxel _____

19. meperidine _____

20. tretinoin _____

INTEGUMENTARY SYSTEM

4

Chapter Outline

Structure and Function

You may not think of the skin as an organ, but it is actually the largest organ of the body. Let's take a look at the structure and function of the integumentary system.

The skin consists of three layers (Fig. 4-1). The **epidermis** is the thin outer layer that is constructed mostly of nonliving, keratinized (hardened) cells. It is waterproof and provides protection for the deeper layers. The epidermis is thickest on the palms of the hands and the soles of the feet. The base of this layer, aptly named the **basement membrane**, is where new, living epidermal cells are produced. These cells are pushed upward as even newer cells form beneath them. Eventually, they rise to the top, away from blood vessels and nerve endings, and die, thus becoming keratinized tissue. This is why cells on the top layer of your skin can be scraped away without causing pain.

Flashpoint

The prefix *epi-* means *above* or *upon;* so the name *epidermis,* which means *above or upon the dermis,* tells you exactly where it is located.

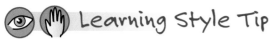 Learning Style Tip

Look carefully at the illustrations and photos in this book. Draw and label what you see.

The **dermis** lies just beneath the epidermis and is much thicker. It is made of fibrous connective tissue containing elastin, which provides elasticity, and collagen, which provides strength. It also contains a good blood supply and numerous other structures, including hair follicles, nerves, sweat glands, oil glands, and sensory receptors.

Beneath the dermis is the **subcutaneous layer.** This layer contains fat tissue as well as deeper blood vessels, nerves, the lower part of hair follicles, elastin, and collagen. The subcutaneous layer provides insulation for deeper structures.

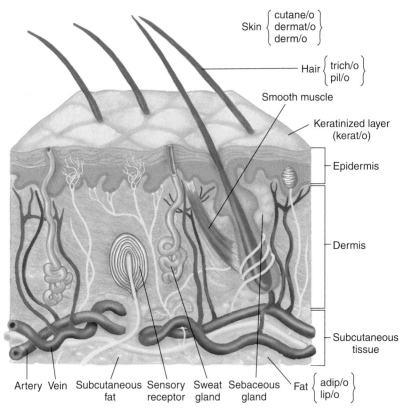

FIGURE 4-1 **The skin.**

Accessory structures of the skin include the **sudoriferous (sweat) glands, sebaceous (oil) glands,** hair, and nails. Sudoriferous glands are located throughout the body but are more concentrated in some areas, such as the soles of the feet and palms of the hands. Sebaceous glands are found at the base of hair follicles all over the body; they secrete an oily substance called **sebum.**

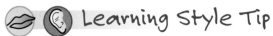 Learning Style Tip

It can be helpful to *speak* and *hear* the information you are learning multiple times. Find a study partner or join a study group whenever possible. Take turns "teaching" each other the information by saying it aloud. Listeners should pay close attention and be prepared to discuss information they feel is incorrect or incomplete.

The **skin** (and its accessory structures) serve several important functions in the body. Its major functions are protection and temperature regulation. The skin protects your body from bacteria and other microorganisms, harmful ultraviolet light from the rays of the sun, and extreme temperatures. Because the outer layer of your skin is waterproof, it keeps pathogens (tiny disease-causing organisms) from entering even when it gets wet, unless there is a break in the skin. Sebum discourages bacterial growth; it also lubricates your skin to keep it soft and supple. If pathogens do get in through a **laceration** (a cut or tear in the flesh) or an **abrasion** (an area where skin or mucous membranes are scraped away), infection may occur. However, as the tissue becomes irritated, a natural inflammatory response occurs. When this happens, the body increases circulation of blood to the injured area. This is responsible for the **edema** (swelling) and **erythema** (redness) that appear. Increased numbers of **leukocytes** (white blood cells) arrive to fight off the invaders and, quite literally, gobble them up. The increased circulation also helps speed the process of healing, as debris is cleared away and healthy new cells fill in the injured area, along with scar tissue.

The skin also contains **melanocytes,** which are pigment-producing skin cells. The pigment they produce, **melanin,** gives skin its colors. In response to ultraviolet light from the sun, melanocytes produce more melanin, causing a suntan. Melanin helps filter ultraviolet light and protect the skin from damage. The amount of melanin in your skin varies depending on your heredity and ethnicity.

Flashpoint
A suntan is the body's way of protecting the skin from damage caused by ultraviolet light.

Pressure, Pain, and Temperature Perception

Because the skin contains a number of different specialized nerves and sensory receptors, it plays a vital role in our ability to perceive pressure as well as pain and temperature. Messages from the receptors allow us to sense when we are being touched and recognize objects we are touching. They signal us to take measures to increase physical comfort, such as rolling over in bed or shifting in our chair to relieve excessive pressure (Box 4-1). We are able to manage our pain by receiving a massage or by applying an ice pack (IP) or moist hot pack (MHP) to the skin. In addition, sensory receptors also provide an important protective function: If you accidentally touch a very hot surface, your heat and pain receptors immediately send a message to your central nervous system, and you respond by pulling your hand away. Such a response is a protective **reflex,** which happens so quickly that you don't have time to think about it.

Box 4-1 Pressure Ulcers

When soft tissue is compressed between a bony prominence and an external surface for a prolonged period of time, a pressure ulcer can develop. Pressure ulcers are integumentary system wounds that are also known as decubitus ulcers and bedsores. They can range in severity from a stage I ulceration with intact skin, to a stage IV ulcer in which muscle, tendon, or bone is visible in the wound. They can appear on various areas of the body, but it is common for them to be found on the back of the heel or on the sacrum. This is especially true when an individual has a decreased level of consciousness or is too weak to move themselves into a different position. Other risk factors for the development of pressure ulcers include inactivity, poor nutrition, incontinence, and impaired sensation. Individuals with prosthetic limbs are also prone to pressure ulcers as weight fluctuations can interfere with proper fit of the limb.

Techniques to prevent pressure ulcers, or to facilitate healing of existing ulcerations, include utilizing turning and repositioning schedules and using pressure relief devices such as cushions, wedges, or mattress overlays. A small rolled up towel under the ankle is a great way to keep the heel off of the bed. Forces such as shear and friction should also be minimized. The head of the bed should not be raised to a point that the person slides downward, and body parts should not be dragged across surfaces. In addition, excessive moisture should be eliminated by keeping clothing dry and using skin sealants or moisture barriers.

The integumentary system also plays an important role in body-temperature regulation. It provides insulation to keep you warm when the external environment is too cold. As your environment becomes colder, your hands and fingers become pale in color, because the blood vessels near your skin's surface constrict in order to give off less heat and thus conserve it for deeper organs. The opposite also occurs: When your environment is too hot, these same blood vessels dilate (expand) in order to give off more heat. This response may cause you to have a flushed appearance. In addition, your sweat glands secrete moisture, which evaporates on your skin's surface and provides even more cooling.

Hair and Nails

Hair and nails are also accessory structures of the integumentary system. Hair is found on most parts of the body and is especially prominent on the head, in the nose and ears, and on the face as eyebrows and eyelashes. It serves a protective function, as it filters out dust and debris from the air. The part of the hair that you can see is the **hair shaft.** The part buried in the skin is the **hair follicle,** which contains the root. Hair is made up of a protein called keratin; it gets its color from melanin. With aging, the amount of melanin may decrease, leading to graying of hair. As new cells are formed in the hair root, older keratinized cells are pushed up and become part of the hair shaft.

Nails help to protect the ends of our fingers and toes. The nail forms in the nail root and is made up of keratinized squamous epithelial cells. As nails grow in a flattened shape, they slide very slowly over a layer of epithelial tissue called the **nailbed.** The area at the base of the nail, sometimes called the half-moon, is the **lunula.** This is where new growth occurs. Figure 4-2 shows the structure of the nail.

Flashpoint

Sensory receptors in the skin help us to interact with our environment and protect us from harm.

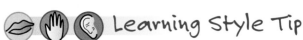 Learning Style Tip

Be sure to recite the new combining forms aloud so you benefit from saying and hearing them. Have fun being overly dramatic with your expressions, pronunciation, and body movements as you say the terms. You may feel silly doing this, but you will remember the terms better later on.

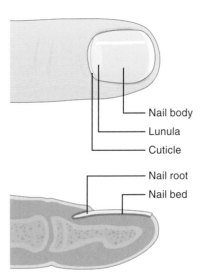

FIGURE 4-2 **Nail structure.**

Structure and Function Practice Exercises

Fill in the Blanks

Choose the term that matches the description.

Exercise 1

Epidermis	Skin	Melanin
Basement membrane	Laceration	Reflex
Dermis	Abrasion	Hair shaft
Subcutaneous layer	Edema	Hair follicle
Sudoriferous glands	Erythema	Nailbed
Sebaceous glands	Leukocytes	Lunula
Sebum	Melanocytes	

1. _____ Area where skin has been scraped away

2. _____ Sweat glands

3. _____ Largest organ of the body with major functions of protection and temperature regulation

4. _____ White blood cells

5. _____ Pigment that gives skin its color

6. _____ Part of the hair that you can see which functions to filter dust and debris from the air

7. _____ Layer of skin that contains hair follicles, nerves, sweat glands, and sensory receptors

8. _____ Redness

9. _____ Action, or response, that happens so quickly that you don't have time to think about it

10. _____ Layer of skin that contains fat and provides insulation for deeper structures

11. _____ Nails slide slowly over this layer of epithelial tissue as they grow

12. _____ Place where new, living epidermal cells are produced

13. _____ Half-moon area at the base of the nail where new growth occurs

14. _____ Substance secreted by oil glands

15. _____ Swelling

16. _____ Part of the hair that is buried in the skin

17. _____ Thin, outer layer of the skin

18. _____ Pigment-producing skin cells

19. _____ Glands found at the base of hair follicles all over
the body

20. _____ Cut or tear in the flesh

Fill in the Blanks

Label Figure 4-3 with the appropriate anatomical terms and combining forms.

Exercise 2

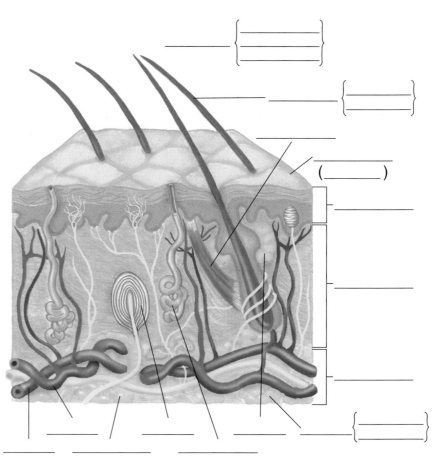

FIGURE 4-3 **Skin with blanks.**

Combining Forms and Abbreviations

Combining Forms

Table 4-1 lists combining forms that pertain to the integumentary system. Table 4-2 lists combining forms related to color.

TABLE 4-1
COMBINING FORMS RELATED TO THE INTEGUMENTARY SYSTEM

Combining Form	Meaning	Example (Pronunciation)	Meaning of New Term
adip/o	fat	adipoid (Ă-dĭ-poyd)	resembling fat
lip/o		lipoma (lĭ-PŌ-mă)	tumor of fat
cutane/o	skin	cutaneous (kū-TĀ-nē-ŭs)	pertaining to the skin
derm/o		dermoplasty (DĔR-mō-plăs-tē)	surgical repair of the skin
dermat/o		dermatologist (dĕr-mă-TŎ-lō-jĭst)	specialist in the study of the skin
cyt/o	cell	cytology (sī-TŎ-lō-jē)	study of cells
eti/o	cause	etiology (ē-tē-Ŏ-lō-jē)	study of causes
hidr/o	sweat	hidrosis (hī-DRŌ-sĭs)	abnormal condition of sweat
hydr/o	water	hydrotherapy (hī-drō-THĔR-ă-pē)	water therapy
idi/o	unknown, peculiar	idiopathic (ĭd-ē-ō-PĂTH-ĭk)	pertaining to an unknown disease
kerat/o	keratinized tissue, cornea	keratotomy (kĕr-ă-TŎ-tō-mē)	cutting into or incision of the cornea
morph/o	shape	morphology (mōr-FŎ-lō-jē)	study of shapes
myc/o	fungus	mycosis (mī-KŌ-sĭs)	abnormal condition of fungus
necr/o	dead	necrosis (nĕ-KRŌ-sĭs)	abnormal condition of dead (tissue)
onych/o	nail	onychomalacia (ŏn-ĭ-kō-mă-LĀ-sē-ă)	softening of the nail
path/o	disease	pathologist (pă-THŎ-lō-jĭst)	specialist in the study of disease
pil/o	hair	depilous (DĔP-ĭl-ŭs)	absence of hair
trich/o		trichopathy (trĭk-ŎP-ă-thē)	disease of the hair
rhytid/o	wrinkle	rhytidectomy (rĭt-ĭ-DĔK-tō-mē)	surgical removal of wrinkles
scler/o	hardening, sclera	sclerosis (sklĕ-RŌ-sĭs)	abnormal condition of hardening
seb/o	sebum	seborrhea (sĕ-bō-RĒ-ă)	flow or discharge of sebum
son/o	sound	sonogram (SŎ-nō-grăm)	record of sound
xer/o	dry	xeroderma (zĕr-ō-DĔR-mă)	dry skin

TABLE 4-2

COMBINING FORMS RELATED TO COLOR

Combining Form	Meaning	Example	Meaning of New Term
albin/o	white	albinism (ĂL-bǐ-nǐ-zum)	condition of whiteness
leuk/o		leukorrhea (loo-kō-RĒ-ǎ)	white flow or discharge
chromat/o	color	chromatic (krō-MĂ-tǐk)	pertaining to color
cirrh/o	yellow	cirrhosis (sǐ-RŌ-sǐs)	abnormal condition of yellowness
xanth/o		xanthoderma (zăn-thō-DĔR-mǎ)	yellow skin
cyan/o	blue	cyanosis (sī-ă-NŌ-sǐs)	abnormal condition of blueness
erythem/o	red	erythematous (ĕr-ǐ-THĒM-ǎt-us)	pertaining to redness
erythr/o		erythrocyte (ĕ-RǏTH-rō-sīt)	red (blood) cell
melan/o	black	melanoma (mě-lǎ-NŌ-mǎ)	black tumor

  Learning Style Tip

Use colored markers or pens to highlight or underline terms with their associated colors (e.g., highlight *cyan/o* in blue) and draw silly pictures to associate with other terms (e.g., draw a wrinkly face next to *rhytid/o*).

IN A FLASH!

Remove the Combining Form Flash Cards for Chapter 4 from the back of this book and run through them at least three times before you continue.

Abbreviations

Flashpoint

Using abbreviations can save you time and lengthy documentation; but, to avoid miscommunication, it is important to use only accurate, facility-approved abbreviations.

Abbreviations are used extensively in the world of health care. The primary reason is to save time in both written and verbal communications. As you will see, some medical terms are quite lengthy and difficult to pronounce. This is yet another reason for the use of abbreviations. Imagine having to say *endoscopic retrograde cholangiopancreatography* more than once in a conversation!

Table 4-3 lists some of the most common abbreviations pertaining to the integumentary system, as well as some that are commonly used for documentation or medication orders.

IN A FLASH!

Go to the Davis*Plus* website to print out the Abbreviation Flash Cards for Chapter 4 and run through them at least three times before you continue.

TABLE 4-3
ABBREVIATIONS

BCC	basal cell carcinoma	IV	intravenous
Bx, bx	biopsy	MM	malignant melanoma
C&S	culture and sensitivity	OTC	over-the-counter
decub	decubitus ulcer; also called *pressure ulcer*	PE	physical examination
derm	dermatology	SCC	squamous cell carcinoma
FH	family history	STM	soft tissue mobilization; also called *massage*
Hx	history	SubQ, Sub-Q	subcutaneous
I&D	incision and drainage	Sx	symptom(s)
ID	intradermal (injection)	Tx	treatment
IP	ice pack	ung	ointment
MHP	moist hot pack		

Combining Forms and Abbreviations Practice Exercises

Fill in the Blanks

Fill in the blanks below using Tables 4-1 and 4-2.

Exercise 3

1. condition of whiteness _____

2. surgical removal of wrinkles _____

3. yellow skin _____

4. black tumor _____

5. abnormal condition of blueness _____

6. study of causes _____

7. white flow or discharge _____

8. pertaining to redness _____

9. red (blood) cell _____

10. study of shapes _____

11. specialist in the study of disease _____

12. pertaining to color _____

13. dry skin _____

14. flow of sebum _____

15. resembling fat _____

16. abnormal condition of hardening _____

17. tumor of fat _____

18. absence of hair _____

19. water therapy _____

20. disease of the hair _____

21. pertaining to the skin _____

22. specialist in the study of the skin _____

23. study of cells _____

24. incision into the cornea _____

25. surgical repair of the skin _____

26. abnormal condition of fungus _____

27. abnormal condition of dead (tissue) _____

28. softening of the nail _____

29. abnormal condition of yellowness _____

30. abnormal condition of sweat _____

31. record of sound _____

32. pertaining to an unknown disease _____

Fill in the Blanks

Write the correct term next to each abbreviation using Table 4-3.

Exercise 4

1. STM _____

2. IV _____

3. ung _____

4. OTC _____

5. Hx _____

6. MHP _____

7. C&S _____

8. decub _____

9. BCC _____

10. SubQ _____

 Learning Style Tip

If you are self-conscious about speaking aloud while studying, then find a private, secluded area like the back corner of the library, an empty classroom, or even your car.

Pathologies, Procedures, and Pharmacology

Pathology Terms

Table 4-4 lists many of the pathology terms that pertain to the integumentary system.

TABLE 4-4	
PATHOLOGY TERMS	
abrasion (ă-BRĀ-zhŭn)	scraping away of skin or mucous membranes
acne (ĂK-nē)	disease of the sebaceous (oil) glands and hair follicles in the skin, marked by plugged pores, pimples, cysts, and nodules on the face, neck, chest, back, and other areas
actinic keratosis (ăk-TĬ-nĭk kĕr-ă-TŌ-sĭs)	precancerous condition in which rough, scaly patches of skin develop, most commonly on sun-exposed areas such as the scalp, neck, face, ears, lips, hands, and forearms; also known as *solar keratosis*

Continued

TABLE 4-4
PATHOLOGY TERMS—cont'd

alopecia (ă-lō-PĒ-shē-ă)	autoimmune disease that results in loss of hair; alopecia areata causes patchy hair loss from the scalp; alopecia totalis causes total scalp hair loss; alopecia universalis causes total body hair loss

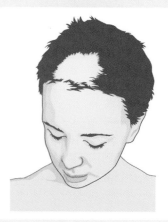

Alopecia.

basal cell carcinoma (BĀ-săl sĕl kăr-sĭ-NŌ-mă)	common type of skin cancer that typically appears as a small, shiny papule and eventually enlarges to form a whitish border around a central depression or ulcer that may bleed
bulla (BŬ-lă)	large blister or skin vesicle filled with fluid
burn (bŭrn)	type of thermal injury to the skin caused by a variety of heat sources; classified according to severity as first-degree (superficial), second-degree (partial-thickness), and third-degree (full-thickness)

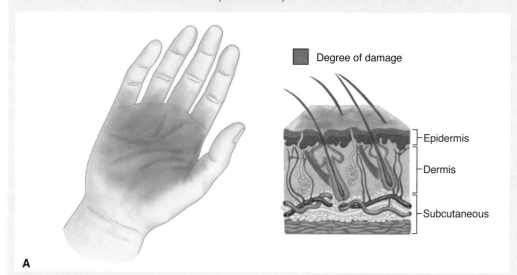

Degree of damage

Epidermis

Dermis

Subcutaneous

A

Burn: (A) first-degree burn,

TABLE 4-4
PATHOLOGY TERMS—cont'd

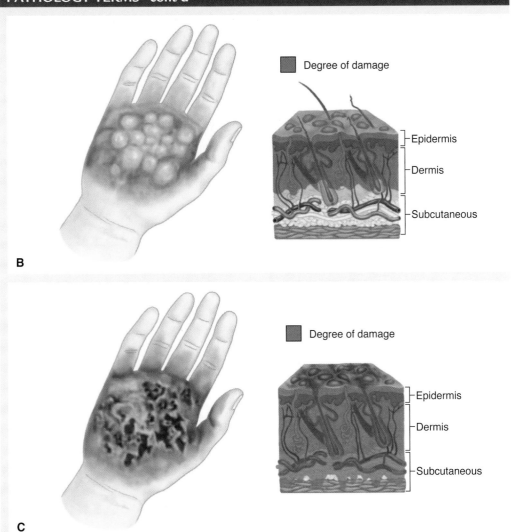

(B) second-degree burn, (C) third-degree burn. (From Eagle, S., et al. [2009]. *The professional medical assistant.* Philadelphia, PA: F.A. Davis Company, p. 984; with permission)

callus (KĂ-lŭs)	thickened, hardened, toughened area of skin caused by frequent or chronic pressure or friction

Continued

TABLE 4-4
PATHOLOGY TERMS—cont'd

carbuncle (KĂR-bŭng-kul)	very large furuncle or cluster of connected furuncles

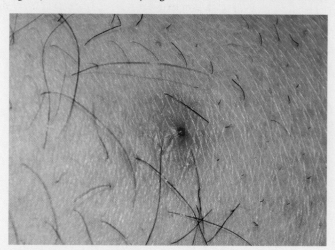

Carbuncle. (Photograph © Thinkstock)

cellulitis (sĕl-ū-LĪ-tĭs)	potentially serious bacterial skin infection marked by pain, redness, edema, warmth, and fever
comedo (KŎ-mē-dō)	blackhead
corn (kōrn)	small callus that develops on smooth, hairless skin surfaces, such as the backs of fingers or toes, in response to pressure and friction; hard corns typically develop on the sides of feet and tops of toes; soft corns usually develop between toes

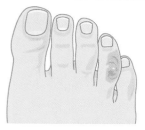

Corn.

cyst (sĭst)	fluid- or solid-containing pouch in or under the skin

TABLE 4-4
PATHOLOGY TERMS—cont'd

decubitus ulcer (dē-KŪ-bĭ-tŭs ŬL-sĕr)	area of injury and tissue death caused by unrelieved pressure that impedes circulation in the skin and underlying tissues; also called *pressure ulcer* or *bedsore*

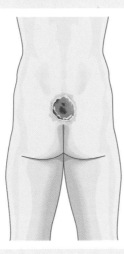

Decubitus ulcer.

ecchymosis, contusion (ĕ-kĭ-MŌ-sĭs, kŏn-TOO-zhŭn)	discoloration of the skin, bruise

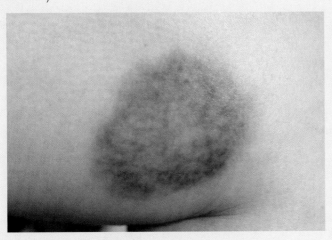

Ecchymosis. (Photograph © Thinkstock)

Continued

TABLE 4-4
PATHOLOGY TERMS—cont'd

eczema (ĔK-zĕ-mă)	inflammatory skin condition marked by red, hot, dry, scaly, cracked, and itchy skin or blisters

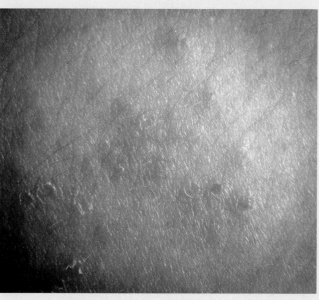

Eczema. (Photograph © Thinkstock)

epidermoid cyst (ĕ-pĭ-DĔR-moyd sĭst)	small sac or pouch below the skin surface containing a thick, cheesy substance; appears pale white or yellow but can be darker in dark-skinned people
fissure (FĬSH-ūr)	small, cracklike break in the skin
folliculitis (fō-lĭ-kū-LĪ-tĭs)	inflammation of hair follicles, marked by rash with small red bumps, pustules, tenderness, and itching; common on the neck, armpit, and groin area
frostbite (FRŎST-bīt)	injury that occurs when skin tissues are exposed to temperatures cold enough to cause them to freeze

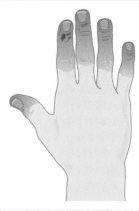

Frostbite.

furuncle (FŪR-ŭng-kul)	infection of a hair follicle and nearby tissue, also called a *boil*; more invasive than folliculitis because it involves the sebaceous gland

TABLE 4-4

PATHOLOGY TERMS—cont'd

impetigo (ĭm-pĕ-TĪ-gō)	bacterial skin infection marked by yellow to red weeping, crusted, or pustular lesions; common in children

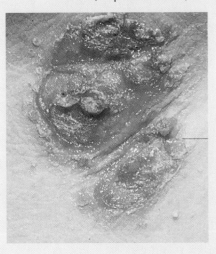

Impetigo.

incision (ĭn-SĬ-zhŭn)	surgical cut in the flesh
laceration (lăs-ĕ-RĀ-shŭn)	cut or tear in the flesh
Lyme disease (līm dĭ-ZĒZ)	bacterial infection transmitted by ticks, marked by erythema chronicum migrans, a red, circular rash that slowly expands and enlarges; untreated disease causes multisystem symptoms
macule (MĂ-kūl)	flat, discolored spot on the skin, such as a freckle

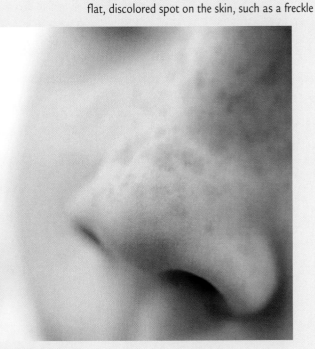

Macule. (Photograph © Thinkstock)

Continued

TABLE 4-4

PATHOLOGY TERMS—cont'd

malignant melanoma (mă-LĬG-nănt mĕ-lă-NŌ-mă)	aggressive form of skin cancer that often begins as various-colored, asymmetrical lesions larger than 6 mm in diameter
melasma (mĕ-LĂZ-mă)	development of irregular areas of darker-pigmented skin on the forehead, nose, cheek, and upper lip; also called *chloasma* or the *mask of pregnancy*
papule (PĂP-ūl)	small, raised spot or bump on the skin, such as a mole

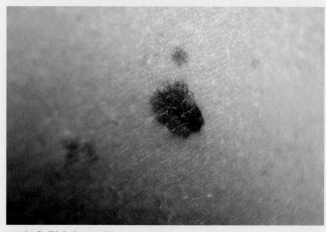

Papule. (Photograph © Thinkstock)

paronychia (păr-ō-NĬK-ē-ă)	acute or chronic infection of the margins of the fingernail or toenail, marked by warmth, erythema, edema, pus, throbbing, pain, or tenderness; causes the nail to become discolored and thickened
pediculosis (pĕ-dĭk-ū-LŌ-sĭs)	infestation of head, body, or pubic lice, marked by itching, the appearance of lice on the body, and eggs (nits) attached to hair shafts
petechiae (pĕ-TĔ-kē-ē)	tiny red or purple hemorrhagic spots (singular *petechia*)

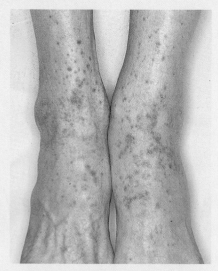

Petechiae. (From Goldsmith, L.A., et al. [1997]. *Adult and pediatric dermatology: a color guide to diagnosis and treatment.* Philadelphia, PA: F.A. Davis Company, p. 61; with permission)

TABLE 4-4

PATHOLOGY TERMS—cont'd

psoriasis (sō-RĪ-ă-sĭs)	chronic, inflammatory skin disorder marked by the development of silvery-white scaly plaques or patches with sharply defined borders and reddened skin beneath

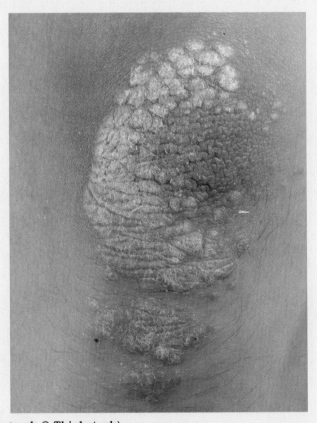

Psoriasis. (Photograph © Thinkstock)

puncture (PŬNGK-chūr)	hole or wound made by a sharp, pointed instrument
pustule (PŬS-tūl)	small, pus-filled blister
rosacea (rō-ZĀ-sē-ă)	chronic condition that causes flushing and redness of the face, neck, and chest

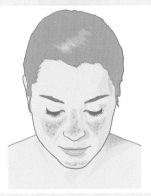

Rosacea.

Continued

TABLE 4-4
PATHOLOGY TERMS—cont'd

scabies (SKĀ-bēz)	contagious skin disease transmitted by the itch mite, with symptoms of itching, scaly papules, insect burrows, and secondary infected lesions most prevalent in skin folds at the wrists and elbows, between the fingers, under the arms, in the groin, and under the beltline
scales (skālz)	area of skin that is excessively dry and flaky

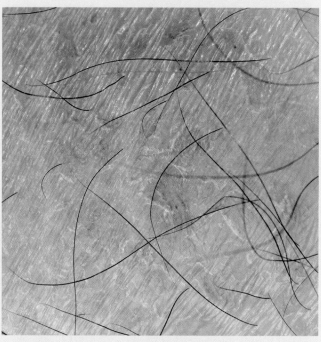

Scales. (Photograph © Thinkstock)

sebaceous cyst (sē-BĀ-shŭs sĭst)	small sac or pouch below the skin surface filled with a thick fluid or semisolid oily substance called sebum
seborrheic keratosis (sĕ-bō-RĒ-ĭk kĕr-ă-TŌ-sĭs)	benign, flat, irregularly shaped skin growths of various colors with a warty, waxy, "stuck-on" appearance
squamous cell carcinoma (SKWĀ-mŭs sĕl kăr-sĭ-NŌ-mă)	type of cancer that usually appears in the mouth, esophagus, bronchi, lungs, or vagina and uterine cervix, marked by a firm, red nodule or a scaly appearance; may ulcerate
tinea (TĬ-nē-ă)	fungal skin disease occurring on various parts of the body, also called *dermatophytosis* or *ringworm*; forms include tinea capitis (scalp), tinea corporis (trunk), tinea cruris (genital area; also called *jock itch*), tinea nodosa (mustache and beard), tinea pedis (feet; also called *athlete's foot*), and tinea unguium (nails)

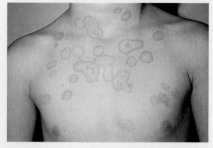

Tinea. (From *Taber's cyclopedic medical dictionary* [21st ed.; 2009]. Philadelphia, PA: F. A. Davis Company, p. 2324; with permission)

TABLE 4-4
PATHOLOGY TERMS—cont'd

ulcer (ŬL-sĕr)	lesion of the skin or mucous membranes, marked by inflammation, necrosis, and sloughing of damaged tissues
vesicle (VĔS-ĭ-kul)	clear, fluid-filled blister
vitiligo (vĭt-ĭl-Ī-gō)	chronic skin disease that results in patchy loss of skin pigment; may also affect hair color and cause white patches or streaks

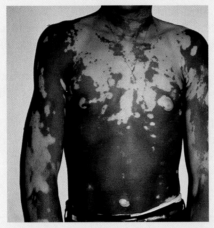

Vitiligo. (From Goldsmith, L.A., et al. [1997]. *Adult and pediatric dermatology: a color guide to diagnosis and treatment.* Philadelphia, PA: F.A. Davis Company, p. 121; with permission)

wart (wōrt)	small, benign skin tumor caused by various strains of the human papillomavirus (HPV); appearance varies from tiny to moderate-sized bumps or cauliflower-shaped growths
wheal (hwēl)	rounded, temporary elevation in the skin, white in the center with a red-pink periphery and accompanied by itching

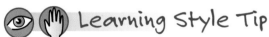 Learning Style Tip

Collect photos and illustrations of pathological conditions from journals, Internet image search engines, and other sources to create a poster or collage. Be sure to write the name of each disorder and a brief description next to each image. Tape the poster somewhere that you will see it daily, and review the information on it at least once each day.

IN A FLASH!
Go to the DavisPlus website to print out the Pathology Term Flash Cards for Chapter 4 and run through them at least three times before you continue.

Flashpoint
An easy way to remember the difference between a papule and a macule is that you can **p**alpate (touch or feel) a **p**apule but not a macule.

Common Diagnostic Tests and Procedures

Biopsy: Removal of a tissue sample for microscopic examination

Cosmetic Enhancement Procedures

Dermabrasion: Removal of small scars, nevi (moles), tattoos, or fine wrinkles with a wire brush or burr impregnated with diamond particles, leaving a smoother surface

Dermaplaning: Removal of small scars, nevi (moles), tattoos, or fine wrinkles with a dermatome (a device resembling an electric razor), leaving a smoother surface

Microdermabrasion: Similar to dermabrasion but less invasive, involving multiple treatments of gentle abrasion; useful in reducing fine lines, nevi (moles), age spots, and acne scars

Chemical peel: Application of a chemical solution to the skin to improve appearance by removing blemishes, fine wrinkles, uneven pigmentation, scars, and tattoos

Laser resurfacing: Use of short pulses of light to remove fine lines and damaged skin and to minimize scars and even out areas of uneven pigmentation; sometimes called a *laser peel*

BOTOX (botulinum toxin): An injection into selected muscles of the face that interferes with muscle contraction, thereby reducing the appearance of wrinkles

Pharmacology

Table 4-5 provides a list of common integumentary system medications.

TABLE 4-5			
PHARMACOLOGY			
Therapeutic Classification	**Generic Name**	**Brand Name**	**Common Use**
Anti-acne agent	benzoyl peroxide	Benoxyl, Benzac, Desquam, Fostex, Triaz, Vanoxide, Zoderm	Reduce amount of acne-causing bacteria
Antibacterial	mupirocin	Bactroban, Centany	Kill bacteria or prevent its growth
	clindamycin	Cleocin	Kill bacteria or prevent its growth
Antifungal agent	ketoconazole	Nizoral	Kill fungus or prevent its growth
	terbinafine	Lamisil	
	clotrimazole	Lotrimin	Interfere with the formation of the fungal cell membrane
	fluconazole	Diflucan	
Antipsoriatic	anthralin	Drithocreme, Micanol, Psoriatec, Zithranol	Slow down the growth of skin cells
Immunosuppressant	adalimumab	Humira	Block tumor necrosis factor (TNF)
	etanercept	Enbrel	

TABLE 4-5

PHARMACOLOGY—cont'd

Therapeutic Classification	Generic Name	Brand Name	Common Use
	ustekinumab	Stelara	
	methotrexate	Trexall	Interfere with the growth of skin cells
Keratolytic	salicylic acid	Duofilm, Virasil	Dissolve the substance that causes skin cells to stick together
Retinoid	tazarotene	Tazorac	Decrease inflammation and other skin changes
	tretinoin	Atralin, Renova, Retin-A	Keep skin pores clear; treat sun damage

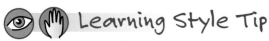 Learning Style Tip

Locate images from journals or websites and glue them to 3-by-5-inch cards to make flash cards for any pathological condition or procedure for which you don't have cards. Review them daily.

Pathologies, Procedures, and Pharmacology Practice Exercises

Deciphering Terms

Write the correct meaning of these medical terms.

Exercise 5

1. cyanoderma _____

2. sclerotic _____

3. hyperkeratosis _____

4. leukocytopenia _____

5. hypodermic _____

6. erythrocyte _____

7. dermatology _____

8. melanocyte _____

9. trichomycosis _____

10. hypertrophy _____

11. xeroderma _____

12. xanthoma _____

13. lipolysis _____

14. adiposis _____

15. onychoma _____

Fill in the Blanks

Fill in the blanks below using pathology terms from Table 4-4.

Exercise 6

1. The term that means *scraping away of skin* is _____.

2. Terms that mean *discoloration of the skin* or *bruise* are
   _____. and_____.

3. The term that means *tiny hemorrhagic spot* is _____.

4. _____ is a skin infection marked by yellow to red crusted or pustular lesions.

5. _____ causes patchy loss of skin pigmentation.

6. A _____ is a clear, fluid-filled lesion, such as a blister.

7. A _____ is a small, pus-filled blister.

8. The medical name for a blackhead is _____.

9. _____ is a contagious skin disease transmitted by the itch mite.

10. A small raised spot or bump, such as a mole, is a _____.

11. _____ results in loss of body hair.

12. A _____ is a cut or tear in the flesh.

13. A _____ is a small, cracklike break in the skin.

14. _____ is an inflammatory skin disease that causes redness, itching, and blisters.

15. A _____ is a flat, discolored spot on the skin, such as a freckle.

16. A bacterial skin infection marked by pain, redness, edema, warmth, and fever is called _____.

17. The medical name for the fungal infection of the skin commonly known as ringworm is _____.

18. _____ describes an area of the skin that is excessively dry and flaky.

19. A _____ is a fluid- or solid-containing pouch in or under the skin.

20. A _____ is a thickened, hardened, toughened area of skin caused by frequent or chronic pressure or friction.

Multiple Choice

Select the one best answer to the following multiple-choice questions.

Exercise 7

1. Which of the following terms is **not** paired with the correct meaning?

   a. erythr/o: red

   b. xanth/o: white

   c. melan/o: black

   d. cyan/o: blue

2. Which of the following abbreviations is **not** paired with the correct meaning?

   a. Bx: biopsy

   b. Tx: treatment

   c. PE: physical examination

   d. FA: family history

3. Which of the following pathology terms is **not** paired with the correct meaning?

   a. abrasion: scraping away of skin or mucous membranes

   b. contusion: bruise

   c. macule: small, raised spot or bump on the skin

   d. cellulitis: bacterial skin infection

4. Which of the following pathology terms is **not** paired with the correct meaning?

   a. comedo: blackhead

   b. cyst: fluid- or solid-containing pouch in or under the skin

   c. pustule: small, pus-filled blister

   d. fissure: surgical cut in the flesh

5. Which of the following pathology terms is **not** paired with the correct meaning?

   a. eczema: inflammatory skin disease with redness, itching, and blisters

   b. scabies: contagious skin disease transmitted by the itch mite

   c. impetigo: patchy loss of skin pigmentation

   d. tinea: fungal skin disease occurring on various parts of the body

Fill in the Blanks

Using Table 4-5, write the therapeutic classification of the medication next to each generic or brand name.

Exercise 8

1. etanercept _____

2. clindamycin _____

3. salicylic acid _____

4. Stelara _____

5. Retin-A _____

6. Lamisil _____

7. methotrexate _____

8. benzoyl peroxide _____

9. fluconazole _____

10. Drithocreme _____

CASE STUDY

Read the case study and answer the questions that follow. Most of the terms are included in this chapter. Refer to your medical dictionary for the other terms.

Cellulitis

Herbert Marshall is a 56-year-old man admitted to the hospital with a severe case of cellulitis. Mr. Marshall has a history of chronic tinea pedis, which he usually treats with OTC medications. When he awoke yesterday, his left foot was erythematous, hot, and tender. He applied an OTC antifungal cream, hoping that would improve his condition. However, today he presented at the clinic complaining of throbbing pain in his foot. The Sx of inflammation have worsened, including increased erythema and edema of the foot and lower leg. After completing a PE, the physician made a diagnosis of cellulitis and admitted Mr. Marshall to the hospital for IV antibiotic Tx.

Cellulitis is an infection of the skin, usually caused by streptococcal or staphylococcal bacteria entering through a break in the skin. Common symptoms include erythema, heat, edema, and tenderness. Treatment for mild cases is oral antibiotics. Severe cases usually require IV antibiotic therapy. Surgical debridement, medical removal of dead tissue, may also be necessary.

Case Study Questions

Exercise 9

1. Mr. Marshall's foot has become more:
   a. blue
   b. red
   c. dry
   d. yellow

2. Mr. Marshall's foot has also become:
   a. swollen
   b. hardened
   c. bruised
   d. scaly

3. The physician performed a:
   a. biopsy
   b. treatment
   c. physical examination
   d. incision and drainage

4. Mr. Marshall was admitted to the hospital for:
   a. treatment
   b. a biopsy
   c. surgery
   d. a subcutaneous injection

5. The antibiotics will be administered to Mr. Marshall by:
   a. subcutaneous injection
   b. intradermal injection
   c. intramuscular injection
   d. intravenous injection

6. Mr. Marshall has a history of chronic:
   a. dry, flaky skin
   b. blackheads
   c. loss of skin pigmentation
   d. athlete's foot

7. The abbreviation Sx stands for:
   a. symptom(s)
   b. biopsy
   c. treatment
   d. injection

8. Cellulitis is usually an infection of the:
   a. hair
   b. skin
   c. fingernails or toenails
   d. glands

9. Cellulitis is caused by:
   a. a virus
   b. poor hygiene
   c. bacteria
   d. exposure to cold temperatures

10. Cellulitis may be treated with:
    a. oral antibiotics
    b. intravenous antibiotics
    c. surgery
    d. all of these

11. If you had a painful, tender, and swollen foot, it is likely that you would hesitate to use the foot or put any weight on it. Discuss how this would affect activities of daily living (ADLs) for you and for others around you. What if you lived alone?

End-of-Chapter Practice Exercises

Word Building

*Using **only** the word parts in the lists provided, create medical terms with the indicated meanings.*

Exercise 10

Prefixes	Combining Forms	Suffixes
circum-	adip/o	-al
epi-	albin/o	-cyte
hypo-	cyan/o	-derma
	cyt/o	-ectomy
	dermat/o	-emia
	derm/o	-ic
	erythr/o	-ism

kerat/o   -oid
leuk/o   -oma
lip/o   -osis
melan/o   -penia
myc/o   -tic
necr/o
onych/o
trich/o
scler/o
xanth/o
xer/o

1. resembling fat _____

2. pertaining to dry skin _____

3. condition of whiteness _____

4. abnormal condition of yellowness _____

5. pertaining to the skin _____

6. pertaining to above or upon the skin _____

7. abnormal condition of skin fungus _____

8. deficiency of red (blood) cells _____

9. abnormal condition of blueness of the skin _____

10. hardening of the skin _____

11. abnormal condition of hair fungus _____

12. abnormal condition of keratinized tissue _____

13. white (condition of) blood _____

14. abnormal condition of nail fungus _____

15. black tumor _____

16. pertaining to death _____

17. pertaining to beneath the skin _____

18. surgical removal of fat _____

19. fat cell _____

20. dry skin _____

True or False

Decide whether the following statements are true or false.

Exercise 11

1. True   False   **Laser resurfacing** involves the use of short pulses of light to remove fine lines and damaged skin and to minimize scars.

2. True   False   In **dermaplaning,** a surgeon scrapes away the outermost layer of skin using a wire brush or burr impregnated with diamond particles.

3. True   False   In a **BOTOX** procedure, a small amount of toxin is injected into selected muscles of the face.

4. True   False   A **biopsy** involves the removal of a tissue sample for microscopic examination.

5. True   False   The abbreviation for **biopsy** is BSY.

6. True   False   The abbreviation **ID** stands for *incision and drainage.*

7. True   False   The abbreviation for **physical examination** is Px.

8. True   False   The abbreviation **Tx** stands for *treatment.*

9. True   False   The abbreviation **FH** stands for *family history.*

10. True   False   The abbreviation **SubQ** stands for *sclerosis.*

Deciphering Terms

Write the correct meaning of these medical terms.

Exercise 12

1. hidrotic _____

2. morphogenesis _____

3. hydrous _____

4. mycoid _____

5. cirrhotic _____

6. chromatogram _____

7. leukopenia _____

8. sonography   _____

9. rhytidoplasty   _____

10. pathophobia   _____

Multiple Choice

Select the one best answer to the following multiple-choice questions.

Exercise 13

1. Which of the following terms is matched with the correct definition?

    a. adip/o: acne

    b. cutane/o: cell

    c. necr/o: dead

    d. myc/o: macule

2. Which of the following terms is matched with the correct definition?

    a. seb/o: sweat

    b. son/o: shape

    c. cyan/o: cause

    d. xanth/o: yellow

3. Which of the following terms is matched with the correct definition?

    a. dermat/o: dead

    b. cyt/o: cell

    c. idi/o: cause

    d. leuk/o: large

4. Which of the following terms is matched with the correct definition?

    a. xer/o: white

    b. albin/o: hardening

    c. chromat/o: cornea

    d. erythr/o: red

5. Which of the following terms is matched with the correct definition?

    a. hidr/o: water

    b. morph/o: malignant

    c. onych/o: nail

    d. rhytid/o: hair

6. Which of the following terms is matched with the correct definition?
   a. SCC: subcutaneous
   b. Bx: treatment
   c. ID: incision and drainage
   d. ung: ointment

7. Which of the following terms is matched with the correct definition?
   a. cirrh/o: blue
   b. xer/o: dry
   c. melan/o: malignant
   d. trich/o: treatment

8. Which of the following terms is matched with the correct definition?
   a. PE: probable etiology
   b. Sx: treatment
   c. FH: hair fungus
   d. MM: malignant melanoma

9. Which of the following terms is matched with the correct definition?
   a. lip/o: skin
   b. eti/o: unknown
   c. hydr/o: sweat
   d. pil/o: hair

10. Which of the following terms is matched with the correct definition?
    a. kerat/o: cyst
    b. dermat/o: skin
    c. path/o: papule
    d. scler/o: scales

11. Which of the following terms means *abnormal condition of nail softening*?
    a. cyanoderma
    b. onychomycosis
    c. hyperhidrosis
    d. none of these

12. The term *rhytidoplasty* means:

    a. examination of the nasal passages

    b. abnormal condition of excessive wrinkles

    c. plastic surgery of the nose

    d. elimination of wrinkles by plastic surgery

13. A patient is most likely to visit a dermatologist to undergo dermaplaning for which of the following disorders?

    a. acne

    b. alopecia areata

    c. carbuncle

    d. cyst

14. Which of the following is a malignant condition?

    a. actinic keratosis

    b. bulla

    c. folliculitis

    d. basal cell carcinoma

15. Which of the following is the result of accidental injury?

    a. callus

    b. melasma

    c. paronychia

    d. abrasion

16. All of the following skin problems are related to excess pressure except:

    a. corn

    b. callus

    c. fissure

    d. decubitus ulcer

17. All of the following are infections of the skin **except:**

    a. petechiae

    b. furuncle

    c. impetigo

    d. pustule

18. All of the following procedures involve removal of tissue **except:**

   a. biopsy

   b. dermaplaning

   c. dermabrasion

   d. BOTOX

19. Which of the following helps to remove fine lines or wrinkles?

   a. laser resurfacing

   b. microdermabrasion

   c. dermaplaning

   d. all of these

20. Which of the following is done to aid in diagnosis?

   a. microdermabrasion

   b. BOTOX

   c. biopsy

   d. none of these

NERVOUS SYSTEM 5

Chapter Outline

Structure and Function

The nervous system plays a key role in maintaining **homeostasis,** the state of dynamic equilibrium in the internal environment of the body. More complex than the most advanced computer, the nervous system is capable of storing vast amounts of data as well as receiving and sending thousands of messages throughout the body instantly and simultaneously.

While the nervous system functions as a total system, you may find it more easily understood if we divide it into its two major parts: the central nervous system (CNS) and the peripheral nervous system (PNS). However, we first begin by looking at the most essential element: the neuron.

A nerve cell, known as a **neuron,** is illustrated in Figure 5-1. Neurons vary in size and shape, but they all have the following key parts: cell body, axon, and dendrites. The **cell body** houses all of the microscopic structures that keep the cell energized and functioning. The **dendrites,** which resemble the branches of a tree, are responsible for receiving information from the internal and external environment and bringing this information to the cell body. The **axon** sends electrical impulses and transmits signals to other cells. The axon may be short or quite long and is sometimes covered in a special protective layer called the **myelin sheath.**

> Flashpoint
> Your brain is something like a very complex computer with infinite data-storage capabilities.

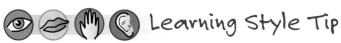 Learning Style Tip

Use the illustrations by tracing them with your fingertip, naming the various parts aloud, and describing their functions as you do so. This is useful for visual, auditory, verbal, and kinesthetic learners.

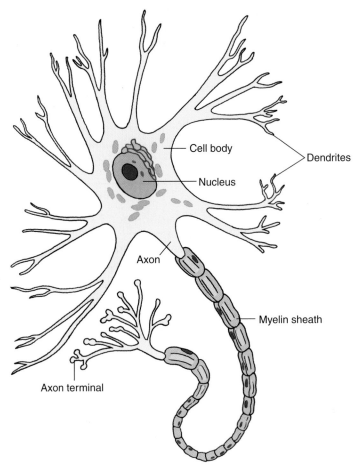

FIGURE 5-1 Neuron.

The **central nervous system (CNS)** comprises the brain and spinal cord (Fig. 5-2). This is where data storage and information processing occurs. The brain is made up of three major divisions: the **cerebrum,** which makes up the largest portion; the cerebellum; and the brainstem. The cerebrum is divided into two hemispheres sometimes called the left and right brains. They are connected by a structure called the **corpus callosum.**

The surface of the cerebrum, called the **cortex,** is characterized by deep folds and shallow grooves, which increase its surface area and maximize function. The cortex is full of neurons as well as specialized support cells that carry nutrients to the neurons called **glia.** It is divided into four areas known as the frontal, temporal, parietal, and occipital lobes. Each of these areas is responsible for specific functions such as sensory perception, movement, emotions, memory, and behavior. The **cerebellum** is sometimes called the "little brain." It is located inferior and posterior to the rest of the brain. It is about the size of your fist and is shaped like a walnut. It also has folds and grooves, similar to the cerebrum. It is responsible for posture, balance, and coordination.

The **brainstem** sits anterior to the cerebellum and includes the medulla oblongata and the pons. It is an essential pathway that conducts impulses between the brain and spinal cord and controls autonomic functions, such as breathing. The brain is enclosed and protected by the hard bones of the skull, known as the **cranium** (Box 5-1). The **spinal cord** extends from the base of the brain down to the second lumbar vertebra and is surrounded and protected by the vertebral column. It is divided into sections that correspond to the vertebrae and paired spinal nerves. The spinal cord provides the pathway for **sensory impulses** going to the brain from the rest of the body and **motor impulses** coming from the brain to the rest of the body.

Protecting both the brain and the spinal cord are three membranes called the **meninges.** The meninges provide a supportive structure for many small blood vessels on the brain's surface. They also protect the brain and spinal cord, housing cerebrospinal fluid that continuously circulates and provides a cushion against injury from impact and sudden movement.

A nerve cell in the human body functions somewhat like an electrical cord in your home. In an electrical cord, the wires are protected by a rubber coating of insulation; so too, your nerves are protected by the myelin sheath. The electrical cord sends electricity from the energy source to the refrigerator, television, or other device so that it can operate. Your nerve cells send electrical impulses down the axon to muscles, organs, or other tissues in the periphery so that they can function. When the insulating layer of an electrical extension cord becomes frayed or otherwise damaged, the cord may "short out"; as a result, signal transmission may be temporarily or permanently lost, and the device may no longer work. Similarly, if the myelin sheath on the axon degenerates or is damaged, the electrical impulse may be temporarily or permanently lost. As a

Flashpoint

Many people believe that they are either "left-brained" (logical and analytical) or "right-brained" (intuitive and creative). While the two hemispheres have somewhat different functions, dominance is related to the task we are trying to accomplish, not to the type of person we are.

Brain

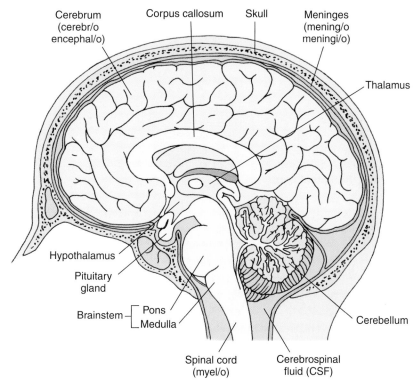

FIGURE 5-2 Central nervous system: (A) brain,

Spinal cord

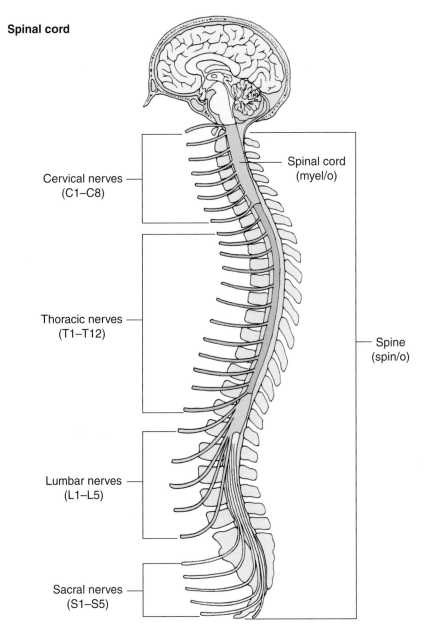

FIGURE 5-2—cont'd **(B)** spinal cord.

result, the organ or muscle that it innervates may not function properly. This explains some of the symptoms caused by degenerative neuromuscular diseases such as *multiple sclerosis.*

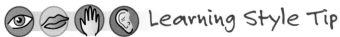 Learning Style Tip

Use Figure 5-2A to create a 3-D model of the brain out of clay. Include the key parts as described in this chapter and make each out of a different color. Name them and describe their function aloud as you make them. It's okay if you aren't a great sculptor—the point is to learn and remember!

Box 5-1 Traumatic Brain Injury Facts and Prevention

Traumatic brain injuries (TBIs) are most commonly caused by falls, being hit by an object, or by motor vehicle accidents. According to the Centers for Disease Control and Prevention (CDC), 138 people in the United States die every day from injuries that include TBI. Survivors can have impairments that may last for a few days or for the rest of their lives. There are many ways a TBI can affect an individual, depending upon where the brain was injured. For example, an injury to the front of the brain, or frontal lobe, may cause problems with decision making, problem solving, behavior, and self-control. An injury to the cerebellum, at the back of the brain, may cause problems with balance and coordination. Other areas of the brain control emotions, memory, speech, language comprehension, object recognition, and much more. Many TBI survivors require long-term rehabilitation. Their injuries may be life-changing events that also impact their families, their job, and their ability to interact in the community.

The CDC reports that from 2006 to 2010, 40% of TBIs in the United States were caused by falls. In children 0 to 14 years old, 55% of TBIs were fall related. A helmet should be worn by anybody who is participating in activities such as skiing, snowboarding, or skateboarding and when riding on open, unrestrained, vehicles such as a bicycle, motorcycle, or snowmobile.

Motor vehicle accidents (MVAs) are the leading cause of TBI-related death for children and young adults ages 5 to 24. When riding in cars, child safety seats should be used, seat belts should be worn, and drivers should not operate the vehicle under the influence of alcohol or drugs. Even some prescription medications can affect a person's ability to drive safely.

In adults aged 65 and older, 81% of TBIs are caused by falls, and falls are the leading cause of TBI-related death in this age group. More than half of these falls occur in the home. It is a myth that falling is a normal part of aging! Communities throughout the United States are offering comprehensive falls prevention programs such as "Stepping On" that teach older adults how to recognize and remove hazards in their homes and how to decrease the risk of falls through regular vision checks, medication reviews, use of assistive devices, and regular exercise. For more information about falls prevention or "Stepping On" programs, visit the CDC website at www.cdc.gov or the National Council on Aging (NCOA) website at www.ncoa.org.

Central and Peripheral Nervous Systems

The central nervous system (brain and spinal cord) is located in the middle, or most *central*, part of the body. The **peripheral nervous system (PNS)** is located outside of, or *peripheral* to, the CNS and includes the nerves in the arms and legs.

The PNS includes 31 pairs of spinal nerves, 12 cranial nerves, and the nerves in the arms and legs. Almost all nerves are part sensory and part motor. Some cranial nerves are all sensory or all motor. **Sensory nerves** gather information from the skin, the muscles, and the joints. The information includes sensations such as temperature, touch, pressure, movement sense, position sense, and pain. These sensations also allow us to distinguish between sharp and dull and to recognize different weights, shapes, and textures of objects. This sensory information is sent to the brain, and the brain responds by sending messages back out to the body via the **motor nerves,** which control body movement. The message may be a conscious one that prompts you to action, such as putting on a coat if you are cold, or it may be unconscious, causing you to reflexively lift your foot if you step on something sharp.

A key function of the 31 pairs of spinal nerves is innervation of the skin and muscles of the limbs. Areas of the skin associated with specific spinal nerve roots are called **dermatomes** (Fig. 5-3). Groups of muscles associated with specific spinal nerve roots are called **myotomes.**

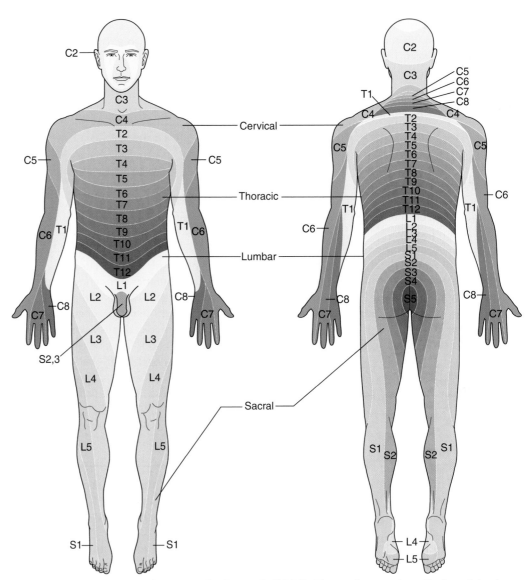

FIGURE 5-3 Dermatomes. (From Eagle, S., et al. (2009). *The professional medical assistant.* Philadelphia, PA: F.A. Davis Company, p. 441; with permission)

In injuries such as compression of a spinal nerve root, pain is felt along the associated dermatome rather than at the actual site of injury. This **referred pain** and other symptoms such as numbness or tingling are felt in your arms or legs rather than in your neck or back. Injury to spinal nerve roots may also cause muscle weakness in a group of muscles away from the site of injury. An injury to a spinal nerve root in the neck may cause weakness of wrist muscles, and an injury to a spinal nerve root in the low back may cause weakness of ankle muscles.

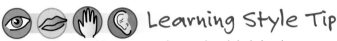 Learning Style Tip

Using masking tape and a marker, label the dermatomes on a study partner. Name them aloud as you do so. Then change roles and let your partner do the same with you.

An important part of the PNS is the **autonomic nervous system (ANS),** which controls involuntary functions. It consists of motor nerves to smooth muscle, cardiac muscle, and glands such as sweat glands and salivary glands. It is further divided into the sympathetic and parasympathetic nervous systems (Fig. 5-4). The **sympathetic nervous system** is responsible for the survival response known as the fight-or-flight response. This response prepares a person for action, whether it is to fight in self-defense or to run from danger. Physical changes within the body caused by this response include increased heart rate and force, increased blood pressure and glucose levels, bronchodilation, and decreased intestinal peristalsis. These changes provide the body with increased energy and oxygen while slowing some functions (such as digestion) which are less important at the time. The **parasympathetic nervous system** essentially creates an opposite response and dominates during nonstressful times. Some of its effects include decreased heart rate, bronchoconstriction, and increased peristalsis.

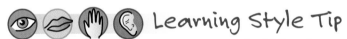 Learning Style Tip

Use Figure 5-4 to create your own colorful flowchart on a whiteboard or poster that illustrates the various branches of the nervous system. Doing this yourself will help to clarify the information in your mind and in your memory. Speak aloud as you do so to benefit from verbalizing and hearing the information.

Flashpoint

To remember the functions of the autonomic nervous system, think *autonomic = automatic.*

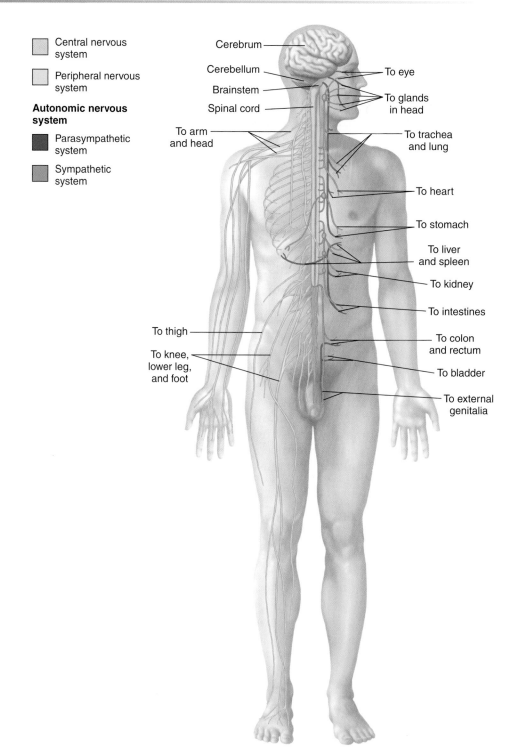

Central nervous system

Peripheral nervous system

Autonomic nervous system

Parasympathetic system

Sympathetic system

Cerebrum

Cerebellum

Brainstem

Spinal cord

To arm and head

To eye

To glands in head

To trachea and lung

To heart

To stomach

To liver and spleen

To kidney

To intestines

To thigh

To knee, lower leg, and foot

To colon and rectum

To bladder

To external genitalia

FIGURE 5-4 Central and peripheral nervous systems, along with the autonomic nervous system. (From Eagle, S., et al. (2009). *The professional medical assistant.* Philadelphia, PA: F.A. Davis Company, p. 438; with permission)

Structure and Function Practice Exercises

Fill in the Blanks

Choose the term that matches the description.

Exercise 1

Homeostasis	Glia	Sensory nerves
Neuron	Corpus callosum	Motor nerves
Cell body	Cerebellum	Dermatomes
Dendrites	Brainstem	Myotomes
Axon	Cranium	Referred pain
Myelin sheath	Spinal cord	Autonomic nervous system
Central nervous system	Sensory impulses	Sympathetic nervous system
Cerebrum	Motor impulses	Parasympathetic nervous system
Cortex	Meninges	
	Peripheral nervous system	

1. _____ A special protective layer on the axon

2. _____ Support cells that carry nutrients to neurons

3. _____ The essential pathway that conducts impulses between the brain and spinal cord

4. _____ Areas of skin associated with specific spinal nerve roots

5. _____ The state of dynamic equilibrium in the internal environment of the body

6. _____ The system responsible for the physical changes of the fight-or-flight response

7. _____ The pathway for sensory impulses going to the brain and motor impulses coming from the brain

8. _____ Divides the cerebrum into two hemispheres

9. _____ The system that includes nerves in the arms and legs

10. _____ Houses all of the microscopic structures that keep the cell energized and functioning

11. _____ Information from the rest of the body that travels to the brain

12. _____ Nerves that control body movement

13. _____ The brain and the spinal cord

14. _____ Gather information from the skin, muscles, and joints

15. _____ Deep folds and shallow grooves on the surface of the cerebrum which increase its surface area

16. _____ The system that dominates during nonstressful times

17. _____ The hard bones of the skull

18. _____ A nerve cell

19. _____ The system that controls involuntary functions

20. _____ Receives information and brings it to the cell body

21. _____ Pain that is felt at an area of the body away from the actual injury site

22. _____ Groups of muscles associated with specific spinal nerve roots

23. _____ The largest portion of the brain

24. _____ Information from the brain that travels to the rest of the body

25. _____ Three membranes that protect the brain and spinal cord

26. _____ Sends electrical impulses and transmits signals to other cells

27. _____ Responsible for posture, balance, and coordination

Fill in the Blanks

Label Figure 5-5A with the appropriate anatomical terms and combining forms.

Exercise 2

Brain

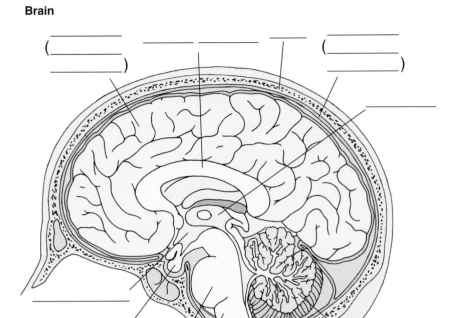

FIGURE 5-5 Central nervous system, with blanks: (A) brain,

Fill in the Blanks

Label Figure 5-5B with the appropriate anatomical terms and combining forms.

Exercise 3

Spinal cord

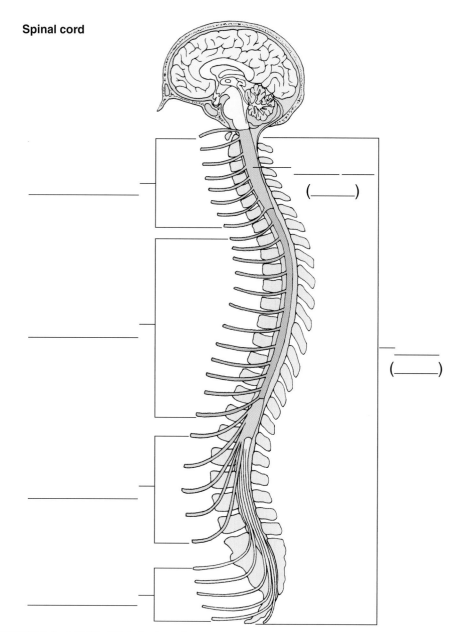

FIGURE 5-5—cont'd (B) spinal cord.

Fill in the Blanks

Label Figure 5-6 with the appropriate anatomical terms and combining forms.

Exercise 4

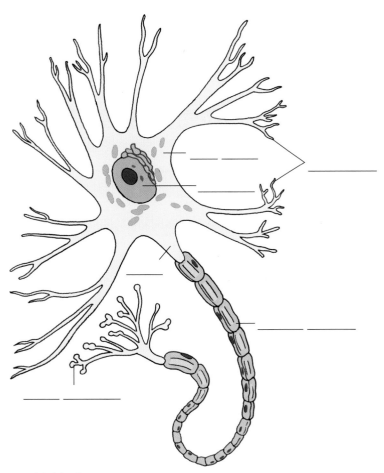

FIGURE 5-6 **Neuron with blanks.**

Combining Forms and Abbreviations

Combining Forms

Table 5-1 contains combining forms that pertain to the nervous system, examples of terms that utilize the combining form, and a pronunciation guide. Read aloud to yourself as you move from left to right across the table. Be sure to use the pronunciation guide so that you can learn to say the terms correctly.

TABLE 5-1

COMBINING FORMS RELATED TO THE NERVOUS SYSTEM

Combining Form	Meaning	Example	Meaning of New Term
cephal/o	head	cephalalgia (sĕf-ă-LĂL-jē-ă)	pain of the head
cerebell/o	cerebellum	cerebellitis (sĕr-ĕ-bĕ-LĪT-ĭs)	inflammation of the cerebellum
cerebr/o	brain	cerebrovascular (sĕ-rĕ-brō-VĂS-kū-lăr)	pertaining to the brain and vessels
encephal/o		encephalocele (ĕn-SĔF-ă-lō-sēl)	hernia of the brain
gangli/o	ganglion	ganglioma (găng-glē-Ō-mă)	tumor of a ganglion
gli/o	glue, gluelike	glioma (glī-Ō-mă)	gluelike tumor
lex/o	word, phrase	dyslexia (dĭs-LĔK-sē-ă)	bad, painful, or difficult words or phrases
mening/o	meninges	meningitis (mĕn-ĭn-JĪT-ĭs)	inflammation of the meninges
meningi/o		meningioma (mĕ-nĭn-JĒ-ō-mă)	tumor of the meninges
myel/o	spinal cord, bone marrow	myelography (mī-ĕ-LŎG-ră-fē)	process of recording the spinal cord or bone marrow
narc/o	sleep, stupor	narcolepsy (NĂR-kō-lĕp-sē)	seizure of sleep or stupor
neur/o	nerve	neurocytoma (nūr-ō-sī-TŌ-mă)	tumor of a nerve cell
phas/o	speech	aphasia (ă-FĀ-zē-ă)	absence of speech
psych/o	mind	psychiatry (sī-KĪ-ă-trē)	field of medicine of the mind
radicul/o	nerve root	radiculopathy (ră-dĭ-kū-LŎ-pă-thē)	disease of a nerve root
spin/o	spine	spinal stenosis (SPĪ-năl stĕ-NŌ-sĭs)	abnormal condition of narrowing or stricture of the spinal cord
sthen/o	strength	myasthenia (mī-ăs-THĒ-nē-ă)	condition of absence of muscle strength
thalam/o	thalamus	thalamotomy (thăl-ă-MŎT-ō-mē)	cutting into or incision of the thalamus
ton/o	tension, tone	tonometer (tō-NŎM-ĕt-ĕr)	measuring instrument for tension
ventricul/o	ventricle	ventriculoscopy (vĕn-trĭk-ū-LŎS-kō-pē)	visual examination of a ventricle

IN A FLASH!

Go to the Davis*Plus* website to print out the Combining Forms Flash Cards for Chapter 5 and run through them at least three times before you continue.

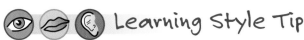 Learning Style Tip

Try this silly exercise: Study with a group or a friend and take turns "selling" each other combining forms. Here's an example of a sales pitch: "Have I got a deal for you! A handy, dandy, multipurpose combining form by the name of *neur/o*. This versatile little combining form is useful if you happen to have nerve pain (neuralgia) caused by nerve inflammation (neuritis), and you need to see a doctor (neurologist) who specializes in disorders pertaining to the nerves (neurology). If you need an operation (neurosurgery), then you'll need a special doctor (neurosurgeon). And if none of that is true, but you are simply feeling neurotic (pertaining to nerves)—well, it's handy for that too."

Abbreviations

Table 5-2 lists some of the most common abbreviations related to the nervous system, as well as others often used in medical documentation.

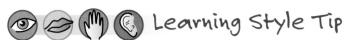 Learning Style Tip

Use multiple learning styles by reading the definitions of terms and abbreviations followed by writing them out and reading them aloud several times as you do so.

TABLE 5-2			
ABBREVIATIONS			
ADHD	attention-deficit hyperactivity disorder	LOC	level of consciousness, loss of consciousness
ALS	amyotrophic lateral sclerosis (Lou Gehrig's disease)	LP	lumbar puncture
ANS	autonomic nervous system	MRI	magnetic resonance imaging
CNS	central nervous system	MVA	motor vehicle accident
CP	cerebral palsy	MS	multiple sclerosis
CSF	cerebrospinal fluid	OCD	obsessive-compulsive disorder
CT	computed tomography	PNS	peripheral nervous system
CVA	cerebrovascular accident	SCI	spinal cord injury
EEG	electroencephalography	TBI	traumatic brain injury
EMG	electromyogram	TGA	transient global amnesia
GBS	Guillain-Barré syndrome	TIA	transient ischemic attack
ICP	intracranial pressure	TN	trigeminal neuralgia

IN A FLASH!
Go to the Davis*Plus* website to print out the Abbreviations Flash Cards for Chapter 5 and run through them at least three times before you continue.

Combining Forms and Abbreviations Practice Exercises

Fill in the Blanks

Fill in the blanks below using Table 5-1.

Exercise 5

1. pain of the head _____

2. tumor of the meninges _____

3. cutting into or incision of the thalamus _____

4. gluelike tumor _____

5. pertaining to the brain and vessels _____

6. inflammation of the meninges _____

7. visual examination of a ventricle _____

8. inflammation of the cerebellum _____

9. process of recording the spinal cord or bone marrow _____

10. tumor of a nerve cell _____

11. measuring instrument for tension _____

12. bad, painful, or difficult words or phrases _____

13. tumor of a ganglion _____

14. seizure of sleep or stupor _____

15. disease of a nerve root _____

16. condition of absence of muscle strength _____

17. hernia of the brain _____

18. absence of speech _____

19. abnormal condition of narrowing or stricture of the spinal cord _____

20. field of medicine of the mind _____

Fill in the Blanks

Write the correct term next to each abbreviation using Table 5-2.

Exercise 6

1. CSF _____

2. ICP _____

3. CT _____

4. LOC _____

5. SCI _____

6. TN _____

7. ADHD _____

8. OCD _____

9. TBI _____

10. CVA _____

Pathologies, Procedures, and Pharmacology

Pathology Terms

Table 5-3 lists terms that relate to diseases or abnormalities of the nervous system. Use the pronunciation guide and say the terms out loud as you read them. This will help you get in the habit of saying them properly.

> ### IN A FLASH!
> Go to the DavisPlus website to print out the Pathology Terms Flash Cards for Chapter 5 and run through them at least three times before you continue.

TABLE 5-3
PATHOLOGY TERMS

Alzheimer's disease (ĂLTS-hī-mĕrz dĭ-ZĒZ)	form of chronic, progressive dementia caused by the atrophy of brain tissue
amyotrophic lateral sclerosis (ALS) (ă-mī-ō-TRŌ-fĭk LĂ-tĕr-ăl sklĕ-RŌ-sĭs)	chronic, progressive, degenerative neuromuscular disorder that destroys motor neurons of the body; also called *Lou Gehrig's disease*
Bell's palsy (bĕlz PAWL-zē)	form of facial paralysis, usually unilateral and temporary; also known as *facial palsy*

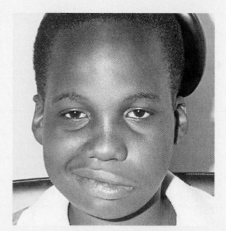

Bell's palsy. (From Dillon, P. M. [2008]. Nursing health assessment. Philadelphia, PA: F.A. Davis Company, p. 218; with permission. Courtesy of Wills Eye Hospital)

brain abscess (brān ĂB-sĕs)	collection of pus anywhere within the brain
brain tumor (brān TŪ-mŏr)	any type of abnormal mass growing within the cranium
cerebral concussion (sĕ-RĒ-brăl kŏn-KŬ-shŭn)	vague term referring to a brief loss of consciousness or brief episode of disorientation or confusion following a head injury

TABLE 5-3

PATHOLOGY TERMS—cont'd

cerebral contusion (sĕ-RĒ-brăl kŏn-TOO-zhŭn)   bruising of brain tissue

Cerebral
contusion

A   Contrecoup

Cerebral
contusion

B   Coup

Cerebral contusion. (From Eagle, S., et al. [2009]. *The professional medical assistant.* Philadelphia, PA: F.A. Davis Company, p. 448; with permission)

cerebral palsy (CP) (sĕ-RĒ-brăl PAWL-zē)   group of motor-impairment syndromes caused by lesions or abnormalities of the brain arising in the early stages of development

Continued

TABLE 5-3
PATHOLOGY TERMS—cont'd

cerebrovascular accident (CVA) (sĕ-rĕ-brō-VĂS-kū-lăr ăk'sĭ-dĕnt)	damage or death of brain tissue caused by interruption of blood supply due to a clot or vessel rupture; also known as *stroke*

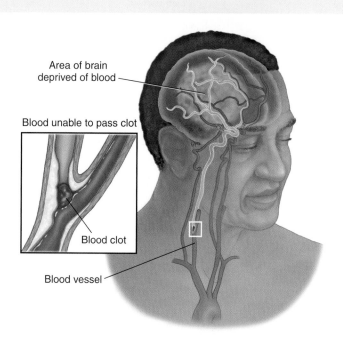

Area of brain deprived of blood

Blood unable to pass clot

Blood clot

Blood vessel

Cerebrovascular accident (CVA). (From Eagle, S., et al. [2009]. *The professional medical assistant.* Philadelphia, PA: F.A. Davis Company, p. 444; with permission)

delirium (dĕ-LĬR-ē-ŭm)	acute, reversible state of agitated confusion, marked by disorientation, hallucinations, or delusions
dementia (dē-MĔN-shē-ă)	progressive neurological disorder, with numerous causes, in which an individual suffers an irreversible decline in cognition due to disease or brain damage; sometimes called *senility*
depression (dē-PRĔSH-ŭn)	mood disorder marked by loss of interest or pleasure in living
encephalitis (ĕn-sĕf-ă-LĪ-tĭs)	inflammation of the brain; often combined with meningitis and then called *encephalomeningitis*
epidural hematoma (ĕp-ĭ-DŪR-ăl hē-mă-TŌ-mă)	collection of blood between the dura mater and the skull
epilepsy (ĔP-ĭ-lĕp-sē)	chronic disorder of the brain marked by recurrent seizures, which are repetitive abnormal electrical discharges within the brain
Guillain-Barré syndrome (GBS) (gē-YĂ-băr-RĀ SĬN-drōm)	acute inflammatory disorder that causes rapidly progressing paralysis (which is usually temporary) and sometimes also sensory symptoms; also known as *inflammatory polyneuropathy and acute infective polyneuritis.* A variant of GBS is *Miller Fisher Syndrome.*

TABLE 5-3
PATHOLOGY TERMS—cont'd

Huntington's disease (HUN-ting-tunz dĭ-ZĒZ)	hereditary, progressive, degenerative nervous disorder that leads to bizarre, involuntary movements and dementia; also called *Huntington disease or Huntington chorea*
meningitis (mĕn-ĭn-JĪT-ĭs)	infection and inflammation of the meninges, the spinal cord, and CSF, usually caused by an infectious illness; often combined with encephalitis and then called *encephalomeningitis*
migraine headache (MĪ-grān HED-āk)	familial disorder marked by episodes of severe throbbing headache that is commonly unilateral and sometimes disabling
multiple sclerosis (MS) (MŬL-tĭ-pul sklĕ-RŌ-sĭs)	disease involving progressive myelin degeneration, which results in loss of muscle strength and coordination
neural tube defect (NUR-ul TŪB dē-fekt)	incomplete closure of the spinal canal, which may allow protrusion of the spinal cord and meninges at birth, leading to paralysis; also known as *spina bifida*

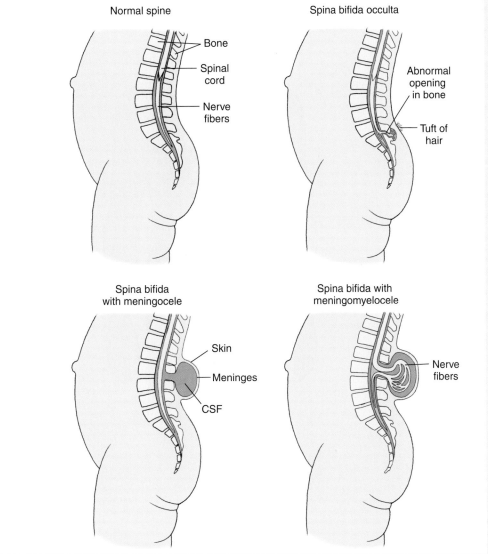

Neural tube defect (spina bifida).

Continued

TABLE 5-3
PATHOLOGY TERMS—cont'd

Parkinson's disease (PĂR-kĭn-sŏnz dĭ-ZĒZ)	progressive, degenerative disorder that results in tremors, gait changes, and occasionally dementia. *Parkinsonism* is a condition that resembles Parkinson's disease. It has a different cause, such as medications, and symptoms can stabilize or improve.
peripheral neuropathy (pĕr-ĬF-ĕr-ăl nū-RŎP-ă-thē)	dysfunction of nerves that transmit information to and from the brain and spinal cord, characterized by pain, altered sensation, and muscle weakness
poliomyelitis (pōl-ē-ō-mī-ĕl-Ī-tĭs)	inflammation of the spinal cord, caused by a virus, which may result in spinal and muscular deformity and paralysis
Reye's syndrome (rīz SĬN-drōm)	serious disease associated with aspirin use by children with viral illnesses, which may result in permanent brain damage or even death
sciatica (sī-ĂT-ĭ-kă)	pain, numbness, weakness, or tingling that is felt from the lower back along the pathway of the sciatic nerve into the legs

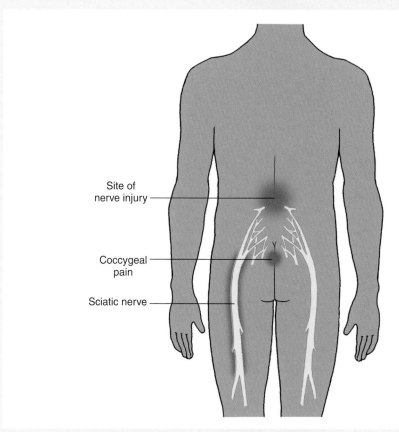

Site of nerve injury

Coccygeal pain

Sciatic nerve

Sciatica.

TABLE 5-3	
PATHOLOGY TERMS—cont'd	
shingles (SHĬNG-gulz)	unilateral painful vesicles occurring on the upper body, caused by the herpes zoster virus; also called *herpes zoster* or *zona*

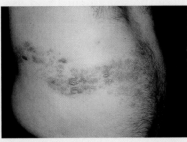

Shingles. (From Goldsmith, L.A., et al. [1997]. *Adult and pediatric dermatology: a color guide to diagnosis and treatment.* Philadelphia, PA: F.A. Davis Company, p. 307; with permission)

spinal cord injury (SCI) (SPĪ-năl kord IN-jă-rē)	traumatic bruising, crushing, or tearing of the spinal cord
spinal stenosis (SPĪ-năl stĕ-NŌ-sĭs)	narrowing of an area of the spine that puts pressure on the spinal cord and spinal nerve roots
subdural hematoma (sub-DUR-ul hē-mă-TŌ-mă)	collection of blood between the dura and the arachnoid layer (middle or second layer of the meninges)
tension headache (TĔN-shŭn HED-āk)	non-migraine headache in which pain is felt in all or part of the head
tetanus (TĔT-ă-nŭs)	noncontagious illness marked by severe, prolonged spasm of skeletal muscle fibers; also known as *lockjaw*
transient global amnesia (TGA) (TRĂNZ-ē-ĭnt GLŌ-băl ăm-NĒ-zē-ă)	rare disorder, not caused by a neurological event or injury, that causes sudden, temporary loss of recent memory
transient ischemic attack (TIA) (TRĂNZ-ē-ĭnt ĭs-KĒ-mĭk ă-TĂK)	temporary strokelike symptoms caused by a brief interruption of blood supply to a part of the brain
traumatic brain injury (TBI) (traw-MĂT-ĭk brān IN-jă-rē)	injury to the brain following a blow to the head, commonly caused by a fall or motor vehicle accident (see Box 5-1)
trigeminal neuralgia (TN) (trī-JĔM-ĭn-ăl nū-RĂL-jē-ă)	neurological disorder that causes severe, episodic facial pain along the pathway of the fifth cranial (trigeminal) nerve; also called *tic douloureux*

Common Diagnostic Tests and Procedures

Cerebrospinal fluid (CSF) analysis: Analysis of CSF for blood, bacteria, and other abnormalities
Computed tomography (CT): Study of the brain and spinal cord using radiology and computer analysis

Electroencephalography (EEG): Study of electrical activity of the brain
Electromyogram (EMG): Record of muscle activity from electrical stimulation
Lumbar puncture (LP): Puncture of subarachnoid layer at the fourth intervertebral space to obtain CSF for analysis (Fig. 5-7)
Magnetic resonance imaging (MRI): Use of an electromagnetic field and radio waves to create visual images on a computer screen
Myelography: Radiography of the spinal cord and associated nerves after intrathecal injection (into the spinal canal) of a contrast medium

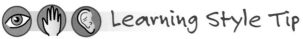 Learning Style Tip

Take the time to view assigned videos and complete online activities. They provide great audiovisual information that may help you gain a greater understanding of the material.

Pharmacology

Table 5-4 provides a list of some common CNS medications. There are numerous nervous system medications used to treat disorders such as anxiety, convulsions, depression, insomnia, mania, pain, and schizophrenia that are not included in this table.

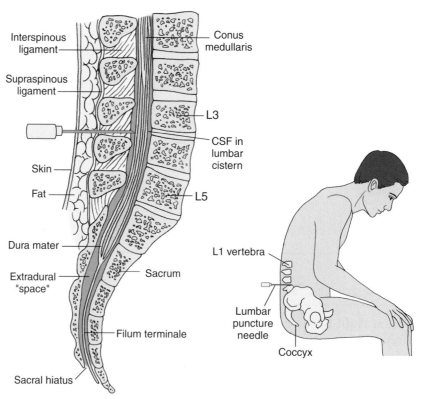

FIGURE 5-7 **Lumbar puncture.**

TABLE 5-4
PHARMACOLOGY

Therapeutic Classification	Generic Name	Brand Name	Common Use
Anticholinergic antiparkinson agent	biperiden	Akineton	Compensate for lack of dopamine in Parkinson's disease
	benztropine	Cogentin	
	diphenhydramine	Benadryl, Nytol, Sominex, Twilite, Unisom	
	procyclidine	Kemadrin	
	trihexyphenidyl	Artane	
Calcium channel blocker	nimodipine	Nimotop, Nymalize	Treat subarachnoid hemorrhage
Cholinesterase inhibitor	donepezil	Aricept	Treat dementia associated with Alzheimer's disease
	galantamine	Razadyne	
	rivastigmine	Exelon	
	tacrine	Cognex	
Coumarins and indandiones	warfarin	Coumadin, Jantoven	Thromboembolic stroke prophylaxis
Dopaminergic antiparkinson agent	carbidopa/ levodopa	Parcopa, Sinemet	Replace or prevent degradation of dopamine in Parkinson's disease
	pramipexole	Mirapex	
	ropinirole	Requip	
Manufactured protein	interferon beta	Avonex, Betaseron, Extavia, Rebif	Slow the progression of multiple sclerosis
Miscellaneous antipsychotic agent	haloperidol	Haldol	Treat dementia
Miscellaneous CNS agent	memantine	Namenda	Treat dementia associated with Alzheimer's disease
Platelet aggregation inhibitor, salicylates	aspirin	Ascriptin, Bayer, Bufferin, Ecotrin, St. Joseph 81 mg	Prevent thrombus formation, reduce pain and inflammation
	clopidogrel	Plavix	
Platelet aggregation inhibitor	ticlopidine	Ticlid	Prevent thrombus formation
Thrombolytic	alteplase	Activase	Dissolve a thrombus

Pathologies, Procedures, and Pharmacology Practice Exercises

Deciphering Terms

Write the correct meaning of these medical terms.

Exercise 7

1. cerebrospinal _____
2. neuropathy _____
3. myeloma _____
4. meningitis _____
5. encephalography _____
6. gliocyte _____
7. cerebrosclerosis _____
8. hemiplegia _____
9. paraplegic _____
10. quadriparesis _____

Fill in the Blanks

Fill in the blanks below using Table 5-3.

Exercise 8

1. The term that refers to a seizure disorder is _____.

2. A form of facial paralysis that is usually unilateral and temporary is _____.

3. A _____ results in the death of brain cells.

4. Incomplete closure of the spinal canal is known as _____.

5. A _____ causes mild, temporary strokelike symptoms.

6. _____ is a hereditary nervous disorder that results in bizarre, involuntary movements and dementia.

7 _____ is defined as bruising of brain tissue.

8. _____ is a serious disease, associated with aspirin use by children with viral illnesses, which may result in permanent brain damage or even death.

9. _____ is an acute, reversible state of agitated confusion marked by disorientation, hallucinations, or delusions.

10. _____ is a collection of blood between the dura mater, also known as the outermost covering of the brain, and the skull.

Multiple Choice

Select the one best answer to the following multiple-choice questions.

Exercise 9

1. Mrs. Fritz was hospitalized with a CVA. She is currently comatose and unresponsive. To determine whether she still has meaningful brain activity, the physician will most likely order:

   a. an EMG

   b. an LP

   c. a CFS

   d. an EEG

2. Ms. Yee sustained a TIA. Because of this, she currently has diminished sensation and movement on only the right side of her body. Ms. Yee is experiencing:

   a. quadriplegia

   b. aphasia

   c. hemiplegia

   d. quadriparalysis

3. Mr. Stutzman is recovering from a stroke but still has difficulty speaking. The proper term for this is:

   a. dysphasia

   b. dysphagia

   c. aphasia

   d. aphagia

4. Mrs. Villanueva is recovering from a CVA but is still struggling with swallowing. The proper term for this is:

   a. dysphasia

   b. dysphoria

   c. euphagia

   d. dysphagia

5. Mr. Washington was brought to the emergency department with a high fever, confusion, and a headache. The physician wants to obtain a specimen of cerebrospinal fluid to study it for the presence of blood, bacteria, or other abnormalities. What procedure is the physician most likely to perform?

    a.   MRI

    b.   LP

    c.   EMG

    d.   CT

Fill in the Blanks

Using Table 5-4, write the common use of the medication next to each generic or brand name.

Exercise 10

1. Activase _____

2. aspirin _____

3. Sinemet _____

4. Aricept _____

5. benztropine _____

6. Mirapex _____

7. interferon beta _____

8. Namenda _____

9. diphenhydramine _____

10. haloperidol _____

 Learning Style Tip

Completing chapter activities gives you the chance to review information in a way that uses your visual and kinesthetic senses. Reading questions aloud helps verbal and auditory learners comprehend and process them better; consequently, you will be more likely to get them correct.

CASE STUDY

Read the case study and answer the questions that follow. Most of the terms are included in this chapter. Refer to your medical dictionary for the other terms.

Shingles

Nicole Daniels is a 25-year-old mother of two young children. She developed a rash several days ago and described it as a narrow strip of "tiny bumps" on the right side of her chest. Initially she noticed pruritus. Today she presented with a strip of herpetic vesicles that she describes as "exquisitely painful," with a sensation like a "fiery itch." She complained of sensitivity so severe that wearing clothing was painful because she could barely tolerate anything touching her skin. After completing a Hx and PE, her physician diagnosed her with shingles. He prescribed acyclovir to reduce the viral shedding and neuralgia. He also gave Ms. Daniels a prescription for acetaminophen with codeine to help relieve her pain.

Shingles is caused by the reactivation of the herpes varicella-zoster virus years after an initial outbreak of chickenpox. A painful eruption of vesicles occurs along the course of a segment of a spinal or cranial peripheral nerve. The lesions are nearly always unilateral. The trunk is most often affected, but the face and head may also be involved. After an outbreak of chickenpox, the virus lies dormant in the nerve cells. Individuals with a weakened immune system are more vulnerable to outbreaks. Pain may continue for months after the lesions heal; this is known as *postherpetic neuralgia*. Fortunately, recurrent outbreaks of shingles are rare. Shingles is contagious to people who have not previously had chickenpox. If infected, these people would not develop shingles; they would develop chickenpox.

Case Study Questions

Exercise 11

1. What did Ms. Daniels first notice on the side of her chest?
   a. papules
   b. scales
   c. macules
   d. vesicles

2. After a few days, the "tiny bumps" turned into:
   a. scales
   b. bigger bumps
   c. blisters
   d. scabs

3. Ms. Daniels has neuralgia, which is:
   a. itching
   b. nerve pain
   c. fatigue
   d. nerve paralysis

4. Chickenpox is caused by:
   a. the herpes varicella-zoster virus
   b. a bacterial infection from chickens
   c. AIDS
   d. a fungus

5. The pattern of the outbreak is usually unilateral. This means that it is:
   a. on both sides of the body
   b. on one side of the body
   c. all over the body
   d. on the upper half of the body

6. People who are most vulnerable to shingles outbreaks are:
   a. those with strong immune systems
   b. those with weakened immune systems
   c. those who have had rubella
   d. those who have had measles

7. Discuss how the outbreak of shingles may affect Nicole Daniels' activities of daily living (ADLs). How might it impact her family?

End-of-Chapter Practice Exercises

Word Building

*Using **only** the word parts in the lists provided, create medical terms with the indicated meanings.*

Exercise 12

Prefixes	Combining Forms	Suffixes
hemi-	electr/o	-al
infra-	encephal/o	-algia
iso-	gli/o	-cele
para-	mening/o	-ic
poly-	myel/o	-itis
quadri-	neur/o	-oma
	spin/o	-ous
		-paresis
		-pathy
		-plegia

1. much nerve inflammation _____

2. pertaining to positioned beneath the spine _____

3. herniation of the spinal cord and meninges _____

4. inflammation of the brain and meninges _____

5. pertaining to near the spine _____

6. tumor of nerve glue _____

7. pertaining to the same electricity _____

8. partial paralysis of half (the body) _____

9. paralysis of four (extremities) _____

10. paralysis of two (extremities) _____

True or False

Decide whether the following statements are true or false.

Exercise 13

1. True   False   **CT** stands for *craniothoracic.*

2. True   False   **CNS** stands for *central nervous system.*

3. True   False   **Epilepsy** is a brain disorder characterized by recurrent seizures.

4. True   False   A form of facial paralysis affecting one or both sides of the face, which is usually temporary, is known as **Bell's palsy.**

5. True   False   A **transient ischemic attack (TIA)** causes death of the affected brain cells.

6. True   False   A **shingles** outbreak is caused by the herpes varicella-zoster virus.

7. True   False   A **CVA** is also known as a brain attack.

8. True   False   **Sciatica** causes nerve pain in the buttocks and legs.

9. True   False   **Spina bifida**, or neural tube defect, may cause paralysis.

10. True   False   **Huntington's disease** causes inflammation of the spinal cord by a virus that may result in spinal and muscle deformity and paralysis.

Deciphering Terms

Write the correct meaning of these medical terms.

Exercise 14

1. myelomeningocele _____

2. myelosclerosis _____

3. cerebrospinal _____

4. myasthenic _____

5. cerebroventricular _____

6. narcosis _____

7. thalamotomy _____

8. myelogram _____

9. neurotomy _____

10. gliocytic _____

Multiple Choice

Select the one best answer to the following multiple-choice questions.

Exercise 15

1. Which of the following terms is matched to the correct definition?
   a. cephal/o: brain
   b. gangli/o: glue, gluelike
   c. narc/o: nerve
   d. ton/o: tension

2. Which of the following terms is matched to the correct definition?
   a. thalam/o: strength
   b. myel/o: meninges
   c. phas/o: speech
   d. cerebr/o: cranium

3. Which of the following terms is matched to the correct definition?
   a. lex/o: word, phrase
   b. radicul/o: reflex
   c. mening/o: brain
   d. ventricul/o: vertebrae

4. Which disorder is caused by lesions or abnormalities of the brain arising in the early stages of development?
   a. ALS
   b. Bell's palsy
   c. Huntington's disease
   d. cerebral palsy

5. Which of the following causes progressive confusion?
   a. delirium
   b. dementia
   c. TIA
   d. cerebral concussion

6. Which of the following causes an acute form of progressive paralysis?
   a. GBS
   b. Bell's palsy
   c. Huntington's disease
   d. spinal stenosis

7. A chronic, progressive, degenerative neuromuscular disorder that destroys motor neurons of the body is:

   a. ALS

   b. MS

   c. Parkinson's disease

   d. spina bifida

8. Which of the following causes temporary memory loss?

   a. MS

   b. TIA

   c. TGA

   d. OCD

9. Delirium is:

   a. an acute, reversible state of agitated confusion marked by disorientation, hallucinations, or delusions

   b. a mood disorder marked by loss of interest or pleasure in living

   c. a progressive neurological disorder that causes irreversible decline in cognition due to disease or brain damage

   d. none of these

10. A collection of blood between the dura and the arachnoid is known as:

    a. a cerebral concussion

    b. a subdural hematoma

    c. a cerebral contusion

    d. spina bifida

11. A serious disease associated with aspirin use by children with viral illnesses is:

    a. trigeminal neuralgia

    b. tetanus

    c. Reye's syndrome

    d. cerebral palsy

12. Which of the following abbreviations refers to a diagnostic procedure?

    a. CVA

    b. ICP

    c. LP

    d. LOC

13. All of the following abbreviations indicate diagnostic procedures **except:**

 a.   CT

 b.   EEG

 c.   EMG

 d.   PNS

14. Which of the following terms means *brain tumor?*

 a.   cephaloma

 b.   encephaloma

 c.   ganglioma

 d.   meningioma

15. Which of the following terms means *pertaining to a seizure (episode) of sleep or stupor?*

 a.   narcoleptic

 b.   tonic

 c.   glial

 d.   neuralgia

16. Which of the following terms means *bad, painful, or difficult speech?*

 a.   dysphagia

 b.   aphrasia

 c.   dysphasia

 d.   aphasia

17. The term *radiculitis* indicates inflammation of the:

 a.   ganglion

 b.   brain

 c.   thalamus

 d.   nerve root

18. A term that indicates a condition of muscle weakness is:

 a.   myasthenia

 b.   myalgia

 c.   myosclerosis

 d.   none of these

19. A term that indicates hardening of the brain is:

    a.   cerebroma

    b.   encephalotome

    c.   cephalodynia

    d.   none of these

20. A term that indicates inflammation of the brain and meninges is:

    a.   cerebritis

    b.   neuroencephalitis

    c.   cerebellitis

    d.   encephalomeningitis

6 CARDIOVASCULAR SYSTEM

Chapter Outline

Structure and Function

The cardiovascular system includes a complex network of arteries, veins, capillaries, and the key structure, the heart, which pumps blood throughout your entire body.

The heart is a hollow, muscular organ about the size of a closed fist that pumps oxygen-rich blood and nutrients to the trillions of cells of the body (Fig. 6-1). To accomplish this, it beats an average of 60 to 100 times a minute for your entire lifetime. Your heart is located in the center of your chest, slightly to the left, in an area called the **mediastinum.** It has three layers: the outer lining, called the **epicardium**; the middle muscular layer, called the **myocardium;** and the inner lining, called the **endocardium.** The heart is enclosed in a fibrous membrane called the **pericardium**, or pericardial sac, which also contains a small amount of **pericardial fluid.** This fluid acts as a lubricant that reduces friction as the heart repeatedly contracts and relaxes.

The heart has two upper chambers, the right and left **atria,** which perform about 30% of the work, and two larger, lower chambers, the right and left **ventricles,** which perform the other 70% of the work. The left ventricle is the largest and most muscular chamber, because it works harder than the others. The right and left sides of the heart are divided by a thick layer of muscle tissue called the **septum.**

There are four valves in the heart that open and close to regulate blood flow. The **tricuspid valve** exits the right atrium into the right ventricle, and the mitral, or **bicuspid valve,** exits the left atrium into the left ventricle. The **pulmonary valve** exits the right ventricle into the pulmonary arteries, and the **aortic valve** exits the left ventricle into the aorta.

Flashpoint
The average person's heart beats 104,000 times per day, which adds up to 38,000,000 times every year!

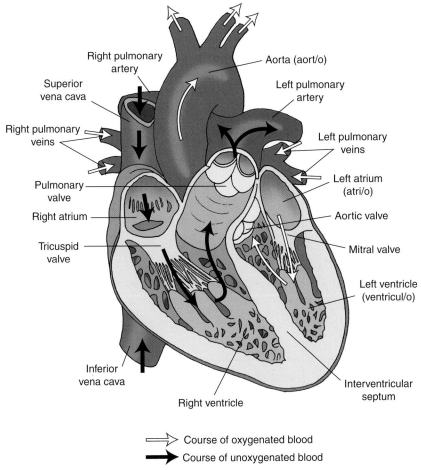

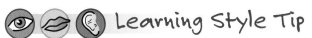

FIGURE 6-1 **The heart.**

Learning Style Tip

Verbally describe photos or illustrations in this book to a real or imaginary friend who cannot see them. Provide all of the details they need to accurately visualize what you are describing. Record your voice as you do this so that you can study, by listening, while doing other things such as household chores or driving.

The largest part of the heart, the lower left area, is known as the **apex.** This site is best for **auscultating** (listening to) sounds from the mitral valve and is where the **apical pulse** is best heard. Listening to the apical pulse for 1 full minute is considered the most accurate method of measuring heart rate and is the preferred method in situations where accuracy is very important.

Blood flows through both sides of the heart at the same time. Blood that is low in oxygen (O_2) but high in carbon dioxide (CO_2) returns from the body to the right atrium via the inferior and superior **venae cavae.** As both atria contract at the same time, they each pump blood to a different area. The right atrium pumps blood downward through the tricuspid valve into the right ventricle. As the right ventricle contracts, it forces blood up and out through the pulmonary valve into the pulmonary arteries. The pulmonary arteries lead to the lungs, where CO_2 is exchanged for O_2. The **pulmonary arteries** are unique in that they are the only arteries in the body that transport oxygen-poor blood. As

Flashpoint

A pulse oximeter is a small noninvasive device that is placed on the end of the finger to quickly measure heart rate and the amount of oxygen in the blood.

the blood circulates through the lungs, it gets rid of CO_2 and picks up O_2. Blood that is now oxygen rich returns through the pulmonary veins to the left atrium (Box 6-1). The **pulmonary veins** are unique in that they are the only veins in the body that transport oxygen-rich blood. As the left atrium contracts, it forces blood downward through the mitral valve into the left ventricle. From there, the blood is pumped by the left ventricle upward and out through the aortic valve into the aorta and out to various parts of the body.

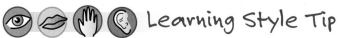 Learning Style Tip

With a study group or a study partner, use sidewalk chalk to draw a giant illustration of the heart on cement or pavement outdoors. Make it as colorful and as accurate as you can. Label and verbally identify all the heart structures. Draw arrows to indicate the direction of blood flow. When the drawing is complete, take turns walking along the circulatory route through the right side of the heart, to the lungs, back through the left side of the heart, out to the body, and then back to where you started. As you follow this route, identify whether you are simulating the path of oxygen-rich or oxygen-poor blood and why. If you have young family members, they may enjoy doing the drawing as you direct them in what to draw.

Box 6-1 The Pulse Oximeter

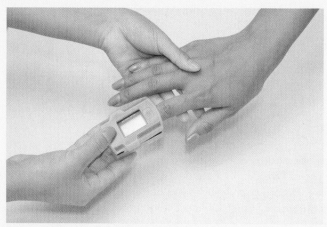

Pulse oximeter. (Photograph © Thinkstock)

If you have been to visit a hospital patient, or seen one on television, you may have noticed a device clipped to the end of the patient's finger. It was probably a pulse oximeter. This device is used to monitor heart rate and to measure the saturation of peripheral oxygen (SpO_2) in the blood. The pulse oximeter is able to differentiate between oxygenated and deoxygenated blood by passing two beams of light, infrared and red, through the finger to a light detector. The oxygenated hemoglobin in blood is a bright red color and absorbs more of the infrared light. The deoxygenated hemoglobin is a dark red color and absorbs more of the red light. The absorption difference is calculated and a measurement of oxygenated blood appears on the screen as a percentage. This helps determine if sufficient oxygen is being supplied to the body. The normal SpO_2 for healthy individuals is 96%–99%. An SpO_2 of lower than 90% may indicate respiratory distress. Pulse oximeters are used in a variety of settings, including outpatient physician offices and home health care. Physical therapists use portable units (see the accompanying photo) to monitor changes in the patient's SpO_2 during exercise.

Coronary Vessels

The heart has its own network of coronary vessels that keep it supplied with oxygen and nutrients. Occasionally, **_arteriosclerosis_** develops in these vessels; in this condition, the vessels become narrowed and hardened due to a number of factors, including **_hypertension_** (high blood pressure). In addition, a fatty, plaque-like substance composed of **cholesterol** may build up on the inside surfaces of the coronary vessels, causing further narrowing or even blockage. This is known as **_atherosclerosis_** and contributes to the development of **_coronary artery disease (CAD)_**. It is also sometimes called _atherosclerotic heart disease (ASHD)_. If a vessel becomes completely **occluded** (blocked), then the heart muscle downstream dies from a lack of oxygen. This is known as a **_myocardial infarction (MI)_** or a **_heart attack._**

As oxygen-rich blood is pumped from the heart, it travels to all parts of the body through an intricate network of arteries (Fig. 6-2). The arteries vary in size, from the very large aorta to very tiny **arterioles**. From the arterioles, blood enters numerous microscopic-sized **capillaries** with walls that are just one cell thick. This allows O_2 and nutrients to easily leave the capillaries and enter the tissues and cells. It also allows waste products and CO_2 to easily move from the cells and tissues back into the capillaries. Blood that is now low in O_2 and high in CO_2 and waste leaves the capillaries and enters microscopic-sized **venules**

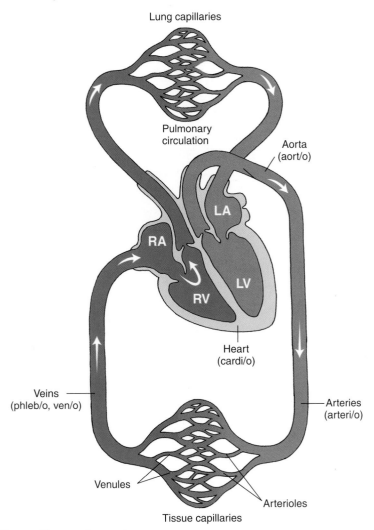

FIGURE 6-2 **The cardiovascular system.**

(tiny veins). As it continues on its return journey, the blood travels through larger and larger veins until it reaches the heart. Blood is drained from the head and upper body via the superior vena cava and from the lower body via the inferior vena cava. Venous blood travels under much less pressure than arterial blood. Because of this, it cannot easily flow against gravity to ascend the legs and return to the heart. Fortunately, veins contain one-way valves that facilitate circulation by preventing the backflow of blood. The pumping action created by the contraction and relaxation of leg muscles also helps to propel the blood upward.

Have you ever wondered what makes your heart beat? Your heart has its own special pacemaker that has been working since before you were born (Fig. 6-3). A cluster of specialized cells in your right atrium called the **sinoatrial (SA) node** serves as a natural pacemaker for the heart, initiating an electrical impulse about 60 to 100 times per minute. Each of these impulses is transmitted throughout all the muscle cells of your heart, resulting in an electrical charge called depolarization. When this occurs, the inside of the cardiac muscle cells becomes electrically positive in relation to the outside. In response, all of the individual cardiac muscle cells in your atria contract in unison. The name given to the normal rhythm of the heart is *normal sinus rhythm,* named for the SA node (Fig. 6-4).

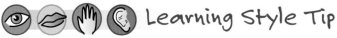 Learning Style Tip

Trace the conduction pathway of the heart with your finger as you verbally identify all of its structures and describe their function.

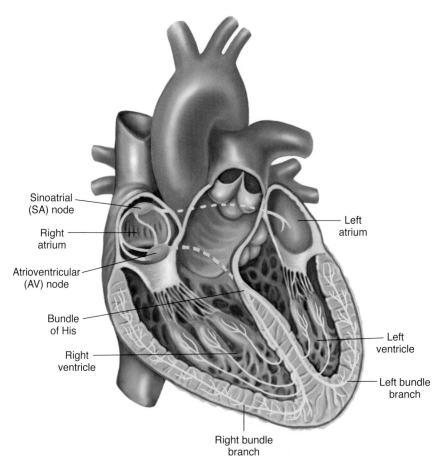

FIGURE 6-3 Electrical conduction system of the heart.

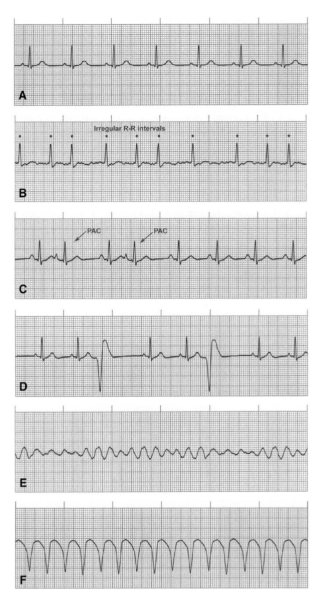

FIGURE 6-4 Cardiac rhythm (normal and abnormal rhythms): **(A)** normal sinus rhythm (NSR); **(B)** atrial fibrillation (AF, A-fib); **(C)** sinus rhythm with premature atrial contractions (PACs); **(D)** sinus rhythm with premature ventricular contractions (PVCs); **(E)** ventricular fibrillation (V-fib); **(F)** ventricular tachycardia (VT, V-tach). (From Eagle, S., et al. [2009]. *The professional medical assistant.* Philadelphia, PA: F. A. Davis Company, p. 465; with permission)

Within the floor of the right atrium is another pacemaker, the **atrioventricular (AV) node.** It is sometimes thought of as a backup pacemaker. It receives the impulse from the SA node and transmits it downward to both ventricles via the bundle of His located within the septum and the Purkinje fibers distributed through the septum and throughout the ventricles. As the electrical impulse is transmitted throughout your ventricles, all ventricular muscle fibers contract in unison. This contraction occurs just slightly after the contraction of the atria, and the combination of the two results in one complete heartbeat. This entire process is repeated with each heartbeat.

Flashpoint

Blood-pressure readings reflect the amount of pressure exerted against the arterial walls during the ventricular contraction and ventricular relaxation phases of the cardiac cycle. A reading of 140/90 or higher is considered high blood pressure by the American Heart Association.

The contraction and relaxation of the four heart chambers, known as the **cardiac cycle,** creates each heartbeat. Each cardiac cycle is quite rapid, taking an average of just 0.8 second. Blood pressure, created by the pumping of blood, is written as two numbers, one over the other: 120/80. The upper number, the systolic pressure, reflects the highest pressure exerted against artery walls during ventricular contraction, or **systole.** The lower number, the diastolic pressure, reflects the lowest pressure exerted against artery walls during ventricular relaxation, or **diastole.** Large arteries in the body that have a strong pulse and are easily palpated are known as **pulse points.** These points, sometimes called pressure points, may be compressed to slow bleeding in the case of hemorrhage (Fig. 6-5).

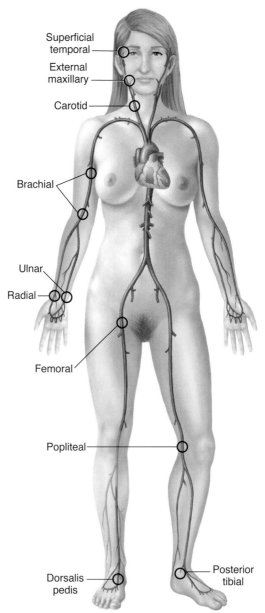

Superficial
temporal

External
maxillary

Carotid

Brachial

Ulnar

Radial

Femoral

Popliteal

Dorsalis
pedis

Posterior
tibial

FIGURE 6-5 **Pulse points.** (From Eagle, S., et al. [2009]. *The professional medical assistant.* Philadelphia, PA: F. A. Davis Company, p. 330; with permission)

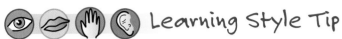 Learning Style Tip

Practice locating pulse points on one another as identified in Figure 6-5 and name each as you palpate (feel) it. Use the pads of your first two fingers to press firmly on the area but not too hard. Different areas may require different amounts of pressure. Count how many beats you feel in one minute. Try finding a pulse after your partner has been sitting quietly and again after they have exercised for a few minutes. Compare the two results.

Structure and Function Practice Exercises

Fill in the Blanks

Choose the term that matches the description.

Exercise 1

Mediastinum	Bicuspid valve	Occluded
Epicardium	Pulmonary valve	Arterioles
Myocardium	Aortic valve	Capillaries
Endocardium	Apex	Venules
Pericardium	Auscultating	Sinoatrial node
Pericardial fluid	Apical pulse	Atrioventricular node
Atria	Venae cavae	Cardiac cycle
Ventricles	Pulmonary arteries	Systole
Septum	Pulmonary veins	Diastole
Tricuspid valve	Cholesterol	Pulse points

1. _____ The fibrous membrane that encloses the heart

2. _____ Exits the left atrium into the left ventricle

3. _____ Tiny veins

4. _____ The area slightly left of the center of the chest

5. _____ Blood returns from the body to the right atrium through these inferior and superior structures.

6. _____ The contraction and relaxation of the four heart chambers

7. _____ A lubricant that reduces friction as the heart contracts and relaxes

8. _____ Blood enters these after leaving the arterioles. Their walls are just one cell thick.

9. _____ The natural pacemaker for the heart

10. _____ The middle, muscular layer of the heart

11. _____ A fatty, plaque-like substance that can narrow or block coronary vessels

12. _____ The two lower chambers of the heart

13. _____ They transport oxygen-rich blood to various parts of the body.

14. _____ Tiny arteries

15. _____ The term that means "listening to"

16. _____ Exits the left ventricle into the aorta

17. _____ The outer lining of the heart

18. _____ Large arteries with a strong pulse that are easily palpated

19. _____ The largest part of the heart; the lower left area

20. _____ The thick layer of muscle tissue that divides the left and right sides of the heart

21. _____ The "backup" pacemaker that transmits the SA node impulse to both ventricles

22. _____ The lower blood pressure number which reflects the lowest pressure exerted against artery walls during ventricular relaxation

23. _____ The inner lining of the heart

24. _____ Exits the right ventricle into the pulmonary arteries

25. _____ The term that means "blocked"

26. _____ The upper blood pressure number which reflects the highest pressure exerted against artery walls during ventricular contraction

27. _____ Exits the right atrium into the right ventricle

28. _____ The two upper chambers of the heart

29. _____ They lead to the lungs and transport oxygen-poor blood.

30. _____ Listening to this is considered the most accurate method of measuring heart rate.

Fill in the Blanks

Label Figure 6-6 with the appropriate anatomical terms and combining forms.

Exercise 2

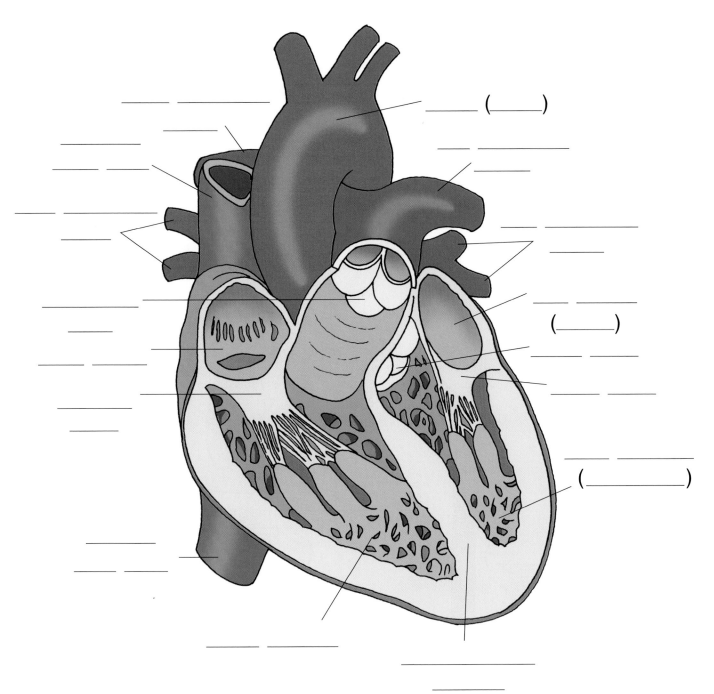

FIGURE 6-6 The heart with blanks.

Fill in the Blanks

Label Figure 6-7 with the appropriate anatomical terms and combining forms.

Exercise 3

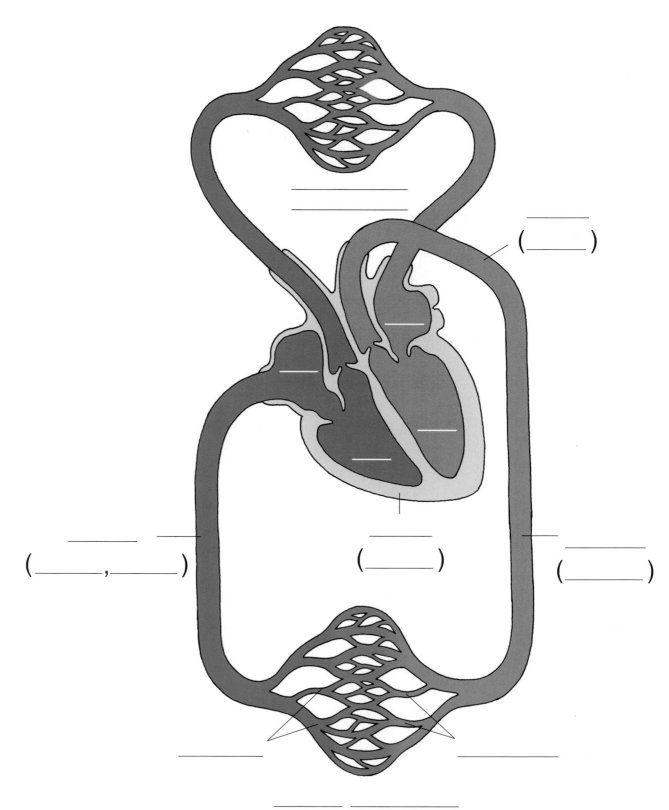

FIGURE 6-7 The cardiovascular system with blanks.

Combining Forms and Abbreviations

Combining Forms

Table 6-1 contains some of the combining forms that pertain to the cardiovascular system, examples of terms that utilize the combining forms, and a pronunciation guide. Read aloud to yourself as you move from left to right across the table. Be sure to use the pronunciation guide so that you can learn to say the terms correctly.

TABLE 6-1

COMBINING FORMS RELATED TO THE CARDIOVASCULAR SYSTEM

Combining Form	Meaning	Example (Pronunciation)	Meaning of New Term
angi/o	vessel	angioedema (ăn-jē-ō-ĕ-DĒ-mă)	swelling of a vessel
vas/o		vasorrhaphy (văs-OR-ă-fē)	suturing of a vessel
aort/o	aorta	aortostenosis (ā-or-tō-stĕ-NŌ-sĭs)	narrowing or stricture of the aorta
arteri/o	artery	arteriosclerosis (ăr-tē-rē-ō-sklĕ-RŌ-sĭs)	abnormal condition of hardening of an artery
ather/o	thick, fatty	atheroma (ăth-ĕr-Ō-mă)	thick, fatty tumor
atri/o	atria	atrioventricular (ā-trē-ō-vĕn-TRĬK-ū-lăr)	pertaining to the atria and the ventricles
cardi/o	heart	tachycardia (tăk-ē-KĂR-dē-ă)	condition of a rapid heart rate
coron/o		coronary (KOR-ō-nă-rē)	pertaining to the heart
electr/o	electricity	electrocardiogram (ē-lĕk-trō-KĂR-dē-ō-grăm)	record of electricity of the heart
hem/o	blood	hemolytic (hē-mō-LĬT-ĭk)	pertaining to the destruction of blood
hemat/o		hematemesis (hĕm-ăt-ĔM-ĕ-sĭs)	vomiting of blood
phleb/o	vein	phleborrhexis (flĕb-ō-RĔK-sĭs)	rupture of a vein
ven/o		venostasis (vē-nō-STĀ-sĭs)	stopping of a vein
thromb/o	thrombus (clot)	thrombophlebitis (thrŏm-bō-flē-BĪ-tĭs)	inflammation of a vein with the presence of a clot
valv/o	valve	valvotomy (văl-VŎT-ō-mē)	cutting into or incision of a valve
valvul/o		valvuloplasty (VĂL-vū-lō-plăs-tē)	surgical repair of a valve
vascul/o	blood vessel	vasculogenesis (văs-kū-lō-JĔN-ĕ-sĭs)	creation of a blood vessel
ventricul/o	ventricle	ventriculostomy (vĕn-trĭk-ū-LŎS-tō-mē)	mouthlike opening into a ventricle

IN A FLASH!

Go to the Davis*Plus* website to print out all of the Combining Form Flash Cards for Chapter 6 and run through them at least three times before you continue.

Flashpoint

Heart disease is the most common cause of death among Americans and stroke is the number four cause. Visit the American Heart Association website at *www.heart.org* to learn more about these conditions.

Abbreviations

Table 6-2 lists some of the most common abbreviations related to the cardiovascular system as well as others often used in medical documentation.

IN A FLASH!

Go to the Davis*Plus* website to print out all of the Abbreviation Flash Cards for Chapter 6 and run through them at least three times before you continue.

TABLE 6-2
ABBREVIATIONS

Cardiovascular System

AF, A-fib	atrial fibrillation	CCU	coronary care unit
ASHD	arteriosclerotic heart disease	CHF	congestive heart failure
AV, A-V	atrioventricular	CP	chest pain
BP	blood pressure	CPR	cardiopulmonary resuscitation
bpm	beats per minute	CV	cardiovascular
CABG	coronary artery bypass graft	DVT	deep-vein thrombosis
CAD	coronary artery disease	ECG, EKG	electrocardiogram
ECHO	echocardiogram	PAC	premature atrial contraction
HF	heart failure	PT	prothrombin time
HR	heart rate		
HTN	hypertension (high blood pressure)	PTCA	percutaneous transluminal coronary angioplasty
ICU	intensive care unit	PTT	partial thromboplastin time
INR	international normalized ratio	PVC	premature ventricular contraction
LA	left atrium	RA	right atrium
LV	left ventricle	RBC	red blood cell
MI	myocardial infarction		
MR	mitral regurgitation	RV	right ventricle
MS	mitral stenosis	V-fib	ventricular fibrillation
MVP	mitral valve prolapse	VT, V-tach	ventricular tachycardia
P	pulse	VTE	venous thromboembolism

Combining Forms and Abbreviations Practice Exercises

Fill in the Blanks

Fill in the blanks below using Table 6-1.

Exercise 4

1. mouthlike opening into a ventricle _____

2. swelling of a vessel _____

3. condition of a rapid heart _____

4. cutting into or incision of a valve _____

5. record of electricity of the heart _____

6. abnormal condition of hardening of an artery _____

7. rupture of a vein _____

8. suturing of a vessel _____

9. thick fatty tumor _____

10. vomiting of blood _____

11. surgical repair of a valve _____

12. creation of a blood vessel _____

13. narrowing or stricture of the aorta _____

14. stopping of a vein _____

15. pertaining to the atria and the ventricles _____

16. pertaining to the destruction of blood _____

17. inflammation of a vein with the presence of a clot _____

18. pertaining to the heart _____

Fill in the Blanks

Fill in the blanks below using Table 6-2.

Exercise 5

1. The abbreviation CABG stands for _____
   _____ _____
   _____ .

2. The names of the two upper chambers of the heart are abbreviated
   _____ and _____
   _____ .

3. The names of the two lower chambers of the heart are abbreviated
   _____ and _____ .

4. After checking Jaemoon's BP, or _____
   _____, the physician diagnosed him with HTN, which
   stands for _____ .

5. The physician ordered an EKG to record Shawn's heart rhythm. This
   stands for _____ .

6. Ventricular tachycardia may be abbreviated _____ or
   _____ .

7. The nurse will give the results of the PT/INR, or _____
   _____ / _____
   _____ _____, test to the physician.

8. HR, or _____ _____, is measured
   in bpm, or _____ _____
   _____ .

9. Atrial fibrillation may be abbreviated _____ or
   _____ .

10. The patient complained of CP, which stands for _____
    _____ .

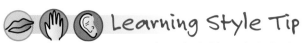 Learning Style Tip

Listen to instrumental music (with no lyrics) when you study and sing key terms, definitions, or phrases to the music. Make up dance moves by using gestures that describe what you are singing.

Pathologies, Procedures, and Pharmacology

Pathology Terms

Table 6-3 includes terms that relate to diseases or abnormalities of the cardio-vascular system. Use the pronunciation guide and say the terms aloud as you read them. This will help you get in the habit of saying them properly.

TABLE 6-3
PATHOLOGY TERMS

anemia (ă-NĒ-mē-ă)	group of disorders generally defined as a reduction in the mass of circulating red blood cells
aneurysm (ĂN-ū-rĭ-zum)	weakening and bulging of part of a vessel wall

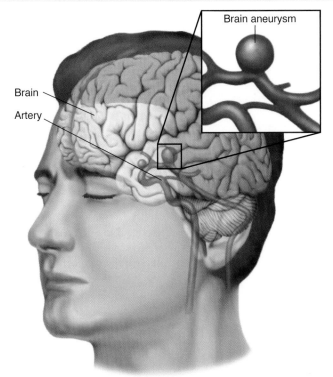

Aneurysm. (From Eagle, S., et al. [2009]. *The professional medical assistant.* Philadelphia, PA: F. A. Davis Company, p. 476; with permission)

Continued

TABLE 6-3
PATHOLOGY TERMS—cont'd

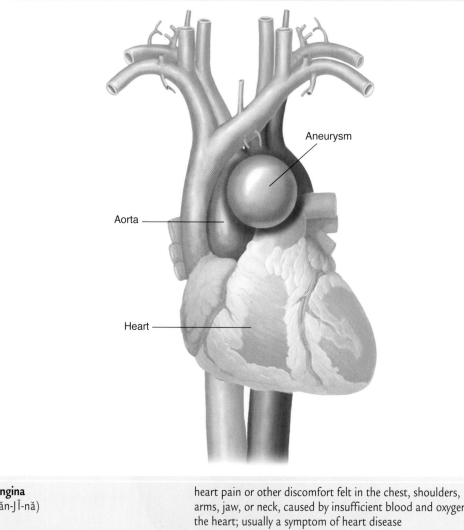

angina (ăn-JĪ-nă)	heart pain or other discomfort felt in the chest, shoulders, arms, jaw, or neck, caused by insufficient blood and oxygen to the heart; usually a symptom of heart disease
arrhythmia (ă-RĬTH-mē-ă)	loss of heart rhythm (rhythmic irregularity)
arteriosclerosis (ăr-tē-rē-ō-sklĕ-RŌ-sĭs)	thickening, loss of elasticity, and loss of contractility of arterial walls; commonly called *hardening of the arteries*
atherosclerosis (ăth-ĕr-ō-sklĕ-RŌ-sĭs)	the most common form of arteriosclerosis, marked by deposits of cholesterol, lipids, and calcium on the walls of arteries, which may restrict blood flow

TABLE 6-3
PATHOLOGY TERMS—cont'd

atrial fibrillation (AF, A-fib) (Ā-trē-ăl fĭ-brĭl-Ā-shŭn)	common irregular heart rhythm marked by uncontrolled atrial quivering and a rapid ventricular response

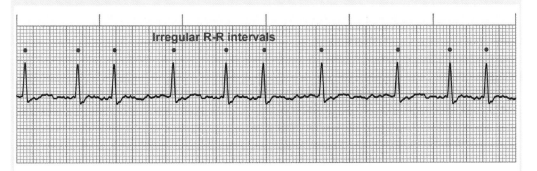

Atrial fibrillation. (From Jones, S. [2008]. *ECG success*. Philadelphia, PA: F. A. Davis Company, p. 32; with permission)

bruit (bruw-ē)	soft blowing sound caused by turbulent blood flow in a vessel
cardiac tamponade (KĂR-dē-ăk tăm-pŏn-ĀD)	serious condition in which the heart becomes compressed from an excessive collection of fluid or blood between the pericardial membrane and the heart
cardiomyopathy (kăr-dē-ō-mī-ŎP-ă-thē)	group of conditions in which the heart muscle has deteriorated and functions less effectively
congestive heart failure (CHF) (kŭn-JES-tĭv hărt FĀL-yĕr)	inability of the heart to pump enough blood to meet the needs of the body, resulting in lung congestion and dyspnea
cor pulmonale (kor pŭl-mă-NĀL-ē)	condition of right ventricular enlargement or dilation from increased right ventricular pressure; also called *pulmonary heart disease* or *right-sided heart failure*

Continued

TABLE 6-3
PATHOLOGY TERMS—cont'd

coronary artery disease (CAD) (KOR-ō-nă-rē ĂR-tĕr-ē dĭ-ZĒZ)	narrowing of the lumen, or inner open space of a vessel, of heart arteries due to arteriosclerosis and atherosclerosis

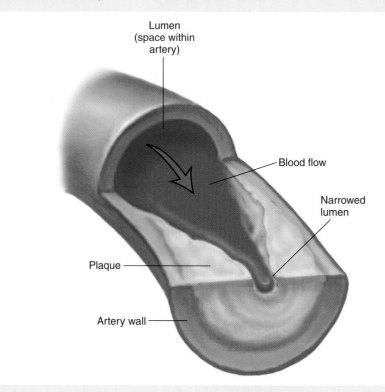

Coronary artery disease. (From Eagle, S., et al. [2009]. *The professional medical assistant.* Philadelphia, PA: F. A. Davis Company, p. 473; with permission)

TABLE 6-3
PATHOLOGY TERMS—cont'd

deep-vein thrombosis (DVT) (dĕp vān thrŏm-BŌ-sĭs)	development of a blood clot in a deep vein, usually in the legs; also known as *thrombophlebitis*

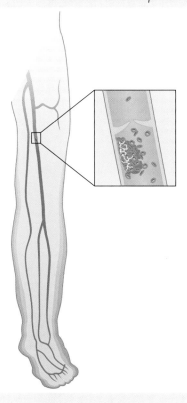

Deep-vein thrombosis.

disseminated intravascular coagulation (DIC) (dĭ-SEM-ĭ-nāt-ĕd ĭn-tră-VĂS-kū-lăr kō-ăg-ū-LĀ-shŭn)	serious condition that arises as a complication of another disorder, in which widespread, unrestricted microvascular blood clotting occurs; primary symptom is hemorrhage
embolus (ĔM-bō-lŭs)	undissolved matter floating in blood or lymph fluid that may cause an occlusion and infarction
endocarditis (ĕn-dō-kăr-DĪ-tĭs)	infection of the inner lining of the heart that may cause vegetation to form within one or more heart chambers or valves

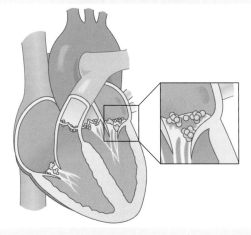

Endocarditis.

Continued

TABLE 6-3
PATHOLOGY TERMS—cont'd

fibrillation (fĭ-brĭl-Ā-shŭn)	quivering of heart muscle fibers instead of an effective heartbeat
hypertension (HTN) (hī-pĕr-TĔN-shŭn)	blood pressure that is consistently higher than 140 systolic, 90 diastolic, or both
ischemia (ĭs-KĒ-mē-ă)	temporary reduction in blood supply to a localized area of tissue
malignant hypertension (mă-LĬG-nănt hī-pĕr-TĔN-shŭn)	rare, life-threatening type of hypertension evidenced by optic-nerve (eye) edema and extremely high systolic and diastolic blood pressure
mitral regurgitation (MĪ-trăl rē-gŭr-jĭ-TĀ-shŭn)	condition in which the mitral valve does not close tightly, allowing blood to flow backward into the left atrium; also called *mitral insufficiency* or *mitral incompetence*

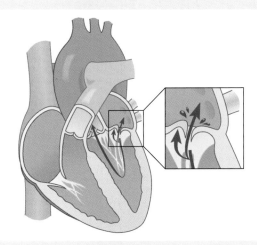

Mitral regurgitation.

mitral stenosis (MĪ-trăl stĕ-NŌ-sĭs)	condition in which the mitral valve fails to open properly, thereby impeding normal blood flow and increasing pressure within the left atrium and lungs

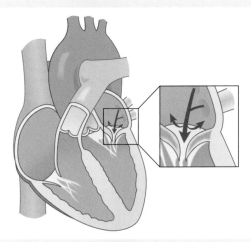

Mitral stenosis.

TABLE 6-3
PATHOLOGY TERMS—cont'd

murmur (MŬR-mŭr)	blowing or swishing sound in the heart, due to turbulent blood flow or backflow through a leaky valve
myocardial infarction (MI) (mī-ō-KĂR-dē-ăl ĭn-FĂRK-shŭn)	death of heart-muscle cells due to occlusion of a vessel; commonly called *heart attack*

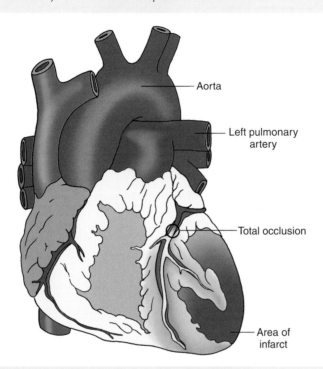

Myocardial Infarction.

myocarditis (mī-ō-kăr-DĪ-tĭs)	condition in which the middle layer of the heart wall becomes inflamed
pericarditis (pĕr-ĭ-kăr-DĪ-tĭs)	acute or chronic condition in which the fibrous membrane surrounding the heart becomes inflamed

Continued

TABLE 6-3
PATHOLOGY TERMS—cont'd

peripheral artery disease (PAD) (pĕr-ĬF-ĕr-ăl ĂR-tĕr-ē dĭ-ZĒZ)	condition of partial or complete obstruction of the arteries of the arms or legs; similar to peripheral vascular disease (PVD), which includes both arteries and veins

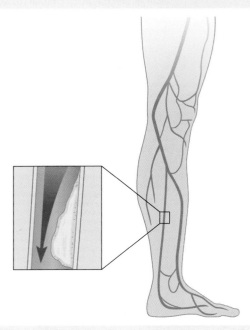

Peripheral artery disease.

polycythemia vera (pŏl-ē-sī-THĒ-mē-ă VĔ-ră)	chronic disorder marked by increased number and mass of all bone marrow cells, especially RBCs, with increased blood viscosity and a tendency to develop blood clots
Raynaud's disease (rĕ-NŌdz dĭ-ZĒZ)	disorder that affects blood vessels in the fingers, toes, ears, and nose, marked by vessel constriction and reduced blood flow in response to triggers such as cold temperature; also known as *Raynaud gangrene* or *Raynaud phenomenon*

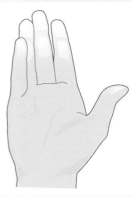

Raynaud's disease.

TABLE 6-3
PATHOLOGY TERMS—cont'd

rheumatic heart disease (roo-MĂT-ĭk hărt dĭ-ZĒZ)	complication of rheumatic fever in which inflammation and damage occur to parts of the heart, usually the valves
shock (shŏk)	syndrome of inadequate perfusion (circulation of blood, nutrients, and oxygen through tissues and organs) as a result of hypotension or low blood pressure
thromboangiitis obliterans (TAO) (thrŏm-bō-ăn-jē-Ī-tĭs ŏb-LĬT-ĕr-ănz)	type of vascular disease associated with tobacco use, marked by inflammation and clot formation within small vessels of the hands and feet, which may lead to gangrene and surgical amputation; sometimes called *Buerger's disease*
varicose veins (VĂR-ĭ-kōs vānz)	bulging, distended veins due to incompetent valves, most commonly in the legs

Normal direction of blood flow

Normal valve

Distended valve

Backflow of blood through incompetent valves

Normal leg veins

Varicose veins of leg

Varicose veins.

IN A FLASH!
Go to the Davis*Plus* website to print out all of the Pathology Term Flash Cards for Chapter 6 and run through them at least three times before you continue.

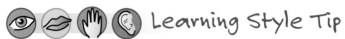 Learning Style Tip

Play Charades or a Pictionary-type game with a study group or study buddy to act out or draw clues for each of the following procedures as your partners guess which one you are demonstrating. It is okay to be silly, laugh, and have fun. In fact, the more fun you have, the better you will remember the procedures.

Common Diagnostic Tests and Procedures

Angiography: Diagnostic or therapeutic radiography (radiological imaging) of the heart and blood vessels

Automated external defibrillator (AED): Small computer-driven defibrillator that analyzes the patient's rhythm, selects the appropriate energy level, charges the machine, and delivers a shock to the patient

Automatic implanted cardioverter defibrillator (AICD): Very small defibrillator, surgically implanted in patients with a high risk for sudden cardiac death, that automatically detects and treats life-threatening arrhythmias

Cardiac catheterization: Evaluation of the heart vessels and valves via the injection of dye that shows up under radiology (Fig. 6-8)

Cardiopulmonary resuscitation (CPR): Emergency procedure that provides manual external cardiac compression and sometimes artificial respiration

Cardioversion: Restoration of normal sinus rhythm (NSR) by chemical or electrical means

Coronary artery bypass graft (CABG): Surgical creation of an alternate route for blood flow around an area of coronary arterial obstruction (Fig. 6-9)

Defibrillation: Delivery of an electric shock with the goal of ending ventricular fibrillation and restoring NSR

Electrocardiography (ECG, EKG): Creation and study of graphic records (electrocardiograms) of electric currents originating in the heart (Fig. 6-10)

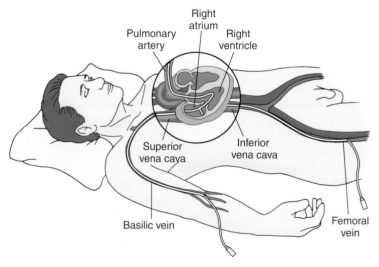

FIGURE 6-8 Cardiac catheterization.

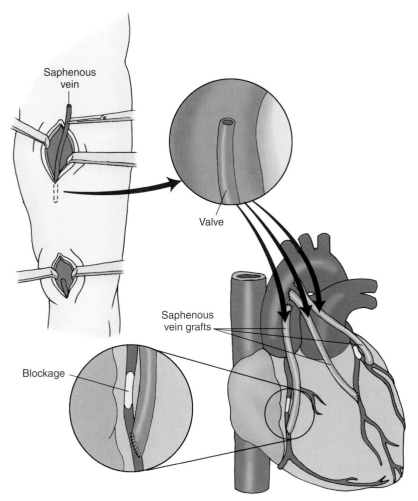

FIGURE 6-9 Coronary artery bypass graft.

Event recorder: Portable monitoring device that transmits heart rhythms by telephone to a central laboratory, where dysrhythmias can be detected and analyzed (Fig. 6-11)

Holter monitor: Portable device worn by a patient during normal activity that records heart rhythm for up to 24 hours (Fig. 6-12)

International normalized ratio (INR): Standardized method of checking the prothrombin time (PT); used to monitor and adjust warfarin (Coumadin) dosage in order to maintain a balance between clot prevention and excessive bleeding

Pacemaker: Device that can trigger the mechanical contractions of the heart by emitting periodic electrical discharges

Partial thromboplastin time (PTT): Measure of blood-clotting time, used to monitor heparin therapy; heparin is an anticoagulant medication that slows the clotting time of blood. A balance must be maintained between clot prevention and excessive bleeding.

Percutaneous transluminal coronary angioplasty (PTCA): Method of treating a narrowed coronary artery via inflation and deflation of a balloon on a double-lumen catheter inserted through the right femoral artery (Fig. 6-13)

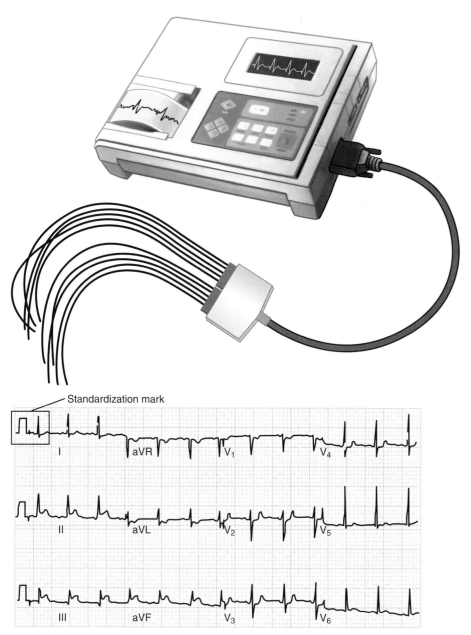

Standardization mark

FIGURE 6-10 **ECG.** (From Eagle, S., et al. [2009]. *The professional medical assistant.* Philadelphia, PA: F. A. Davis Company, pp. 482–483; with permission)

Prothrombin time (PT): Procedure that measures the clotting time of blood; used with the international normalized ratio (INR) to assess levels of anticoagulation in patients taking warfarin (Coumadin). A balance must be maintained between clot prevention and excessive bleeding.

Stress test: Treadmill test that can show if the blood supply is reduced in the arteries that supply the heart

Transesophageal echocardiography (TEE): Study of the heart via a probe placed in the esophagus

Troponin: Protein released into the body by damaged heart muscle, considered the most accurate blood test to confirm the diagnosis of an MI

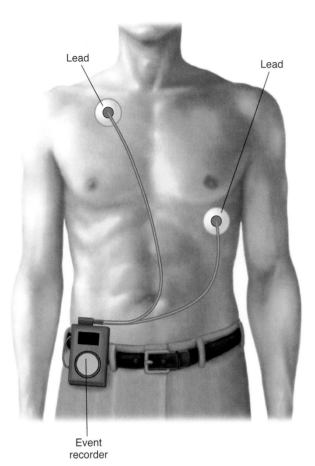

FIGURE 6-11 **Event recorder.** (From Eagle, S., et al. [2009]. *The professional medical assistant.* Philadelphia, PA: F. A. Davis Company, p. 493; with permission)

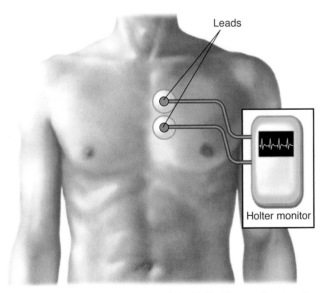

FIGURE 6-12 **Holter monitor.** (From Eagle, S., et al. [2009]. *The professional medical assistant.* Philadelphia, PA: F. A. Davis Company, p. 493; with permission)

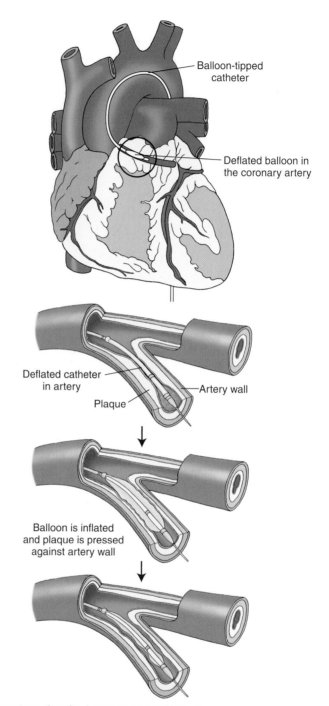

FIGURE 6-13 **Percutaneous transluminal coronary angioplasty.**

Pharmacology

Table 6-4 provides a list of common cardiovascular medications.

TABLE 6-4
PHARMACOLOGY

Therapeutic Classification	Generic Name	Brand Name	Common Use
Anticoagulant	dalteparin	Fragmin	Decrease the clotting ability of the blood
	danaparoid	Orgaran	
	enoxaparin	Lovenox	
	heparin	None	
	tinzaparin	Innohep	
	warfarin	Coumadin	
Antiplatelet agent	aspirin	Bayer, Bufferin, Ecotrin	Prevent blood clot formation
	clopidogrel	Plavix	
	dipyridamole	Persantine	
	ticlopidine	Ticlid	
Angiotensin-converting enzyme (ACE) inhibitors	benazepril	Lotensin	Lower angiotensin II levels; expand blood vessels and decrease resistance
	captopril	Capoten	
	enalapril	Vasotec	
	fosinopril	Monopril	
	lisinopril	Prinivil, Zestril	
	moexipril	Univasc	
	perindopril	Aceon	
	quinapril	Accupril	
	ramipril	Altace	
	trandolapril	Mavik	
Angiotensin II receptor blockers/ inhibitors	candesartan	Atacand	Prevent effects of angiotensin II; keep blood pressure from rising
	eprosartan	Teveten	
	irbesartan	Avapro	
	losartan	Cozaar	
	telmisartan	Micardis	
	valsartan	Diovan	
Beta blockers/ Beta-adrenergic blocking agents	acebutolol	Sectral	Decrease heart rate and cardiac output
	atenolol	Tenormin	
	betaxolol	Kerlone	
	bisoprolol / hydrochlorothiazide	Ziac	

Continued

TABLE 6-4

PHARMACOLOGY—cont'd

Therapeutic Classification	Generic Name	Brand Name	Common Use
	bisoprolol	Zebeta	
	carteolol	Cartrol	
	metoprolol	Lopressor, Toprol XL	
	nadolol	Corgard	
	propranolol	Inderal	
	sotalol	Betapace	
	timolol	Biocadren	
Calcium channel blockers	amlodipine	Norvasc, Lotrel	Interrupt movement of calcium into cells; decrease the heart's pumping strength and relax blood vessels
	bepridil	Vascor	
	diltiazem	Cardizem, Tiazac	
	felodipine	Plendil	
	nifedipine	Adalat, Procardia	
	nimodipine	Nimotop	
	nisoldipine	Sular	
	verapamil	Calan, Isoptin, Verelan	
Diuretics (water pills)	amiloride	Midamor	Remove excess fluids and sodium from the body; relieve the heart's workload
	bumetanide	Bumex	
	chlorothiazide	Diuril	
	chlorthalidone	Hygroton	
	furosemide	Lasix	
	hydrochlorothiazide	Esidrix, Hydrodiuril	
	indapamide	Lozol	
	spironolactone	Aldactone	
Vasodilators	isosorbide dinitrate	Isordil	Relax blood vessels and increase blood supply and oxygen to the heart; reduce the heart's workload
	nesiritide	Natrecor	
	nitroglycerin		
	hydralazine	Apresoline	
	nitrates		
Digitalis preparations	digitoxin		Increase the force of the heart's contractions
	digoxin		
	lanoxin		

TABLE 6-4			
PHARMACOLOGY—cont'd			
Therapeutic Classification	**Generic Name**	**Brand Name**	**Common Use**
Cholesterol lowering	atorvastatin	Lipitor	Lower LDL (bad) cholesterol, raise HDL (good) cholesterol, lower triglyceride levels
	fluvastatin	Lescol	
	lovastatin	Altoprev, Mevacor	
	pitavastatin	Livalo	
	pravastatin	Pravachol	
	rosuvastatin	Crestor	
	simvastatin	Zocor	
	simvastatin and ezetimibe	Vytorin	

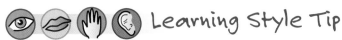 Learning Style Tip

It is easy to use a search engine on your computer, tablet, or smartphone to find websites or videos that will provide additional information about any cardiac topics that you find especially interesting. As always, if you hear key concepts or read and verbalize them aloud, you engage your verbal, auditory, and visual senses, which will greatly increase the chance that you will understand, and later remember the information.

Pathologies, Procedures, and Pharmacology Practice Exercises

Deciphering Terms

Write the correct meaning of these medical terms.

Exercise 6

1. microcardia _____

2. venule _____

3. hemogram _____

4. angiography _____

5. aortoplasty _____

6. arteriole _____

7. atherocyte _____

8. atriodynia _____

9. electrocardiogram _____

10. hematuria _____

11. valvular _____

12. phlebitis _____

13. venostasis _____

14. vasculopathy _____

15. thrombolysis _____

Fill in the Blanks

Fill in the blanks below using Table 6-3.

Exercise 7

1. Jim's heart no longer beats in a regular rhythm. Therefore, he has an _____.

2. When the physician listened to Martha's carotid arteries with a stethoscope, he heard a soft blowing sound caused by turbulent blood flow. This is known as a _____.

3. Ismael has a heart condition that results in lung congestion and dyspnea. The medical term for this condition is _____ _____.

4. Victor was treated with an anticoagulant medication called heparin because of a blood clot in a deep vein of his legs. This condition is known as _____ _____ _____.

5. Cristobalina has bulging, distended veins in her legs. This condition is known as _____ _____.

6. _____ _____ is a group of disorders generally defined as a reduction in the mass of circulating red blood cells.

7. Martha is suffering from _____, which is heart pain and usually a symptom of heart disease.

8. _____ is a group of conditions in which the heart muscle has deteriorated and functions less effectively.

9. Harold has vegetation growing on the inner lining of his heart. The doctor says this is probably caused by _____.

10. An acute or chronic condition in which the fibrous membrane surrounding the heart becomes inflamed is called _____.

Multiple Choice

Select the one best answer to the following multiple-choice questions.

Exercise 8

1. Which of the following disorders does **not** involve an interference in blood flow?
   a. ischemia
   b. myocardial infarction
   c. mitral stenosis
   d. arrhythmia

2. Which of the following does **not** involve the heart rhythm?
   a. V-tach
   b. PAC
   c. V-fib
   d. TIA

3. Which of the following abbreviations stands for the name of a chamber of the heart?
   a. BP
   b. EKG
   c. RA
   d. PCP

4. All of the following refer to a part of the heart **except:**

    a. RA

    b. RV

    c. MI

    d. LV

5. Which of the following may cause temporary stroke-like symptoms?

    a. CHF

    b. TIA

    c. LA

    d. CPR

Fill in the Blanks

Using Table 6-4, write the therapeutic classification of the medication next to each generic or brand name.

Exercise 9

1. Lipitor _____

2. propranolol _____

3. lisinopril _____

4. Coumadin _____

5. atenolol _____

6. Lasix _____

7. perindopril _____

8. Plavix _____

9. aspirin _____

10. Cardizem _____

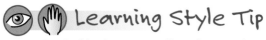 Learning Style Tip

Don't skip the case studies. They are designed to engage your brain as well as your senses. To correctly answer the questions, you must reflect on what you just read and apply it. This type of application forces you to think about the terms in a meaningful (real-world) way. This greatly increases the chances that you will remember the material later.

CASE STUDY

Read the case study and answer the questions that follow. Most of the terms are included in this chapter. Refer to your medical dictionary for the other terms.

Deep-Vein Thrombosis

Arturo Espinoza is a 72-year-old retired cook with a history of ASHD and HTN. He also had an MI a year ago. He is 5´9˝, weighs 220 pounds, and has been a pack-a-day smoker for 45 years. He recently noticed a deep, intense aching in his right lower leg but does not recall having injured it. Over the next few days, his right calf became tender and erythematous. In addition, his right lower leg, from the knee down, has become edematous.

After being evaluated by his family physician, Mr. Espinoza was diagnosed with deep-vein thrombosis (DVT) and started on SubQ heparin injection therapy twice each day (bid). After several days of heparin therapy, Coumadin was started as well. Both PTT and INR levels were monitored. Once Mr. Espinoza achieved a therapeutic level of his Coumadin, he was able to discontinue the heparin. Coumadin therapy is planned for the next 3 to 6 months, and he will return on a monthly basis for monitoring.

Venous thromboembolism (VTE) is a condition in which a thrombus, or blood clot, develops within a vein. When inflammation also develops, the condition is known as **deep-vein thrombosis (DVT)** or *thrombophlebitis*. This condition can occur in any vein but is most common in the deep veins of the legs. Risk factors for DVT include recent surgery, venous stasis from immobility, obesity, increased blood coagulability, and vascular injury. People with an increased risk include the elderly, smokers, and women over 30 years old who use oral contraceptives. If the blood clot breaks off and moves to the lungs it is called a *pulmonary embolism* (PE).

In recent years, increased attention has been paid to the occurrence of DVT among airline passengers. Some have called it *economy-class syndrome* because of the prolonged sitting required of these passengers, which can cause venous stasis. Risk of this syndrome could be minimized if passengers were able to exercise their feet and legs every 1 to 2 hours by walking in the aisles or doing range-of-motion exercises while sitting. Remaining well hydrated and wearing support hose are also helpful.

Treatment goals for DVT are to prevent the blood clot from getting bigger and to prevent it from breaking off and moving to the lungs. Treatment may include rest, elevation of the extremity, compression stockings, and medications such as nonsteroidal anti-inflammatory drugs (NSAIDs) and anticoagulants. A variety of anticoagulant medications are available; some of the most commonly used include heparin, Lovenox, and Fragmin. Heparin levels must be monitored by checking the PTT. After several days, warfarin (Coumadin) therapy is started. Blood levels of this medication are monitored by checking the INR. These medications slow the patient's blood-clotting time, which prevents further clot formation while the body's natural mechanisms dissolve the present clot. A potential side effect of these medications is easy bruising and increased risk of bleeding. Therefore, patients are counseled to watch for signs of bleeding when, for example, passing bowel movements or brushing or flossing the teeth.

Case Study Questions

Exercise 9

1. What known risk factor for DVT does Mr. Espinoza have?
   a. He is a Mexican American.
   b. He is a smoker.
   c. He is a man.
   d. He is a retired cook.

2. Mr. Espinoza has a history of what disorder?
   a. atherosclerotic heart disease
   b. diabetes
   c. epilepsy
   d. *pneumocystis* pneumonia

3. By what route did Mr. Espinoza receive his heparin?
   a. by mouth
   b. intramuscular injection
   c. intradermal injection
   d. subcutaneous injection

4. What lab test was done to determine whether Mr. Espinoza's heparin dose was correct?
   a. PT
   b. PTT
   c. INR
   d. DVT

5. What lab test was done to determine whether Mr. Espinoza's Coumadin dose was correct?
   a. PT
   b. PTT
   c. INR
   d. DVT

6. Treatment of DVT includes which of the following measures?
   a. application of cold therapy
   b. vigorous exercise
   c. nonsteroidal anti-inflammatory medication
   d. topical application of creams or ointments

7. Why has economy-class syndrome become a recent popular name for DVT?
   a. because flying in airplanes at high altitudes causes blood clot formation
   b. because passengers who sit in economy class generally do not move about for the duration of the flight
   c. because all airlines passengers are at high risk for blood-clot formation
   d. because DVT happens only to airline passengers

8. Create a list of ways to decrease the risk for development of DVT.

End-of-Chapter Practice Exercises

Word Building

*Using **only** the word parts in the lists provided, create medical terms with the indicated meanings.*

Exercise 10

Prefixes	Combining Forms	Suffixes
brady-	angi/o	-cele
micro-	aort/o	-cyte
tachy-	arteri/o	-gram
	ather/o	-graphy
	atri/o	-ia
	cardi/o	-ic
	coron/o	-logist
	electr/o	-megaly
	hemat/o	-metry
	phleb/o	-oid
	scler/o	-osis
	thromb/o	-pathy
	valvul/o	-plasty
	vascul/o	-rrhaphy
	ventricul/o	-rrhexis
		-sclerosis
		-tomy
		-version

1. record of a vessel _____

2. pertaining to the aorta _____

3. process of recording an artery _____

4. abnormal condition of hardening of thick, fatty tissue _____

5. rupture of an artery _____

6. condition of a slow heart _____

7. enlargement of the heart _____

8. condition of a rapid heart _____

9. record of heart electricity _____

10. specialist in the study of blood _____

11. incision into a valve _____

12. cutting into a vein _____

13. inflammation of a blood vessel _____

14. cell for clotting _____

15. surgical repair of a vessel _____

16. hernia of a ventricle _____

17. measurement of the ventricle _____

18. condition of a small heart _____

19. rupturing of red blood cells _____

20. softening of the walls of the aorta _____

True or False

Decide whether the following statements are true or false.

Exercise 11

1. True   False   The abbreviation **PTT** stands for platelets.

2. True   False   A **murmur** is an abnormal blowing or swishing sound in the heart caused by turbulent blood flow or backflow through a leaky valve.

3. True   False   An **aneurysm** is a weakened area in the wall of a vessel.

4. True   False   The abbreviation **MI** stands for *muscle injury.*

5. True   False   The abbreviation **PTCA** stands for a type of food.

6. True   False   An **embolus** is a soft blowing sound caused by turbulent blood flow.

7. True   False   The abbreviation **CV** stands for *coronary vessel.*

8. True   False   **Ischemia** refers to a temporary reduction in blood supply to a localized area of tissue.

9. True   False   The abbreviation **ASHD** stands for *arteriosclerotic heart disease.*

10. True   False   **Fibrillation** refers to an abnormal quivering of heart muscle fibers instead of an effective heartbeat.

Deciphering Terms

Write the correct meaning of these medical terms.

Exercise 12

1. macrocardia _____

2. ventriculoscopy _____

3. vasotonic _____

4. vasodilation _____

5. cardiomyopathy _____

6. phleborrhaphy _____

7. thrombolysis _____

8. hematologist _____

9. arteriorrhexis _____

10. vasoconstriction _____

Multiple Choice

Select the one best answer to the following multiple-choice questions.

Exercise 13

1. Which of the following terms is matched to the correct definition?
   a. angi/o: thick, fatty
   b. hem/o: heart
   c. arteri/o: aorta
   d. phleb/o: vein

2. Which of the following terms is matched to the correct definition?
   a. atri/o: atria
   b. vascul/o: valve
   c. hem/o: thrombus
   d. ventricul/o: blood vessel

3. All of the following terms are matched with the correct definition **except:**

   a. aort/o: aorta

   b. cardi/o: heart

   c. hemat/o: blood

   d. vas/o: vascular

4. Which of the following abbreviations represents a test or procedure?

   a. MR

   b. INR

   c. bpm

   d. MVP

5. Which of the following abbreviations represents a type of heart disease?

   a. DVT

   b. ASHD

   c. PT

   d. PVC

6. All of the following terms are matched with the correct definition **except:**

   a. anemia: reduction in the mass of circulating red blood cells (RBCs)

   b. bruit: soft blowing sound caused by turbulent blood flow in a vessel

   c. disseminated intravascular coagulation: serious condition in which widespread, microvascular blood clotting occurs while the patient has symptoms of hemorrhaging

   d. Raynaud's disease: a chronic disorder marked by increased number and mass of all bone marrow cells, especially RBCs, with increased blood viscosity and a tendency to develop blood clots

7. All of the following terms are matched with the correct definition **except:**

   a. aneurysm: weakening and bulging of part of a vessel wall

   b. angina: heart pain or other discomfort felt in the chest

   c. cardiomyopathy: condition in which the heart becomes compressed from an excessive collection of fluid or blood between the pericardial membrane and the heart

   d. endocarditis: infection of the inner lining of the heart that may cause vegetation to form within one or more heart chambers or valves

8. All of the following terms are matched with the correct definition **except:**

   a. embolus: undissolved matter floating in blood or lymph fluid

   b. cor pulmonale: development of a blood clot in a deep vein, usually in the legs

   c. arteriosclerosis: thickening, loss of elasticity, and loss of contractility of arterial walls; commonly called *hardening of the arteries*

   d. ischemia: temporary reduction in blood supply to a localized area of tissue

9. Which of the following is a type of heart-rhythm abnormality?

   a. cardiomyopathy

   b. atrial fibrillation

   c. murmur

   d. thromboangiitis obliterans

10. Coronary artery disease includes which of the following components?

    a. murmur and bruit

    b. atherosclerosis and arteriosclerosis

    c. heart failure and malignant hypertension

    d. mitral regurgitation and mitral stenosis

11. Which of the following is related to incompetent valves?

    a. hypertension

    b. varicose veins

    c. myocardial infarction

    d. myocarditis

12. A surgeon performing a CABG will need to include which of the following?

    a. angiorrhaphy

    b. aortomalacia

    c. valvuloplasty

    d. hematemesis

13. Dr. Emily Shu is studying a piece of paper with the patient's heart-rhythm strip on it. The paper she is studying is an:

    a. electrodiagnosis

    b. electrocardiogram

    c. electrocardiograph

    d. electrocardiophonograph

14. The process of dissolving or destroying a blood clot is called:

    a. thrombocytosis

    b. thrombosclerosis

    c. thrombolytic

    d. thrombolysis

15. A term that indicates narrowing of a vein is:

    a. phlebosclerosis

    b. phleborrhexis

    c. phleborrhagia

    d. phlebostenosis

16. Which of the following terms means *bursting forth of blood?*

    a. hemolysis

    b. hemorrhage

    c. hematoma

    d. hematogenesis

17. If an aortic aneurysm is not repaired, the following may occur:

    a. aortomalacia

    b. aortoclasia

    c. aortocoronary

    d. aortostenosis

18. A test to examine heart vessels is:

    a. a CABG

    b. an angiography

    c. an arterioplasty

    d. a CAD

LYMPHATIC AND IMMUNE SYSTEM

7

Chapter Outline

Structure and Function

As blood circulates throughout the body, fluid leaks out from the blood vessels. The lymphatic system includes an intricate network of vessels that collect the excess tissue fluid, called lymph, and return it to the circulation (Fig. 7-1). **Lymph** is a clear, colorless, alkaline fluid made up mostly of water, along with some protein, salts, fats, white blood cells, and **urea** (a waste product of protein metabolism). **Lymphatic vessels** are found throughout the body alongside arteries, veins, and capillaries.

> ### Flashpoint
> While blood vessels rely on the pumping action of the heart, there is no pump for lymphatic vessels; instead, lymph flow is facilitated by the pumping action of skeletal muscles.

  ### Learning Style Tip

Read twice—slowly and aloud—any key sections of the text that you are struggling to grasp. This sometimes helps to slow down your brain so you can focus on each word and think about what it means before you continue.

The lymphatic system includes **lymph nodes,** commonly called *glands,* which are rich in specialized white blood cells called **phagocytes.** The phagocytes clean debris from lymph through a process called **phagocytosis.** In this process, the white blood cells remove microorganisms, cell debris, and blood cells that are damaged, old, or abnormal by engulfing them and literally gobbling them up. Because of these functions, the **lymphatic system** is also considered part of the immune system. When infection and inflammation occur, the body is able to respond by increasing the production of phagocytes.

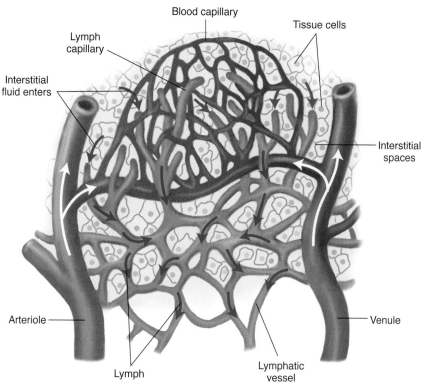

FIGURE 7-1 **Lymphatic vessels.**

Lymphatic vessels are located throughout the body and are connected to the **superior vena cava,** which is where lymph enters the circulatory system and is combined with blood. Lymph nodes are distributed along lymphatic vessels with higher numbers in the **neck, axillae (armpits), groin,** and **abdomen** (Fig. 7-2). There are two sets of lymph nodes in the throat, commonly known as the **tonsils** and **adenoids.** These nodes may become tender and swollen when you have a cold or sore throat; this occurs when the lymph nodes, which have been working to filter lymph in that area, become overwhelmed and inflamed. An inflamed gland may be referred to as _lymphadenitis_ or _lymphadenopathy._ Chronic inflammation may require surgical removal of the gland such as a tonsillectomy. Lymph nodes are also removed for diagnostic purposes. Some of the axillary glands are often removed from the breast cancer patient to determine if the cancer has **metastasized,** or spread, to another part of the body.

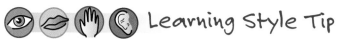 Learning Style Tip

Move your body when you study. This helps even if what you are physically doing has nothing to do with what you are studying. While you flip through flash cards or read, try pacing around a room, going for a walk, running on a treadmill, pedaling on a stationary bicycle, or even working on an arts-and-crafts project. The movement helps keep you awake, keeps your brain engaged, and somehow helps you recall the information later. The same activities can also be done by auditory learners as you listen to taped lectures or audio terminology.

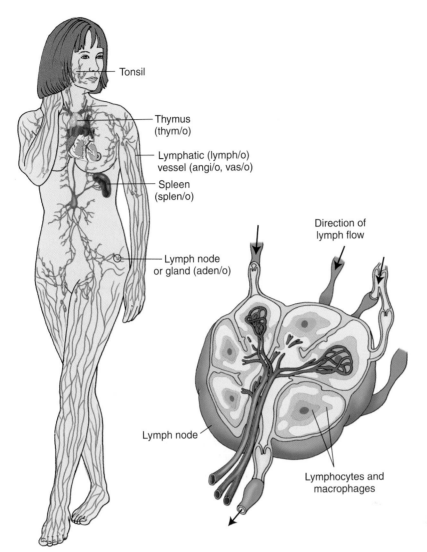

Tonsil

Thymus
(thym/o)

Lymphatic (lymph/o)
vessel (angi/o, vas/o)

Spleen
(splen/o)

Direction of
lymph flow

Lymph node
or gland (aden/o)

Lymph node

Lymphocytes and
macrophages

FIGURE 7-2 **Lymphatic system.**

The Thymus and the Spleen

Other structures involved in the lymphatic system include the thymus and the
spleen. The **thymus gland** is located in the mediastinum above the heart. It
consists of two fused lobes and is divided into an outer part (cortex), mostly
composed of immature **T lymphocytes** (a type of white blood cell), and an inner
part (medulla). The thymus is most active during the prenatal period and early
years of life. It grows until puberty and then gradually shrinks in size as we
age. It plays a role in immunity and is believed to play a role in protecting our
bodies against cancer (Box 7-1). The T lymphocytes are also known as *killer
T* cells because of their ability to seek out and destroy cells that are infected or
have become cancerous. They mature in the thymus and then circulate to other
immune-system structures, including the spleen and lymph nodes.

Box 7-1 Cancer

Cancer is a genetic mutation of cells that causes them to grow and divide abnormally. These abnormal cells originate in a particular organ but can travel to other places of the body through the blood and lymph systems. There are more than 100 types of cancer and cancer is the number two cause of death in the United States. In 2014, it was expected that 1,600 Americans per day would die from this disease. Even though these numbers are alarming, a diagnosis of cancer is not a death sentence. Over the past 20 years, the likelihood of dying from cancer has steadily dropped. Treatments are more effective if the disease is detected early. Research shows that regular screenings for certain types of cancer, such as breast and cervical cancer, increase survival rates.

While genetic and environmental factors may contribute to the development of cancer, it's important to understand that a very large percentage of new cases can be prevented. For example, cancers caused by tobacco or alcohol abuse are entirely preventable. Cancers caused by obesity, inactivity, and poor nutrition could be prevented by lifestyle changes that include healthy eating and exercise. Vaccinations could prevent cancers caused by infectious agents such as the human papillomavirus (HPV), and limiting exposure to the damaging rays of the sun could prevent skin cancer.

Flashpoint

Non-Hodgkin lymphoma is a cancer that affects the organs of the lymphatic system. The American Cancer Society (ACS) estimates that in 2014 there will have been 70,800 new cases and it will have caused nearly 19,000 deaths. Many types of cancer are preventable. For information about all types of cancer, visit the ACS website at *www.cancer.org* or the National Cancer Institute (NCI) at *www.cancer.gov*.

The **spleen** is a dark-red, oval-shaped organ located in the left upper quadrant of the abdomen, just under the ribs. It is surrounded by an outer capsule of connective tissue and is divided into compartments. During prenatal development, the spleen forms red blood cells (RBCs) and white blood cells (WBCs). After birth, the spleen produces RBCs only in cases of severe need; however, it continues creating WBCs as well as antibodies as part of its role in the immune system. It also acts as a type of storage container, generally holding a supply of 100 mL to 300 mL of blood as well as 30% of the body's total platelets. Platelets are important for blood clotting. In the event of hemorrhage, the spleen can return this extra blood and platelets to the circulation to help maintain blood pressure and help with blood clotting. Because of its location and rich blood supply, the spleen may be injured if you suffer a blow to the abdomen. This may require a splenectomy (surgical removal of the spleen) to stop any internal bleeding.

Structure and Function Practice Exercises

Fill in the Blanks

Choose the term that matches the description.

Exercise 1

Lymph
Urea
Lymphatic vessels
Lymph nodes
Phagocytes
Phagocytosis
Lymphatic system

Superior vena cava
Neck, axillae, groin, and abdomen
Tonsils and adenoids
Metastasized
Thymus gland
T lymphocytes
Spleen

1. _____ Lymph enters the circulatory system and combines with blood here

2. _____ Rich in specialized white blood cells; commonly called glands

3. _____ A process in which white blood cells engulf and destroy microorganisms, cell debris, and blood cells that are damaged, old, or abnormal

4. _____ Clear, colorless, alkaline tissue fluid made up mostly of water, along with some protein, fats, white blood cells, and urea

5. _____ Located above the heart and plays a role in immunity and protecting our bodies from cancer

6. _____ Found throughout the body alongside arteries, veins, and capillaries

7. _____ High numbers of lymph nodes are found in these areas

8. _____ A waste product of protein metabolism

9. _____ Lymph nodes in the throat

10. _____ White blood cells that are able to seek out and destroy abnormal cells

11. _____ White blood cells that clean debris from lymph

12. _____ A part of the immune system that collects excess tissue fluid and returns it to circulation

13. _____ Creates white blood cells and antibodies; acts as a type of storage container for blood and platelets

14. _____ Spread to another part of the body

Fill in the Blanks

Label Figure 7-3 with the appropriate anatomical terms and combining forms.

Exercise 2

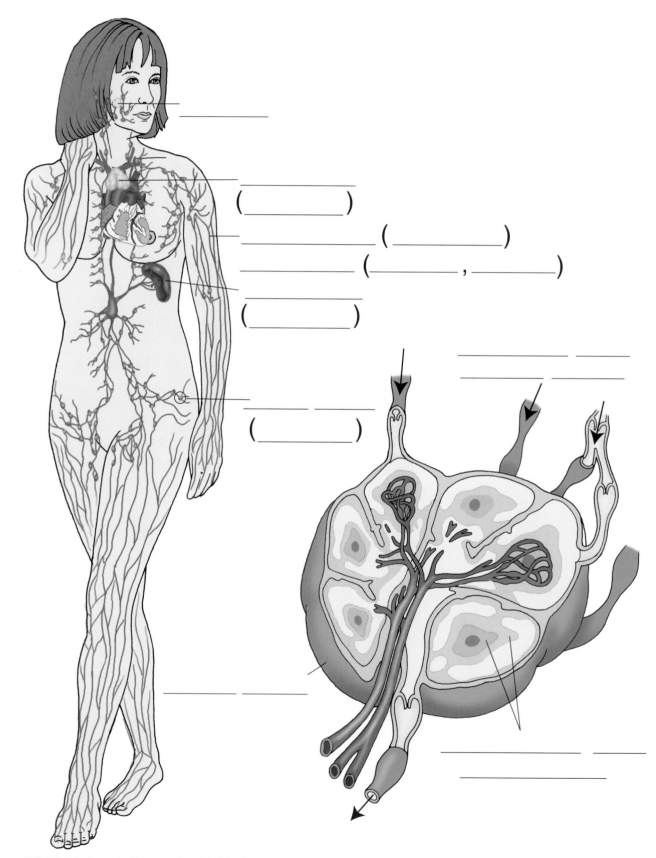

_____

(_____)

_____ (_____)

_____ (_____ , _____)

_____

(_____)

_____ ___

_____ ___

_____ ___

(_____)

_____ ___

_____ ___

_____ ___

FIGURE 7-3 Lymphatic vessels with blanks.

Combining Forms and Abbreviations

Combining Forms

Table 7-1 contains combining forms that pertain to the lymphatic-immune system, examples of terms that utilize the combining forms, and a pronunciation guide. Read aloud to yourself as you move from left to right across the table. Be sure to use the pronunciation guide so that you can learn to say the terms correctly.

TABLE 7-1
COMBINING FORMS RELATED TO THE LYMPHATIC AND IMMUNE SYSTEM

Combining Form	Meaning	Example (Pronunciation)	Meaning of New Term
aden/o	gland	adenoma (Ăd-ĕ-NŌ-mă)	tumor of a gland
adenoid/o	adenoid	adenoidectomy (ăd-ĕ-noyd-ĔK-tō-mē)	excision or surgical removal of an adenoid
angi/o	vessel	angiasthenia (ăn-jē-ăs-THĒ-nē-ă)	absence of vessel strength
vas/o		vasorrhaphy (văs-OR-ă-fē)	suturing of a vessel
bacteri/o	bacteria	bacteriemia (băk-tĕr-Ē-mē-ă)	condition of bacteria in the blood
immun/o	immune	immunopathology (ĭm-ū-nō-pă-THŌL-ō-jē)	study of immune disease
lymph/o	lymph	lymphoma (lĭm-FŌ-mă)	lymph tumor
lymphaden/o	lymph gland	lymphadenocele (lĭm-FĂD-ĕ-nō-sēl)	hernia of a lymphatic vessel
lymphangi/o	lymphatic vessel	lymphangiectasis (lĭm-făn-jē-ĔK-tă-sĭs)	dilation of a lymphatic vessel
lymphocyt/o	lymph cell	lymphocytosis (lĭm-fō-sī-TŌ-sĭs)	abnormal condition of lymph cells
myel/o	bone marrow, spinal cord	myeloma (mī-ĕ-LŌ-mă)	tumor of the bone marrow
path/o	disease	pathophobia (păth-ō-FŌ-bē-ă)	fear of disease
ser/o	serum	serous (SĒR-ŭs)	pertaining to serum
splen/o	spleen	splenomegaly (splĕ-nō-MĔG-ă-lē)	enlargement of the spleen
thym/o	thymus	thymocyte (THĪ-mō-sīt)	thymus cell
tonsill/o	tonsil	tonsillitis (tŏn-sĭl-Ī-tĭs)	inflammation of the tonsil
tox/o	poison, toxin	toxoid (TŎKS-oyd)	resembling poison
toxic/o		toxicogenic (tŏks-ĭ-kō-JĔN-ĭk)	creating poison

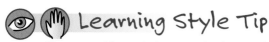 Learning Style Tip

Give yourself permission to write in your book! You will probably be keeping it as a reference tool. Use colorful markers to highlight terms and definitions. Add your own notes, diagrams, or flowcharts.

IN A FLASH!

Go to the Davis*Plus* website to print out all of the Combining Form Flash Cards for Chapter 7 and run through them at least three times before you continue.

Abbreviations

Table 7-2 lists some of the most common abbreviations related to the lymphatic-immune system.

IN A FLASH!

Go to the Davis*Plus* website to print out all of the Abbreviation Flash Cards for Chapter 7 and run through them at least three times before you continue.

Combining Forms and Abbreviations Practice Exercises

Fill in the Blanks

Fill in the blanks below using Table 7-1.

Exercise 3

1. hernia of a lymphatic vessel _____

2. absence of vessel strength _____

3. creating poison _____

TABLE 7-2			
ABBREVIATIONS			
AB, Ab	antibody	GVHD	graft-versus-host disease
AG, Ag	antigen	HIV	human immunodeficiency virus
AIDS	acquired immunodeficiency syndrome	Ig	immunoglobulin
CA	cancer or carcinoma	KS	Kaposi's sarcoma
EBV	Epstein-Barr virus	MET, met	metastasis, metastasize
EIA	enzyme immunosorbent assay	PCP	*Pneumocystis carinii* pneumonia, *Pneumocystis* pneumonia
ESR	erythrocyte sedimentation rate	SLE	systemic lupus erythematosus

4. enlargement of the spleen _____

5. tumor of the bone marrow _____

6. dilation of a lymph vessel _____

7. abnormal condition of lymph cells _____

8. inflammation of the tonsils _____

9. pertaining to serum _____

10. thymus cell _____

11. tumor of a gland _____

12. lymph tumor _____

13. study of immune disease _____

14. a condition of bacteria in the blood _____

15. excision or surgical removal of an adenoid _____

16. fear of disease _____

17. suturing of a vessel _____

18. resembling poison _____

Fill in the Blanks

Fill in the blanks below using Table 7-2.

Exercise 4

1. The abbreviation *SLE* stands for _____

   _____ _____.

2. The abbreviation *ESR* stands for _____

   _____ _____.

3. *Cancer* is often abbreviated as _____.

4. This type of pneumonia is abbreviated PCP, which stands for

   _____ _____

   _____ or _____

   _____.

5. The abbreviations for *antibody* are _____ and

   _____.

6. The abbreviations for *antigen* are _____ and

   _____.

7. Oscar has become very ill with AIDS, which stands for

_____   _____

_____   _____ .

8. The abbreviation MET is used to describe when cancer cells move from one area of the body to another and stands for _____ .

Pathologies, Procedures, and Pharmacology

Pathology Terms

Table 7-3 includes terms that relate to diseases or abnormalities of the lymphatic-immune system. Use the pronunciation guide and say the terms aloud as you read them. This will help you get in the habit of saying them properly.

TABLE 7-3

PATHOLOGY TERMS

acquired immunodeficiency syndrome (AIDS) (ă-KWĬRD ĭm-ūn-ō-dē-FĬSH-ĕn-sē SĬN-drōm)	late-stage infection with the human immunodeficiency virus (HIV) which progressively weakens the immune system
anaphylaxis (ăn-ă-fĭ-LĂK-sĭs)	life-threatening systemic allergic reaction to a substance to which the body was previously sensitized
ankylosing spondylitis (AS) (ăng-kĭ-LŌ-sing spŏn-dĭl-Ī-tĭs)	inflammatory response that causes degenerative changes in the spinal vertebrae; sacroiliac joints; connective tissues such as tendons and ligaments in the hips, shoulders, knees, feet, and ribs; and tissues of the lungs, eyes, and heart valves

Ankylosing spondylitis.

TABLE 7-3
PATHOLOGY TERMS—cont'd

autoimmune hemolytic anemia (aw-tō-ĭm-MŪN hē-mō-LĬT-ĭk ă-NĒ-mē-ă)	group of disorders caused when the immune system misidentifies red blood cells (RBCs) as foreign and creates autoantibodies that attack them
chronic fatigue syndrome (CFS) (KRŎN-ĭk fă-TĒG SĬN-drōm)	complex chronic disorder marked by severe fatigue unrelieved by rest, often worsened by mental or physical activity; sometimes called *chronic fatigue and immune dysfunction syndrome (CFIDS)*
chronic mucocutaneous candidiasis (CMC) (KRŎN-ĭk mū-kō-kū-TĀ-nē-ŭskăn-dĭ-DĪ-ă-sĭs	group of disorders in which persistent or recurrent *Candida* fungal infections develop on the skin, nails, or mucous membranes
Epstein-Barr virus (EBV) (ĔP-stēn-BĂR VĪ-rŭs)	acute infection that causes sore throat, fever, fatigue, and enlarged lymph nodes; also called *mononucleosis* or *gammaherpesviral mononucleosis*
graft-versus-host disease (GVHD) (grăft VĔR-sŭz hōst dĭ-ZĒZ)	complication of bone-marrow transplantation in which lymphoid cells from donated tissue attack the recipient and cause damage to skin, liver, GI tract, and other tissues

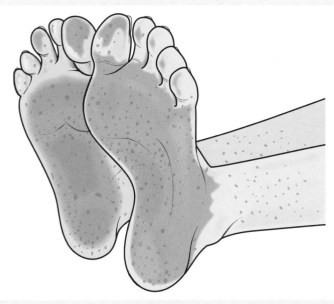

Graft-versus-host disease.

Hodgkin's disease (HŎJ-kĭn dĭ-ZĒZ)	type of lymphatic cancer; also called *Hodgkin lymphoma*

Continued

TABLE 7-3

PATHOLOGY TERMS—cont'd

idiopathic thrombocytopenic purpura (ITP) (ĭd-ē-ō-PĂTH-ĭk thrŏm-bō-sī-tō-PĒ-nĭk PŬR-pū-ră)	disorder in which a deficiency of platelets results in abnormal blood clotting, marked by tiny purple bruises (purpura) that form under the skin

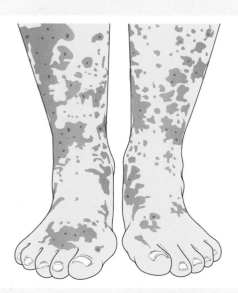

Idiopathic thrombocytopenic purpura (ITP).

lymphosarcoma (lĭm-fō-săr-KŌ-mă)	cancer of lymphatic tissue not related to Hodgkin's disease
non-Hodgkin's lymphoma (nŏn-HŎJ-kĭn lĭm-FŌ-mă)	group of more than 30 types of malignancies of B and T lymphocytes: also called *lymphoma* or *malignant lymphoma*
pernicious anemia (pĕr-NĬSH-ŭs ă-NĒ-mē-ă)	chronic form of megaloblastic anemia (producing many large, immature, dysfunctional RBCs), caused by a deficit in the absorption of vitamin B_{12} that reduces the body's ability to produce sufficient numbers of healthy RBCs
phagocytosis (făg-ō-sī-TŌ-sĭs)	process in which specialized white blood cells (phagocytes) engulf and destroy microorganisms, foreign antigens, and cell debris
Pneumocystis carinii **pneumonia** (nū-mō -SĬS-tĭs kă-RĪ-nē-ī nū-MŌ-nē-ă)	a type of pneumonia associated with AIDS
polymyositis (PM) (pŏl-ē-mī-ō-SĪ-tĭs)	disorder that causes the slow onset of muscle weakness and pain in the muscles of the trunk and progresses to affect muscles of the neck, shoulders, back, hip, and possibly hands and fingers

TABLE 7-3
PATHOLOGY TERMS—cont'd

scleroderma (sklĕr-ă-DĔR-mă)	group of chronic autoimmune diseases that cause inflammatory and fibrotic changes to skin, muscles, joints, tendons, cartilage, and other connective tissues

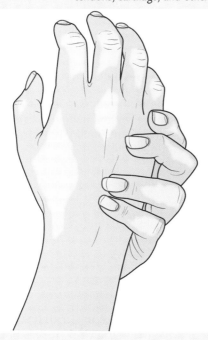

Scleroderma.

Sjögren's syndrome (SS) (SHŌ-grĕn SĬN-drōm)	autoimmune disorder that causes dysfunction of the salivary glands in the mouth and the lacrimal glands in the eyes and affects other areas of the body; also known as *Sicca syndrome*
systemic lupus erythematosus (SLE) (sĭs-TĔM-ĭk LOO-pŭs ĕr-ĭ-thē-mă-TŌ-sŭs)	chronic autoimmune disorder that causes inflammation and degeneration of various connective tissues and organs in the body, such as the skin, lungs, heart, joints, kidneys, blood, or nervous system

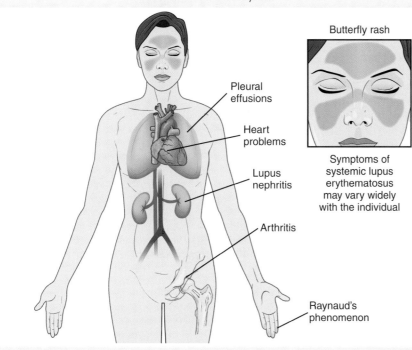

Systemic lupus erythematosus.

Continued

TABLE 7-3

PATHOLOGY TERMS—cont'd

transfusion incompatibility reaction (trănz-FŪ-zhŭn ĭn-kŏm-păt-ĭ-BĬL-ĭ-tē rē-ĂK-shŭn)	reaction of antibodies present in transfused blood to RBCs in the recipient's blood or of antibodies in the recipient's blood to RBCs in the transfused blood
transplant rejection (TRĂNZ-plănt rē-JĔK-shŭn)	identification of transplanted tissue as foreign by the recipient's immune system, which responds by attacking the tissue

  Learning Style Tip

Place sticky notes or tape flash cards around your house with the terms and definitions that you are learning. Recite the terms and definitions aloud or quiz yourself each time you see the notes. Great locations to place the notes or cards include mirrors, cupboard doors, and the front of the refrigerator.

IN A FLASH!

Go to the DavisPlus website to print out all of the Pathology Term Flash Cards for Chapter 7 and run through them at least three times before you continue.

Common Diagnostic Tests and Procedures

Allergy Tests

Patch test: Test in which paper or gauze saturated with an allergen is applied to the skin beneath an occlusive dressing and the response is noted (Fig. 7-4).

Scratch test: Test in which an allergen is placed on a scratched area of the skin and the response is noted (Fig. 7-5).

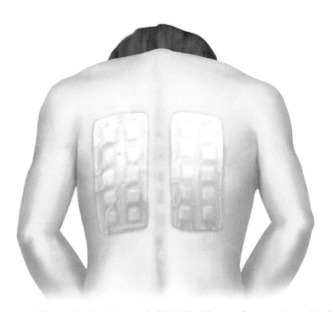

FIGURE 7-4 **Patch test.** (From Eagle, S., et al. [2009]. *The professional medical assistant.* Philadelphia, PA: F. A. Davis Company, p. 430; with permission)

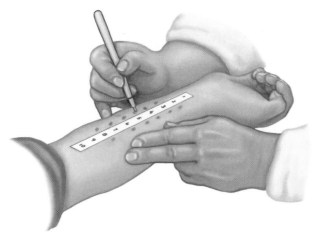

FIGURE 7-5 **Scratch test.** (From Eagle, S., et al. [2009]. *The professional medical assistant.* Philadelphia, PA: F. A. Davis Company, p. 429; with permission)

Tests Used to Diagnose and Monitor HIV and AIDS

CD-4 lymphocyte count: Measurement of the number of specialized WBCs sometimes called *helper T cells;* used to identify whether a person's HIV infection is worsening

Enzyme immunosorbent assay (EIA): Rapid enzyme immunochemical method for identifying the presence of antigens, antibodies, or other substances in the blood; used as a primary diagnostic test for many infectious diseases including syphilis and HIV; formerly called *enzyme-linked immunosorbent assay (ELISA)*

Viral load: Measurement of the number of copies of the HIV in the blood; used to monitor progression of HIV infection and AIDS

Other Tests

Erythrocyte sedimentation rate (ESR, sed rate): Test used in the diagnosis and monitoring of many diseases that cause acute or chronic inflammation; measures the rate at which RBCs settle in plasma or saline over a specific period of time

Monospot (heterophil): Quick test used to screen for the presence of the heterophil antibody that is present in individuals with Epstein-Barr virus infection

Flashpoint

As an individual's HIV worsens, CD-4 count drops and viral load climbs.

Pharmacology

Table 7-4 lists common antiretroviral medications used in the treatment of HIV and immunosuppressive medications used in the treatment of autoimmune disorders. Refer to Chapter 3 for a list of cancer medications that are used to treat the lymphatic system as well as other organ systems.

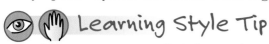 **Learning Style Tip**

Use your computer to find clip art, photos, or graphics to paste into your class notes, homemade flash cards, or any other documents you create as you study.

TABLE 7-4

PHARMACOLOGY

Therapeutic Classification	Generic Name	Brand Name	Common Use
Antiretroviral; nucleoside reverse transcriptase inhibitor (NRTI)	atazanavir	Reyataz	Prevent the HIV virus from spreading
	darunavir	Prezista	
	fosamprenavir	Lexiva	
	indinavir	Crixivan	
	nelfinavir	Viracept	
	ritonavir	Norvir	
	saquinavir	Invirase	
	tipranavir	Aptivus	
Antiretroviral; Non-nucleoside reverse transcriptase inhibitor (NNRTI)	delavirdine	Rescriptor	Prevent the HIV virus from spreading
	efavirenz	Sustiva	
	etravirine	Intelence	
	nevirapine	Viramune	
	rilpivirine	Edurant	
Immunosuppressive	azathioprine	Imuran	Prevent organ transplant rejection and prevent the immune system from attacking the body in autoimmune disorders
	cyclophosphamide	Cytoxan	
	cyclosporine	Sandimmune, Neoral	
	methotrexate	Rheumatrex	

Pathologies, Procedures, and Pharmacology Practice Exercises

Deciphering Terms

Write the correct meaning of these medical terms.

Exercise 5

1. pathologist _____

2. lymphangiogram _____

3. bactericidal _____

4. angiography _____

5. immunology _____

6. lymphocytic _____

7. toxemia _____

8. myelogenous _____

9. splenodynia _____

10. tonsillectomy _____

11. lymphadenopathy _____

12. vasorrhaphy _____

13. serology _____

14. thymotomy _____

15. vasalgia _____

Fill in the Blanks

Fill in the blanks below using Table 7-3.

Exercise 6

1. An autoimmune disorder that causes dysfunction of the salivary glands in the mouth and the lacrimal glands in the eyes and affects other areas of the body is _____ _____.

2. _____ is a life-threatening systemic allergic reaction.

3. Another name for mononucleosis is the _____ _____ virus.

4. _____ disease is a type of lymphatic cancer, also called *lymphoma.*

5. During _____, specialized white blood cells engulf and destroy microorganisms, foreign antigens, and cell debris.

6. A group of chronic autoimmune diseases that cause inflammatory and fibrotic changes to skin, muscles, joints, tendons, cartilage, and other connective tissues is _____.

7. _____ _____ is a group of more than 30 types of malignancies of B or T lymphocytes.

8. Hodgkin's disease is a type of _____

_____ .

9. A complex chronic disorder marked by severe fatigue unrelieved by rest, often worsened by mental or physical activity, is _____

_____ syndrome.

10. Oscar has developed a serious respiratory complication of AIDS,

_____ _____

_____ .

Multiple Choice

Select the one best answer to the following multiple-choice questions.

Exercise 7

1. Which of the following terms means *creating disease?*
   a. pathogenic
   b. pathology
   c. pathologist
   d. pathogen

2. Which of the following is a type of cancer?
   a. Hodgkin's disease
   b. CHF
   c. DVT
   d. TIA

3. A disorder that causes the slow onset of muscle weakness and pain in muscles of the trunk and progresses to affect the muscles of the neck, shoulders, back, and hip is:
   a. plymyositis
   b. scleroderma
   c. Sjögren's syndrome
   d. systemic lupus erythematosus

4. Which of the following is responsible for causing AIDS?
   a. HIV
   b. RV
   c. CAD
   d. LV

5. Which of the following is related to a vitamin B deficit?

    a. pernicious anemia

    b. Hodgkin's disease

    c. polymyositis

    d. graft-versus-host disease

Fill in the Blanks

Using Table 7-4, write the common use of the generic or brand name medication.

Exercise 8

1. fosamprenavir _____

2. cyclosporine _____

3. Viramune _____

4. efavirenz _____

5. Cytoxan _____

6. Methotrexate _____

7. Rescriptor _____

8. Viracept _____

9. rilpivirine _____

10. cyclophosphamide _____

CASE STUDY

Read the case study and answer the questions that follow. Most of the terms are included in this chapter. Refer to your medical dictionary for the other terms.

Epstein-Barr Virus

Cindi is a 17-year-old high school student. She leads an active social life, gets good grades, and is a member of the track team. About 2 weeks ago, she became ill with what she thought was the flu. Her symptoms included sore throat, enlarged and tender lymph nodes in her neck, inflamed tonsils, headache, fever, a brief maculopapular skin rash, and generalized muscle aches. She expected to feel better by now but still has many of her symptoms. Therefore, her mother took her to their family physician for evaluation. He noted that Cindi's spleen is enlarged and that her blood reveals "leukocytosis with atypical lymphocytes and IgM antibodies." Based on these findings, the physician diagnosed Cindi with Epstein-Barr virus. He explained that there is no specific cure but that treatment includes NSAIDs for fever, sore throat, and other discomfort. He also advised her to get plenty of rest and to refrain from vigorous physical activity or contact sports until she has recovered.

The **Epstein-Barr virus (EBV)** is a member of the herpes virus group. It is most common in the United States in people between ages 15 and 25. Beyond that age, most people are immune to it. It is sometimes called the "kissing disease," because it is transmitted in saliva and infects epithelial cells of the oropharynx, nasopharynx, and salivary glands before spreading to the lymphatic system. It typically causes the symptoms that Cindi experienced, including splenic enlargement. Because splenic rupture could result in life-threatening internal hemorrhage, patients are cautioned to refrain from contact sports until they have fully recovered.

Case Study Questions

Exercise 9

1. The illness that Cindi has is also sometimes called:
   a. pernicious anemia
   b. polymyositis
   c. mononucleosis
   d. Sjögren's syndrome

2. Cindi's symptoms include all of the following **except:**
   a. pharyngitis
   b. cervical lymphadenopathy
   c. tonsillitis
   d. jaundice

3. Upon examination, the physician noted that Cindi has:
   a. splenomegaly
   b. gastroenteritis
   c. hepatoma
   d. pharyngostenosis

4. Cindi's blood test revealed:
   a. an abnormal increase in her white blood cells
   b. anemia
   c. bacterial infection
   d. none of these

5. The Epstein-Barr virus is sometimes called the "kissing disease" because:
   a. It is only transmitted through kissing.
   b. It is spread through oral secretions.
   c. Teens should be discouraged from kissing.
   d. None of these

6. Cindi must refrain from vigorous physical activity and contact sports to avoid what life-threatening complication? (Use the proper medical term.)

   _____

7. Create two lists of physical activities that should be avoided while recovering from the Epstein-Barr virus. One list should apply to the younger, 15- to 17-year-old age group, and one list should apply to the older, 23- to 25-year-old age group.

End-of-Chapter Practice Exercises

Word Building

*Using **only** the word parts in the lists provided, create medical terms with the indicated meanings.*

Exercise 10

Prefixes	Combining Forms	Suffixes
eu-	aden/o	-ar
peri-	angi/o	-genic
	adenoid/o	-gram
	bacteri/o	-ic
	immun/o	-logy
	lymph/o	-megaly
	myel/o	-oid
	path/o	-ous
	ser/o	-pathy
	splen/o	-plasty
	thym/o	-sclerosis
	tonsill/o	-tomy
	toxic/o	

1. record of a vessel _____

2. study of bacteria _____

3. creating immunity _____

4. pertaining to serum _____

5. study of poison _____

6. incision into the tonsil _____

7. study of disease _____

8. pertaining to around the tonsil _____

9. hardening of the thymus _____

10. produced by bone marrow _____

11. resembling lymph _____

12. enlarged spleen _____

13. surgical repair of a vessel _____

14. pertaining to a good thymus _____

15. disease of a gland _____

True or False

Decide whether the following statements are true or false.

Exercise 11

1. True   False   **Sjögren's syndrome** is an autoimmune disorder.

2. True   False   **Lymphosarcoma** is a type of cancer of lymphatic tissue not related to Hodgkin's disease.

3. True   False   The abbreviation **CA** stands for *carcinoma* or *cancer.*

4. True   False   **Hodgkin's disease** occurs when the immune system misidentifies RBCs as foreign and creates autoantibodies that attack them.

5. True   False   The abbreviation **Ab** stands for *abnormal.*

6. True   False   **Phagocytosis** is a process in which specialized WBCs engulf and destroy microorganisms, foreign antigens, and cell debris.

7. True   False   **Rejection** occurs when a recipient's immune system identifies transplanted tissue as foreign and begins attacking it.

8. True   False   **Ankylosing spondylitis** affects vertebrae and connective tissue.

9. True   False   The abbreviation **EBV** refers to a test used to diagnose HIV infection.

10. True   False   **Ig** is the abbreviation for *antigen.*

Deciphering Terms

Write the correct meaning of these medical terms.

Exercise 12

1. adenolipoma _____

2. adenoiditis _____

3. angioedema _____

4. vasoconstriction _____

5. myeloma _____

6. immunogen _____

7. lymphadenectasis _____

8. lymphorrhagia _____

9. lymphangioma _____

10. lymphocytopenia _____

Multiple Choice

Select the one best answer to the following multiple-choice questions.

Exercise 13

1. Which of the following terms means *pertaining to bone-marrow cells?*

   a.　lymphocytic

   b.　myelogenous

   c.　myelocytic

   d.　osteoma

2. Which of the following terms means *tumor of a lymphatic vessel?*

   a.　lymphangioma

   b.　lymphadenoma

   c.　lymphadenopathy

   d.　angiomyoma

3. Which of the following terms means *abnormal condition of lymph cells?*

   a.　lymphogenesis

   b.　lymphocytosis

   c.　adenopathy

   d.　lymphokinesis

4. Which of the following terms means *hernia of the spinal cord and meninges?*

   a.　myeloma

   b.　myelocystocele

   c.　myelomeningocele

   d.　myelomalacia

5. Which of the following terms is matched with the correct definition?

    a. tox/o: disease

    b. angi/o: vessel

    c. path/o: poison

    d. aden/o: adenoid

6. All of the following terms are matched with the correct definition **except:**

    a. vas/o: vessel

    b. ser/o: spleen

    c. myel/o: bone marrow

    d. lymphangi/o: lymphatic vessel

7. Which of the following has been called the kissing disease?

    a. EBV

    b. EIA

    c. ESR

    d. SLE

8. Which of the following abbreviations stands for the name of a test used to monitor disorders that cause inflammation in the body?

    a. EBV

    b. EIA

    c. ESR

    d. SLE

9. Which of the following abbreviations represents the name of a disorder that may affect transplant patients?

    a. AIDS

    b. KS

    c. PCP

    d. GVHD

10. Which of the following abbreviations is related to cancer?

    a. MET

    b. Ag

    c. EIA

    d. Ab

11. All of the following terms are matched with the correct definition **except:**

    a. Sjögren's syndrome: autoimmune disorder that causes dysfunction of salivary and lacrimal glands

    b. anaphylaxis: life-threatening systemic allergic reaction

    c. ankylosing spondylitis: inflammatory response that causes degenerative changes in the spinal vertebrae, sacroiliac joints, and other connective tissues

    d. chronic fatigue syndrome: acute infection that causes sore throat, fever, fatigue, and enlarged lymph nodes

12. All of the following terms are matched with the correct definition **except:**

    a. chronic mucocutaneous candidiasis: group of disorders in which persistent or recurrent *Candida* fungal infections develop on the skin, nails, or mucous membranes

    b. lymphosarcoma: cancer of lymphatic tissue not related to Hodgkin's disease

    c. pernicious anemia: group of disorders caused when the immune system misidentifies RBCs as foreign and creates autoantibodies that attack them

    d. phagocytosis: process in which specialized WBCs engulf and destroy microorganisms, foreign antigens, and cell debris

13. All of the following terms are matched with the correct definition **except:**

    a. graft-versus-host disease: complication of bone-marrow transplantation in which lymphoid cells from donated tissue attack the recipient and cause damage to the skin, liver, GI tract, and other tissues

    b. Hodgkin's disease: type of lymphatic cancer; also called *lymphoma*

    c. polymyositis: disorder that causes the slow onset of muscle weakness and pain in the trunk and progresses to affect the muscles of the neck, shoulders, back, and hip

    d. transplant rejection: reaction of antibodies present in transfused blood to RBCs in the recipient's blood or of antibodies in the recipient's blood to RBCs in the transfused blood

14. A chronic autoimmune disorder that causes inflammation and degeneration of various connective tissues and organs in the body such as the skin, lungs, heart, joints, kidneys, blood, or nervous system is:

    a. acquired immunodeficiency syndrome

    b. systemic lupus erythematosus

    c. chronic fatigue syndrome

    d. idiopathic thrombocytopenic purpura

15. A disorder in which a deficiency of platelets results in abnormal blood clotting, marked by tiny purple bruises that form under the skin, is:

    a. ITP

    b. CFS

    c. SS

    d. SLE

16. A group of chronic autoimmune diseases that cause inflammatory and fibrotic changes to skin, muscles, joints, tendons, cartilage, and other connective tissues is:

    a. Sjögren's syndrome

    b. scleroderma

    c. systemic lupus erythematosus

    d. polymyositis

17. Which of the following terms means *skin (disease caused by a) poison?*

    a. toxicoderma

    b. dermopathy

    c. dermatomycosis

    d. toxicopathy

18. Which of the following terms means *suturing of the spleen?*

    a. splenorrhexis

    b. splenolysis

    c. splenodynia

    d. splenorrhaphy

19. Which of the following terms means *condition of a good (healthy) thymus?*

    a. dysthymic

    b. euthymia

    c. thymopathy

    d. endothymic

20. Which of the following terms means *study of serum?*

    a. serologist

    b. serous

    c. serology

    d. seroma

RESPIRATORY SYSTEM

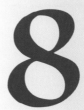

Chapter Outline

Structure and Function

The most basic human need is the need to breathe. We take our first breaths as soon as we are born and continue this vital function through the last moments of our lives. The complex and amazing structures of the respiratory system support this life-sustaining process.

When studying the respiratory system, we often divide it into the upper and lower airways. The **upper airway** consists of the mouth, nose, sinuses, and pharynx. The pharynx is further divided into the **nasopharynx** (back of the nose) and **oropharynx** (back of the mouth). The nose begins with the **nares** (nostrils) and extends back to the nasopharynx. The nasal passages are divided into right and left sides by the **nasal septum.** The **hard palate** divides the nasal cavity from the mouth, which sits beneath it. The **sinus cavities** are air-filled spaces named for the facial bones within which they are located; they include the maxillary, frontal, ethmoidal, and sphenoidal sinuses. Refer to Figure 8-1, which illustrates these structures, as we discuss the path that air takes into and out of the body.

 Learning Style Tip

Go to the campus library or get permission to spend some time in the anatomy and physiology or biology laboratory at your school. Study the anatomical models, in this case the ones representing the respiratory system. Physically touch the various parts, naming them as you do, while you also name their associated combining forms. Make a video of yourself as you do this so you can study the models again from home. Share your videos with your classmates!

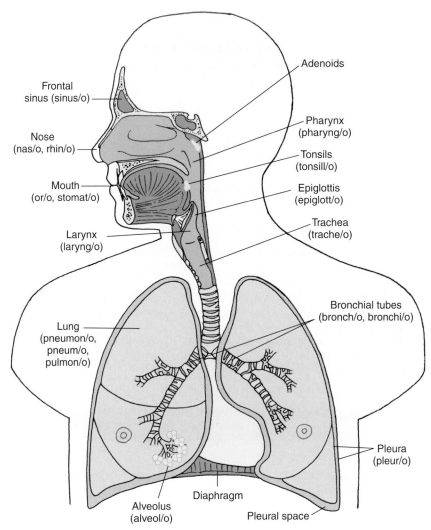

FIGURE 8-1 Sinuses.

Flashpoint

Aspiration is a term that is often used to describe food or fluids being sucked into the lungs.

As air moves through the upper airway, it is warmed, filtered, and humidified. Mucous membranes that line these structures contribute moisture to humidify the air. **Cilia** (tiny hairs) within the nasal cavity help filter the air by removing debris. The rich blood supply of all of these structures warms the air as it passes through. Sinus cavities serve to decrease the weight of the skull, provide resonance for the voice, and produce mucus, which helps eliminate microorganisms as it drains into the nasal cavities.

Air moves to the lower airway as it flows past the **epiglottis** and enters the trachea. The epiglottis acts as a doorway to the trachea and serves a vital protective function by opening to let in air and closing to keep out food and fluid. The **trachea** is approximately 5 inches long and gets its shape and strength from numerous rings of cartilage. It separates the upper and lower airways. As air flows through the tracheal entrance, it passes through the **larynx.** This structure vibrates to create sound when we talk. Air then flows down the trachea and into the **lower airway,** which consists of the bronchi and lungs. The bronchi split off into smaller bronchi and eventually into tiny bronchioles. The composition of the bronchi changes to less cartilage and more smooth muscle as they become smaller. The trachea and bronchi have ciliated mucous-membrane linings, which further moisten air and secrete mucus to trap debris that has been inhaled. Cilia move in a wavelike fashion to propel debris upward. The trachea and bronchi are extremely sensitive, and the presence of foreign particles stimulates a powerful cough reflex that further helps to expel debris.

   ## Learning Style Tip

Use class breaks to get up and physically move. Walk briskly around the building or climb up and down several flights of stairs. As you do so, verbally repeat the definitions of five new terms. The physical activity will stimulate your circulation, wake you up, and energize you. You will return to class readier to learn—and, as an added bonus, you will have just learned five new terms.

The Lungs

The lungs are divided into **lobes;** the right lung has three lobes, and the left lung has two. The lungs are covered with two thin membranes known as the **pleurae.** The term *intrapleural* means within the pleural space in general. The visceral pleura lies directly on the lungs, while the parietal pleura lines the inner wall of the thorax. The term *interpleural* refers to the specific area between the visceral pleura and the parietal pleura. A small amount of **pleural fluid** lies within the space between the two membranes. This space is sometimes referred to as a *potential* space, because there is nothing there other than this tiny amount of fluid. As we breathe in and out, our lungs expand and contract. The elastic quality that allows the lungs to do this is sometimes called **recoil.** As we breathe, the pleural fluid between the visceral and parietal pleurae acts as a sort of lubricant, which helps the process along as the lungs continually expand and contract.

As air continues on its journey into the lungs, it arrives at its final destination, the **alveoli,** which are microscopic-sized air sacs. We have approximately 300 million alveoli in each lung. They are covered with a delicate capillary bed (microscopic blood vessels) that provides a rich blood supply. The alveoli expand somewhat like tiny balloons during inspiration (also called inhalation) as air enters and fills them. They contract and partially deflate during expiration, as much of the air exits the lungs. Because the walls of the alveoli and the capillary beds are each just one cell thick, gases easily move back and forth across them. Excess carbon dioxide (CO_2) leaves the capillaries and moves into the air space within the alveoli and is then exhaled. Oxygen (O_2) moves from the air space in the alveoli into the capillary blood and is then distributed to various parts of the body via the circulatory system.

Flashpoint

Each lung contains approximately 300 million alveoli!

    ## Learning Style Tip

Take several deep, slow breaths. As you do so, visualize the path that oxygen is taking as it moves from your external environment into your respiratory system and finally into your bloodstream. Next, visualize the reverse path that carbon dioxide follows as it leaves your body. Now verbally describe both pathways to a real or imaginary partner.

We take oxygen into our lungs through the act of **inhalation,** or breathing in (also called inspiration), which is usually an unconscious act (Box 8-1). However, we may exert conscious control to take extra-large breaths or even

Box 8-1 The Diaphragm

The diaphragm is a thin, dome-shaped muscle that controls breathing. It separates the thoracic cavity from the abdominal cavity. As the diaphragm contracts, it moves downward, which is why you see your abdomen rise every time you breathe in. As it moves downward, other muscles pull the rib cage upward and outward. Inhalation is caused by this thoracic cavity expansion. The increased size decreases the thoracic pressure, forcing air into the lungs. When the diaphragm and rib cage muscles relax, exhalation occurs. The diaphragm moves upward and the thoracic cavity returns to its smaller size. This increases the thoracic pressure, forcing air out of the lungs. Those with pulmonary diseases may find it easier to breathe when sitting as gravity is able to assist the diaphragm during contraction.

The diaphragm has other functions unrelated to breathing. It also increases pressure in the abdominal cavity, which aids in vomiting, urination, and defecation.

hold our breath for a short time. At some point, however, we feel an overwhelming urge to breathe, which is triggered by a buildup of CO_2. This buildup of CO_2 in the blood causes the blood to become more acidic. To be healthy, our blood must remain slightly alkaline—within the narrow range of 7.35 to 7.45 on the **pH scale,** which is a tool for measuring the acidity or alkalinity of a substance. As blood becomes more acidic, its pH level drops, triggering the urge to breathe. As we inhale, we bring fresh, oxygen-rich air into our lungs, where it can be absorbed into our blood. The act of **exhalation,** or breathing out (or expiration), allows our bodies to eliminate excess CO_2, thus restoring a normal blood pH level. Contrary to what most people think, the drive to breathe is not triggered by lower oxygen levels in the blood but by the lowered pH level caused by CO_2 buildup.

Structure and Function Practice Exercises

Fill in the Blanks

Choose the term that matches the description.

Exercise 1

Upper airway	Sinus cavities	Pleurae
Nasopharynx	Cilia	Pleural fluid
Oropharynx	Epiglottis	Recoil
Nares	Trachea	Alveoli
Nasal septum	Larynx	Inhalation
Hard palate	Lower airway	pH scale
	Lobes	Exhalation

1. _____ Air-filled spaces named maxillary, frontal, ethmoidal, and sphenoidal

2. _____ Separates the upper and lower airways

3. _____ Back of the nose

4. _____ Doorway to the trachea

5. _____ Nostrils

6. _____ Membranes covering the lungs

7. _____ The mouth, nose, sinuses, and pharynx

8. _____ Microscopic-sized air sacs

9. _____ Inspiration

10. _____ Back of the mouth

11. _____ The bronchi and lungs

12. _____ Divides the nasal passages into left and right sides

13. _____ Division of the lungs; the right has three, and the left has two

14. _____ The elastic quality that allows the lungs to expand and contract

15. _____ Divides the nasal cavity from the mouth

16. _____ Tiny hairs within the nasal cavity

17. _____ A tool for measuring the acidity or alkalinity of a substance

18. _____ Vibrates to create sound when we talk

19. _____ Expiration

20. _____ Fluid between the visceral and parietal pleurae that acts as a sort of lubricant

Fill in the Blanks

Label Figure 8-2 with the appropriate anatomical terms and combining forms.

Exercise 2

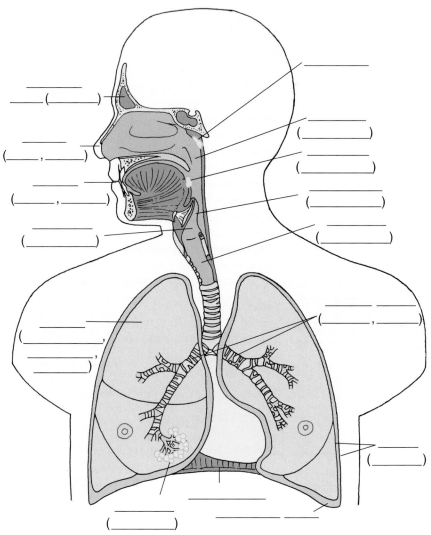

FIGURE 8-2 **The respiratory system with blanks.**

Combining Forms and Abbreviations

Combining Forms

Table 8-1 contains combining forms that pertain to the respiratory system, examples of terms that utilize the combining forms, and a pronunciation guide. Read aloud to yourself as you move from left to right across the table. Be sure to use the pronunciation guide so that you can learn to say the terms correctly.

> ### *IN A FLASH!*
> It's time to print out all of the Combining Forms Flash Cards for Chapter 8 and run through them at least three times before you continue.

TABLE 8-1

COMBINING FORMS RELATED TO THE RESPIRATORY SYSTEM

Combining Form	Meaning	Example (Pronunciation)	Meaning of New Term
aer/o	air	aerophagia (ār-ō-FĂ-jē-ă)	eating or swallowing air
alveol/o	alveoli	alveolitis (ăl-vē-ŏ-LĪ-tĭs)	inflammation of the alveoli
anthrac/o	coal, coal dust	anthracosis (ăn-thră-KŌ-sĭs)	abnormal condition of coal (black lung)
bronch/o	bronchus	bronchitis (brŏng-KĪ-tĭs)	inflammation of the bronchus
bronchi/o		bronchiectasis (brŏng-kē-ĔK-tă-sĭs)	dilation or expansion of the bronchus
bronchiol/o	bronchiole	bronchiolitis (brŏng-kē-ō-LĪ-tĭs)	inflammation of the bronchiole
carcin/o	cancer	carcinoma (kăr-sĭ-NŌ-mă)	cancerous tumor
chondr/o	cartilage	chondroplasty (KŎN-drō-plăs-tē)	surgical repair of the cartilage
coni/o	dust	coniosis (kō-nē-Ō-sĭs)	abnormal condition caused by (inhalation of) dust
diaphragmat/o	diaphragm	diaphragmatocele (dī-ă-frăg-MĂT-ō-sēl)	hernia of the diaphragm
epiglott/o	epiglottis	epiglottal (ĕp-ĭ-GLŎT-ăl)	pertaining to the epiglottis
laryng/o	larynx	laryngitis (lăr-ĭn-JĪ-tĭs)	inflammation of the larynx
lob/o	lobe	lobectomy (lō-BĔK-tō-mē)	excision or surgical removal of a lobe
muc/o	mucus	mucoid (MŪ-koyd)	resembling mucus
nas/o	nose	nasogastric (nā-zō-GĂS-trĭk)	pertaining to the nose and stomach
rhin/o		rhinitis (rī-NĪ-tĭs)	inflammation of the nose
or/o	mouth, mouth-like opening	oral (Ō-răl)	pertaining to the mouth
stomat/o		stomatitis (stō-mă-TĪ-tĭs)	inflammation of the mouth
orth/o	straight	orthopnea (or-THŎP-nē-ă)	breathing in the straight position
ox/i	oxygen	oximeter (ŏk-SĬM-ĕ-tĕr)	measuring instrument for oxygen
ox/o		anoxia (ăn-ŎK-sē-ă)	condition of no oxygen
pharyng/o	pharynx	pharyngeal (făr-ĬN-jē-ăl)	pertaining to the pharynx
phon/o	sound, voice	phonograph (FŌ-nō-grăf)	recording instrument for sound or voice

Continued

TABLE 8-1

COMBINING FORMS RELATED TO THE RESPIRATORY SYSTEM—cont'd

Combining Form	Meaning	Example (Pronunciation)	Meaning of New Term
pleur/o	pleura	pleurodynia (ploo-rō-DĬN-ē-ă)	pain of the pleura
pnea	breathing	apnea (ăp-NĒ-ă)	temporary cessation of breathing
		dyspnea (dĭsp-NĒ-ă)	difficult breathing
pneum/o	lung, air	pneumonia (nū-MŌ-nē-ă)	condition of the lung
pneumon/o		pneumonectomy (nū-mŏn-ĔK-tō-mē)	excision or surgical removal of the lung
pulmon/o	lung	pulmonary (PŬL-mō-nĕ-rē)	pertaining to the lung
sinus/o	sinus	sinusoid (SĪ-nŭs-oyd)	resembling a sinus
spir/o	breathing	spirometer (spī-RŎM-ĕt-ĕr)	measuring instrument for breathing
thorac/o	thorax	thoracentesis (thō-ră-sĕn-TĒ-sĭs)	surgical puncture of the thorax
tonsill/o	tonsil	tonsillitis (tŏn-sĭl-Ī-tĭs)	inflammation of the tonsil
trache/o	trachea	tracheotomy (trā-kē-ŎT-ō-mē)	cutting into or incision of the trachea

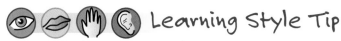 Learning Style Tip

Resist the temptation to skip over practice exercises. Completing them engages your visual and kinesthetic senses; verbalizing the terms as you read and write them engages your verbal and auditory senses. Most importantly, these activities require you to read and review the new terms, which helps you learn and remember them.

Abbreviations

Table 8-2 lists some of the most common abbreviations related to the respiratory system.

IN A FLASH!

It's time to print out all of the Abbreviation Flash Cards for Chapter 8 and run through them at least three times before you continue.

TABLE 8-2

ABBREVIATIONS

ABGs	arterial blood gases
AFB	acid-fast bacillus
ARDS	acute respiratory distress syndrome

TABLE 8-2	
ABBREVIATIONS—cont'd	
CF	cystic fibrosis
CO_2	carbon dioxide
COPD	chronic obstructive pulmonary disease
CPAP	continuous positive airway pressure
CPR	cardiopulmonary resuscitation
CPT	chest physiotherapy
CXR	chest x-ray
DOE	dyspnea on exertion
MDI	metered dose inhaler
O_2	oxygen
OSA	obstructive sleep apnea
PE	pulmonary embolism
PFT	pulmonary function test
pH	potential of hydrogen (measure of acidity or alkalinity)
PND	paroxysmal nocturnal dyspnea
PPD	purified protein derivative
R	respiration
RA	room air
SIDS	sudden infant death syndrome
SOB	short(ness) of breath
stat	immediate(ly)
T&A	tonsillectomy and adenoidectomy
TB	tuberculosis
V_T	tidal volume
URI	upper-respiratory infection
VC	vital capacity

Combining Forms and Abbreviations Practice Exercises

Fill in the Blanks

Fill in the blanks below using Table 8-1.

Exercise 3

1. resembling mucus _____

2. inflammation of the tonsils _____

3. inflammation of the bronchus _____

4. dilation or expansion of the bronchus _____

5. pertaining to the epiglottis _____

6. eating or swallowing air _____

7. pertaining to the pharynx _____

8. surgical repair of the cartilage _____

9. breathing in the straight position _____

10. pertaining to the nose and stomach _____

11. cancerous tumor _____

12. pertaining to the mouth _____

13. condition of no oxygen _____

14. condition of the lung _____

15. inflammation of the nose _____

16. pain of the pleura _____

17. pertaining to the lung _____

18. resembling a sinus _____

19. surgical puncture of the thorax _____

20. excision or surgical removal of the lung _____

21. cutting into or incision of the trachea _____

22. inflammation of the larynx _____

23. inflammation of the mouth _____

24. abnormal condition caused by (inhalation of) dust _____

25. excision or surgical removal of a lobe _____

26. inflammation of the alveoli _____

27. abnormal condition of coal (black lung) _____

28. hernia of the diaphragm _____

29. inflammation of the bronchiole _____

30. measuring instrument for oxygen _____

31. recording instrument for sound or voice _____

32. measuring instrument for breathing _____

Fill in the Blanks

Write the meaning of each abbreviation below using Table 8-2.

Exercise 4

1. VC _____ 2. CPAP _____

3. ABGs _____ 4. MDI _____

5. SOB _____ 6. PE _____

7. CPR _____ 8. TB _____

9. R _____ 10. RA _____

11. COPD _____ 12. ARDS _____

13. CXR _____ 14. PFT _____

15. PND _____ 16. T&A _____

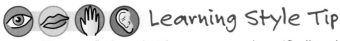 Learning Style Tip

Use your flash cards! They were created specifically to help you engage your visual and kinesthetic styles. Verbal and auditory learners will benefit most by reading the cards aloud as you flip them over. Repetition is the key, so use them every day.

Pathologies, Procedures, and Pharmacology

Pathology Terms

Table 8-3 includes terms that relate to diseases or abnormalities of the respiratory system. Use the pronunciation guide and say the terms aloud as you read them. This will help you get in the habit of saying the terms properly.

IN A FLASH!

It's time to print out all of the Pathology Terms Flash Cards for Chapter 8 and run through them at least three times before you continue.

TABLE 8-3
PATHOLOGIC TERMS

acute bronchitis (ă-KŪT brŏng-KĪ-tĭs)	infection and inflammation of bronchial airways

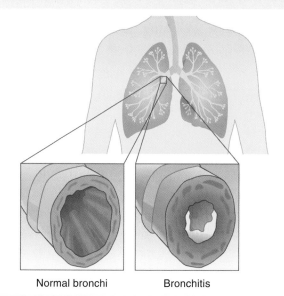

Normal bronchi   Bronchitis

Acute bronchitis.

acute respiratory distress syndrome (ARDS) (ă-KŪT RĔS-pĭr-a-tor-ē dĭs-TRĔS SĬN-drōm)	acute, life-threatening condition of lung injury that develops secondary to some other lung trauma or disorder
allergic rhinitis (ă-LĔR-jĭk rī-NĪ-tĭs	inflammation of the nasal membranes, caused by allergies
asbestosis (ăs-bĕ-STŌ-sĭs)	respiratory disease caused by chronic or repetitive inhalation of asbestos fibers
asthma (ĂZ-mă)	disease marked by episodic narrowing and inflammation of the airways, resulting in wheezing, SOB, and cough

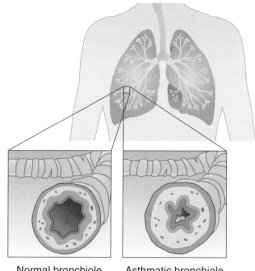

Normal bronchiole   Asthmatic bronchiole

Asthma.

atelectasis (ăt-ĕ-LĔK-tă-sĭs)	partial collapse of the alveoli and tiny airways of the lung

TABLE 8-3

PATHOLOGIC TERMS—cont'd

cardiopulmonary resuscitation (CPR) (KAR-dē-ō-pŭl-mō-nĕ-rēRĒ-su-sĭ-tā-shun)	a skill often taught in first-aid courses that helps restore a victim's breathing and circulation
chronic obstructive pulmonary disease (COPD) (KRŎN-ĭk ŏb-STRŬK-tĭv PŬL-mō-nĕ-rē dĭ-ZĒZ)	group of diseases in which alveolar air sacs are destroyed and chronic, severe SOB results

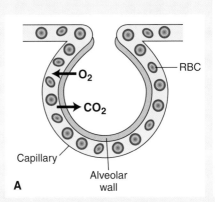 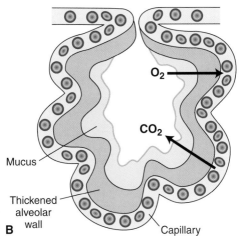

Chronic obstructive pulmonary disease (COPD): (A) normal alveoli, (B) destructive changes of COPD.

coal worker's pneumoconiosis (CWP) (KŌL WER-kerz nū-mō-kō-nē-Ō-sĭs)	respiratory disease caused by chronic or repetitive inhalation of coal dust; often called *black lung* or *anthracosis*
coryza (kŏ-RĪ-ză)	acute inflammation of the nasal mucosa; the common cold
crackles (KRĂ-kuls)	abnormal crackly lung sound—like the sound of Rice Krispies—heard with a stethoscope, caused by air passing over retained secretions or by the sudden opening of collapsed airways
croup (croop)	acute viral disease, usually in children, marked by a barking, "seal-like" cough and respiratory distress
cystic fibrosis (CF) (SĬS-tĭk fĭ-BRŌ-sĭs)	fatal genetic disease that causes frequent respiratory infections, increased airway secretions, and COPD in children
deviated septum (DĒ-vē-ā-tĕd SĔP-tŭm)	condition in which the nasal septum is displaced to the side, causing the two nares (nasal passages) to be unequal

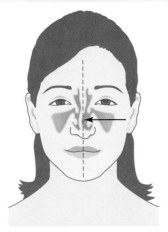

Deviated septum.

Continued

TABLE 8-3
PATHOLOGIC TERMS—cont'd

emphysema (ĕm-fĭ-SĒ-mă)	disorder marked by abnormal increase in the size of air spaces distal to the terminal bronchiole and destruction of the alveolar walls, resulting in loss of normal elasticity and progressive dyspnea
empyema (ĕm-pī-Ē-mă)	collection of infected fluid (pus) between the two pleural membranes that line the lungs
epistaxis (ĕp-ĭ-STĂK-sĭs)	episode of bleeding from the nose; commonly known as a *nosebleed*
hemoptysis (hē-MŎP-tĭ-sĭs)	coughing up blood from the respiratory tract
hemothorax (hē-mō-THŌ-răks)	condition in which blood or bloody fluid has collected within the intrapleural space, causing lung compression and respiratory distress

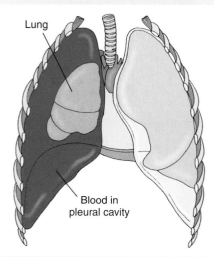

Lung

Blood in pleural cavity

Hemothorax.

histoplasmosis (hĭs-tō-plăz-MŌ-sĭs)	systemic respiratory disease caused by *Histoplasma capsulatum*, a fungus found in soil contaminated with bird droppings
hypercapnia (hī-pĕr-KĂP-nē-ă)	chronic retention of CO_2, causing symptoms of mental cloudiness and lethargy
influenza (ĭn-floo-ĔN-ză)	common, contagious, acute viral respiratory illness; commonly called the *flu*
laryngitis (lăr-ĭn-JĪ-tĭs)	condition of inflammation of the larynx, evidenced by a temporary hoarseness or loss of the voice
legionellosis (lē-jŭ-nĕ-LŌ-sĭs)	bacterial lung infection caused by the bacterium *Legionella pneumophila*

TABLE 8-3
PATHOLOGIC TERMS—cont'd

nasal polyps (NĀ-zul PŎL-ĭps)	rounded tissue growths on the nasal or sinal mucosa

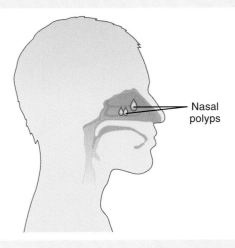

Nasal polyps.

obstructive sleep apnea (OSA) (ŏb-STRŬK-tĭv slēp ăp-NĒ-ă)	dysfunctional breathing that occurs when the upper airway is intermittently blocked during sleep

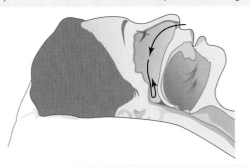

Obstructive sleep apnea.

orthopnea (ōr-THŎP-nē-ă)	labored breathing that occurs when lying flat and improves when sitting up
pharyngitis (făr-ĭn-JĪ-tĭs)	inflammation of the pharynx; commonly called a *sore throat*
pleural effusion (PLOO-răl ĕ-FŪ-zhŭn)	excess collection of fluid in the intrapleural space
pleurisy (PLOO-rĭs-ē)	condition in which the pleurae become inflamed, causing sharp inspiratory chest pain; also called *pleuritis*
pneumoconiosis (nū-mō-kō-nē-Ō-sĭs)	any disease of the respiratory tract caused by chronic or repetitive inhalation of dust particles

Continued

TABLE 8-3

PATHOLOGIC TERMS—cont'd

pneumonia (nū-MŌ-nē-ă)	bacterial or viral infection of the lungs

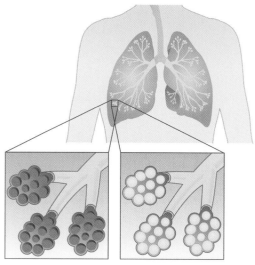

Normal alveoli   Pneumonia

Pneumonia.

pneumothorax (nū-mō-THŌ-răks)	condition in which air collects in the intrapleural space; categorized as open, closed, spontaneous, or tension and commonly called *collapsed lung*

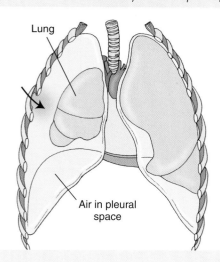

Lung

Air in pleural space

Pneumothorax.

TABLE 8-3

PATHOLOGIC TERMS—cont'd

pulmonary embolism (PE) (PŬL-mō-nĕ-rē ĔM-bō-lĭ-zum)	sudden obstruction of a pulmonary blood vessel by debris, blood clots, or other matter

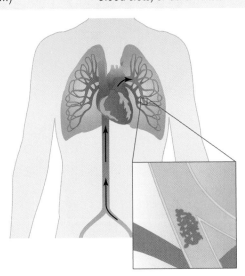

Pulmonary embolism.

pulmonary tuberculosis (TB) (PŬL-mō-nĕ-rē tū-bĕr-kū-LŌ-sĭs)	contagious infection caused by the *Mycobacterium tuberculosis* organism, primarily affecting the lungs but sometimes also spreading to and affecting other organ systems
rhonchi (RŎNG-kī)	coarse, gurgling sound heard in the lungs with a stethoscope, caused by secretions in the air passages
silicosis (sĭl-ĭ-KŌ-sĭs)	respiratory disease caused by chronic or repetitive inhalation of silica (quartz) dust
sinusitis (sī-nŭs-Ī-tĭs)	inflammation of the lining of the sinus cavities

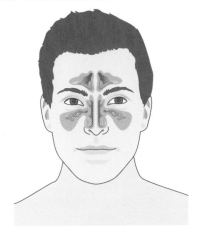

Sinusitis.

stridor (STRĪ-dŏr)	high-pitched upper-airway sound heard without a stethoscope, indicating airway obstruction; a medical emergency
upper-respiratory infection (URI) (ŬP-ĕr RĔS-pĭr-a-tor-ē ĭn-FĔK-shŭn)	infection and inflammation of upper-airway structures, usually caused by a virus; often called the *common cold*
wheeze (hwēz)	somewhat musical sound heard in the lungs, usually with a stethoscope, caused by partial airway obstruction (such as with asthma)

Common Diagnostic Tests and Procedures

Arterial blood gases (ABG): Measurement of O_2 and CO_2 levels and acid-base balance (pH balance) in arterial blood

Bronchoscopy: Visual examination of the airways of the lungs (Fig. 8-3)

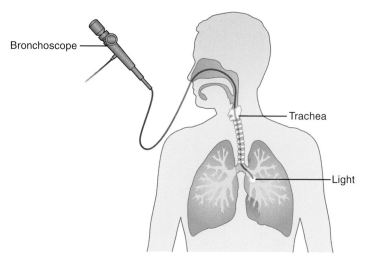

FIGURE 8-3 Bronchoscopy.

Chest x-ray (CXR): Radiological picture of the lungs

Mantoux test: Intradermal injection of tuberculin purified protein derivative (PPD) just beneath the surface of the skin to identify whether the patient has been exposed to tuberculosis

Metered dose inhaler (MDI): Handheld device used to deliver medication to the patient's lower airways (Figs. 8-4 and 8-5)

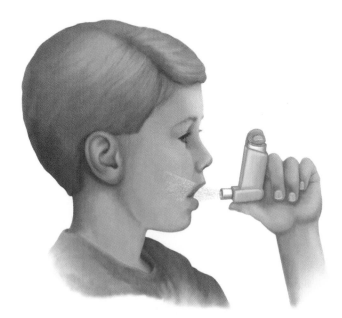

FIGURE 8-4 **Metered dose inhaler.** (From Eagle, S., et al. [2009]. *The professional medical assistant.* Philadelphia, PA: F. A. Davis Company, p. 514; with permission)

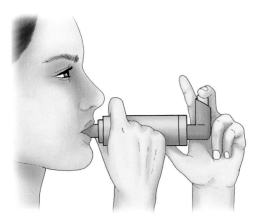

FIGURE 8-5 **Metered dose inhaler with spacer.** (From Eagle, S., et al. [2009]. *The professional medical assistant.* Philadelphia, PA: F. A. Davis Company, p. 514; with permission)

Nebulizer: Device that produces a fine spray or mist to deliver medication to a patient's deep airways (Fig. 8-6)

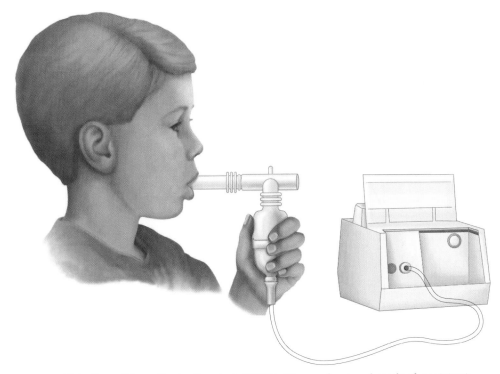

FIGURE 8-6 **Nebulizer.** (From Eagle, S., et al. [2009]. *The professional medical assistant.* Philadelphia, PA: F. A. Davis Company, p. 514; with permission)

Pleurodesis: Infusion of a sterile, irritating substance into the pleural space, causing the pleural linings to fuse to one another by developing scar tissue

Postural drainage: Placement of the patient in various positions that facilitate drainage of secretions from the lungs, often done along with chest physiotherapy (CPT)

Pulmonary angiography: Radiographic examination of pulmonary circulation after injection of a contrast dye

Pulmonary function tests (PFTs): Group of tests that provide information regarding lung capacity; sometimes called *spirometry* (Fig. 8-7)

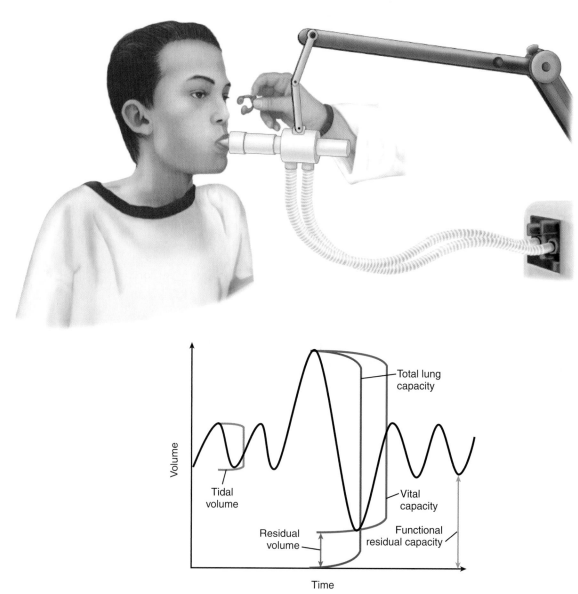

FIGURE 8-7 **Pulmonary function test.** (From Eagle, S., et al. [2009]. *The professional medical assistant.* Philadelphia, PA: F. A. Davis Company, pp. 510–511; with permission)

Pulse oximetry: Indirect measurement of the saturation of peripheral oxygen (SpO_2) to help determine if sufficient oxygen is being delivered to the body; the normal level in a person with healthy lungs is 96% to 99%

Sputum analysis: Examination of mucus or fluid coughed up from the lungs

Thoracentesis: Surgical puncture of the chest wall to remove fluid from the interpleural space; also called *pleurocentesis* (Fig. 8-8)

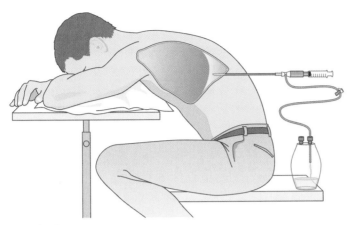

FIGURE 8-8 **Thoracentesis.**

Vital capacity (VC): Measurement of the volume of air that can be exhaled after maximum inspiration

 Learning Style Tip

Sing content you need to remember, like these tests and procedures, using simple, easily remembered tunes such as "Happy Birthday to You" or nursery-school songs.

Pharmacology

Table 8-4 provides a list of common respiratory system medications used to treat coughing, congestion, nasal allergy symptoms, and pathologies such as influenza, asthma, and COPD.

TABLE 8-4

PHARMACOLOGY

Therapeutic Classification	Generic Name	Brand Name	Common Use
Anticholinergic bronchodilator	ipratropium	Atrovent	Relax the smooth muscle of the bronchi
	tiotropium	Spiriva	
Antihistamine	cetirizine	Zyrtec	Relieve allergy symptoms
	diphenhydramine	Benadryl	
	fexofenadine	Allegra	
	loratadine	Claritin	
Anti-influenza agent, antiviral (not a vaccine)	amantadine	Symadine, Symmetrel	Relieve symptoms and reduce the duration of certain types of influenza
	oseltamivir phosphate	Tamiflu	
	rimantadine	Flumadine	
	zanamivir	Relenza	
Antitussive	dextromethorphan	Delsym, PediaCare, Robitussin Cough, Sucrets, Triaminic, Vicks	Suppress cough

Continued

TABLE 8-4			
PHARMACOLOGY—cont'd			
Therapeutic Classification	**Generic Name**	**Brand Name**	**Common Use**
Decongestant	pseudoephedrine	Contac Cold, Drixoral, Neo-Synephrine, Sudafed	Reduce swelling and drainage in the nasal passage
Expectorant	guaifenesin	Guiatuss, Mucinex, Organidin, Robitussin	Relieve congestion by thinning and loosening mucus in the airways
Leukotriene inhibitor	montelukast	Singulair	Prevent asthma attacks
Long-acting beta-adrenergic agonist bronchodilator	budesonide (steroid) and formoterol	Symbicort	Dilate, or open up, bronchi for long-term control of asthma symptoms
	fluticasone (steroid) and salmeterol	Advair	
	formoterol	Foradil, Perforomist	
	salmeterol	Serevent	
Mast cell stabilizer, anti-inflammatory	cromolyn sodium, nedocromil sodium	None	Decrease inflammation, prevent asthma attacks
Short-acting bronchodilator	albuterol	AccuNeb, Proventil, Ventolin	Dilate, or open up, bronchi for quick relief of acute asthma symptoms
	alupent	Metaproterenol	
	isoproterenol	Isuprel	
	levalbuterol	Xopenex	
	pirbuterol	Maxair	
Steroid	fluticasone	Flovent	Prevent inflammation, prevent asthma attack
Steroid	mometasone furoate monohydrate	Nasonex	Relieve nasal allergy symptoms, reduce nasal polyps

Pathologies, Procedures, and Pharmacology Practice Exercises

Deciphering Terms

Write the correct meaning of these medical terms.

Exercise 5

1. laryngeal _____

2. pleuralgia _____

3. pneumatic _____

4. pneumonia _____

5. pulmonary _____

6. sinusotomy _____

7. thoracentesis _____

8. tonsillectomy _____

9. dyspnea _____

10. hemothorax _____

11. pneumothorax _____

12. eupnea _____

13. orthopnea _____

14. rhinitis _____

15. tracheostomy _____

Fill in the Blanks

Fill in the blanks below using Tables 8-2 and 8-3.

Exercise 6

1. Black Lung is a respiratory disease that affects coal-workers. The combining form that means *coal* or *coal dust* is _____.

2. A group of diseases in which the alveoli are destroyed, resulting in chronic SOB, is _____ _____

   _____ _____.

3. The name of the disease in the previous question is abbreviated

   _____.

4. To determine whether he has been exposed to tuberculosis, Victor has a skin test done and is injected with _____

   _____ _____.

5. Julio has _____, which causes him to experience SOB and wheezing in response to various triggers.

6. A medical term for the common cold is _____.

7. A collection of air in the intrapleural space is known as

   _____.

8. Edelia is allergic to bees. If she gets stung, she has a severe reaction known as anaphylaxis and has great difficulty breathing. In addition to sounding wheezy, she develops a high-pitched upper-airway sound caused by obstruction of her airways. This is known as _____.

9. When a physician gives a _____ order, the expectation is that the order will be carried out immediately.

10. Sophie has a cold. This might also be called an _____ _____ _____.

11. The abbreviation for the name of the condition referred to in the previous question is _____.

12. Acute inflammation of the nasal mucosa is known as

    _____.

13. A skill often taught in first-aid courses that helps restore a victim's breathing and circulation is known as _____ _____.

14. The name of the procedure referred to in the previous question is abbreviated _____.

15. Miguel was treated in the urgent-care clinic for epistaxis. This is more commonly known as a _____.

16. A fungus found in soil contaminated with bird droppings can cause a systemic respiratory disease known as _____.

17. Albert has temporarily lost his voice because his larynx is inflamed. He has

    _____.

18. Vaishali has suffered from a partial collapse of the alveoli and tiny airways in her lungs. She has _____.

19. Vita is currently suffering from chronic retention of CO_2 and has symptoms of mental cloudiness and lethargy. She has _____.

20. Missy has had a T&A. Therefore, she has had her _____ and _____ removed.

Multiple Choice

Select the one best answer to the following multiple-choice questions.

Exercise 7

1. A coarse, gurgling sound heard with a stethoscope in the lungs, caused by secretions in the air passages, is known as:

   a. crackles

   b. stridor

   c. rhonchi

   d. wheezes

2. Which of the following tests provides an indirect measure of the level of arterial-blood oxygen saturation?

   a. pulse oximetry

   b. arterial blood gases

   c. vital capacity

   d. sputum analysis

3. Which of the following terms indicates a condition of low oxygen?

   a. apnea

   b. hypoxia

   c. dyspnea

   d. eupnea

4. Which of the following terms means *mouthlike opening in the trachea?*

   a. tracheotomy

   b. tracheotome

   c. tracheostomy

   d. tracheoscopy

5. Mrs. Yachinich sleeps propped up on three pillows so she can breathe better. Which of the following terms best describes this condition?

   a. orthopnea

   b. aerophagia

   c. pneumonitis

   d. aerophobia

Fill in the Blanks

Using Table 8-4, write the therapeutic classification of the medication next to each generic or brand name.

Exercise 8

1. Flovent _____

2. dextromethorphan _____

3. pirbuterol _____

4. zanamivir _____

5. Sudafed _____

6. albuterol _____

7. Serevent _____

8. guaifenesin _____

9. tiotropium _____

10. Nasonex _____

CASE STUDY

Read the case study and answer the questions that follow. Most of the terms are included in this chapter. Refer to the glossary or to your medical dictionary for the other terms.

Chronic Obstructive Pulmonary Disease (COPD)

Helga Freidericks is a 57-year-old woman who came to the urgent-care clinic today complaining of SOB. On admission, her respirations were labored, at a rate of 32 breaths per minute. Her SpO_2 was just 84%, and her VC was decreased. She appeared anxious and stated that she "[couldn't] get enough air." Her lungs had bilateral expiratory wheezes throughout, scattered rhonchi, and bibasilar crackles. She had a frequent cough, productive of thick green sputum.

Stat ABGs were drawn. She was put on O_2 at 2 liters per minute (lpm) per nasal cannula (NC) and given a nebulizer Tx. A sputum specimen was collected and sent for culture and sensitivity (C&S). She was given IV doses of a broad-spectrum antibiotic and a steroid drug. Upon review of her ABGs, it was determined that she was in a state of mild respiratory acidosis.

A short time later, Mrs. Freidericks' respiratory rate had decreased to 20 breaths per minute, her O_2 saturation was 91%, and she stated that she was breathing "much better." She was then transferred to the hospital for further monitoring and continued therapy.

COPD is a chronic disease with several different causes. The most common cause is smoking, because the lungs are subjected to chronic irritation by an inhaled substance 20 to 40 times each day for years on end. As a result, the lung tissue becomes inflamed. Under normal circumstances, body tissue is able to repair itself; however, in the case of smoking, chronic, repeated exposure to the irritants prevents healing and results in chronic inflammation. Over

Flashpoint
COPD affects approximately 24 million Americans. Get more facts at the COPD Foundation website at *www.copdfoundation.org.*

time, permanent damage occurs. The walls of the delicate alveoli lose their elasticity and become permanently distended, like balloons that have been inflated too many times. The walls of the alveoli also erode and thicken and, as a result, function less effectively. They begin to trap air rather than allowing it to escape during expiration. This decreases the amount of oxygen-rich air that can be inhaled in each breath.

As chronic air-trapping occurs, the chest changes dimension, becoming more barrel like. The lungs also flatten on the bottom, robbing the diaphragm (an important respiratory muscle) of its effectiveness. Cilia in the airway normally move debris upward to be coughed out, but, in COPD, cilia become clogged with tar and thus lose their effectiveness. As a result of these physical changes, the COPD patient may begin to experience some or all of the following symptoms:

Orthopnea: The need to remain upright in order to breathe effectively. Physicians often quantify the severity of orthopnea by referring to the number of pillows the patient must recline against while sleeping (e.g., three-pillow orthopnea).

Hypercapnia: The chronic retention of CO_2. In some cases, this changes the way the person's body determines when to breathe. The person may begin to function according to the "hypoxic drive" and feel the urge to breathe when the O_2 level gets too low instead of when the CO_2 level gets too high. This becomes a problem when the person requires supplemental O_2. Too much O_2 can, in some circumstances, actually knock out the urge to breathe, leading to respiratory arrest. Furthermore, hypercapnia can lead to symptoms of mental cloudiness and lethargy.

Chronic hypoxia: A chronic lack of oxygen. As gas exchange becomes less effective, breathing becomes more and more difficult. Eventually the person becomes dependent on oxygen. Yet, in the last stages of the disease, supplemental O_2 is of little help. The person feels chronically short of breath and becomes severely dyspneic with the slightest exertion.

Case Study Questions

Exercise 9

1. Upon admission, Mrs. Freidericks was:
   a. having chest pain
   b. very short of breath
   c. breathing very slowly
   d. unconscious

2. Mrs. Freidericks had:
   a. an increased ability to breathe in
   b. a decreased ability to breathe in
   c. an increased ability to breathe out
   d. a decreased ability to breathe out

3. Mrs. Freidericks' oxygen saturation level was:
   a. checked by pulse oximetry
   b. at a normal level
   c. not known
   d. higher than normal

4. When listening to Mrs. Freidericks' lungs, the physician heard:
   a. normal sounds of air movement
   b. a somewhat musical sound caused by partial airway obstruction
   c. a high-pitched upper-airway sound that indicates airway obstruction
   d. a barking, "seal-like" cough

5. Which of the following statements is true?
   a. Mrs. Freidericks normally slept lying down.
   b. It is always safe to give high levels of oxygen to people with COPD.
   c. Supplemental O_2 effectively relieves dyspnea in the final stages of COPD.
   d. Mrs. Freidericks' chest cavity had most likely become more barrel-like in shape.

6. Which of the following statements is correct?
   a. Cilia continue to work effectively in people with late-stage COPD.
   b. The only cause of COPD is smoking.
   c. People with COPD tend to develop chronic O_2 retention.
   d. Arterial blood was immediately drawn to analyze the levels of O_2, CO_2, and pH.

7. In a person with healthy lungs, the drive to breathe is stimulated by:
   a. low levels of oxygen
   b. a drop in blood pH caused by high levels of CO_2
   c. a feeling of emptiness in the lungs
   d. a neurological message sent from the brain to the lungs

8. Describe how COPD could impact a person's activities of daily living (ADLs).

9. The person with COPD may not be interested in exercise or an active lifestyle due to difficulty with breathing. Identify some consequences of inactivity.

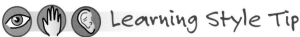 Learning Style Tip

Find videos at *www.youtube.com* that match the information in this chapter. Enter *respiratory system* into the YouTube search bar. Send a couple of your favorite videos to your classmates by clicking on "share." You can copy and paste the highlighted link into an e-mail, upload it onto a class discussion board, or post it on a social media site.

End-of-Chapter Practice Exercises

Word Building

*Using **only** the word parts in the lists provided, create medical terms with the indicated meanings.*

Exercise 10

Prefixes	Combining Forms	Suffixes
dys-	aer/o	-al
eu-	bronch/o	-ary
peri-	carcin/o	-dynia
tachy-	chondr/o	-gen
	cutane/o	-genesis
	epiglott/o	-genic
	laryng/o	-ic
	muc/o	-itis
	myc/o	-malacia

nas/o   -oid
pharyng/o   -oma
pleur/o   -osis
pneum/o   -ous
pulmon/o   -pathy
sinus/o   -pexy
thorac/o   -pnea
tonsill/o   -scopy
trache/o   -stomy
               -tomy

1. pertaining to the bronchus and lung _____

2. tumor of cartilage _____

3. creation of air _____

4. pertaining to mucus and skin _____

5. visual examination of the trachea and bronchus _____

6. disease of the tonsil _____

7. softening of the trachea _____

8. inflammation of the epiglottis _____

9. pertaining to bad, painful, or difficult breathing _____

10. good or normal breathing _____

11. cutting into or incision of the thorax _____

12. fungal infection of the pharynx _____

13. pain of the pleura _____

14. surgical fixation of the lung _____

15. pertaining to the lung _____

16. resembling the sinus _____

17. mouthlike opening in the trachea _____

18. pertaining to causing cancer _____

19. rapid breathing _____

20. visual examination of the larynx _____

True or False

Decide whether the following statements are true or false.

Exercise 11

1. True False   A collection of air in the intrapleural space is known as **hemothorax.**

2. True False   The abbreviation **PND** stands for *pulmonary neoplastic disease.*

3. True False   A collection of pus in the pleural cavity is known as **empyema.**

4. True False   The abbreviation **ARDS** stands for *adult research drug study.*

5. True False   A nosebleed is known as **epistaxis.**

6. True False   The abbreviation **ABG** stands for *arterial blood gases.*

7. True False   Another name for the common cold is **croup.**

8. True False   The abbreviation **VC** stands for *very critical.*

9. True False   A collection of fluid in the intrapleural space is known as **pleural effusion.**

10. True False   An abnormal "Rice Krispies" sound heard in the lungs with a stethoscope is known as **crackles.**

Deciphering Terms

Write the correct meaning of these medical terms.

Exercise 12

1. aerophagia _____

2. alveolar _____

3. pharyngeal _____

4. spirogram _____

5. nasal _____

6. anthracoid _____

7. mucolysis _____

8. phonophobia _____

9. carcinoma _____

10. oxygenic _____

Multiple Choice

Select the one best answer to the following multiple-choice questions.

Exercise 13

1. Which of the following terms is matched with the correct definition?

   a. coni/o: dust

   b. chondr/o: cancer

   c. phon/o: pharynx

   d. spir/o: sinus

2. All of the following terms are matched with the correct definition **except:**

   a. chondr/o: cartilage

   b. rhin/o: nose

   c. stomat/o: mouth

   d. pleur/o: lung

3. Which of the following is related to coryza?

   a. CWP

   b. URI

   c. AFB

   d. ARDS

4. Which of the following indicates a surgical procedure?

   a. T&A

   b. PPD

   c. PND

   d. MDI

5. All of the following terms refer to abnormal breathing sounds **except:**

   a. crackles

   b. stridor

   c. orthopnea

   d. wheeze

6. Which of the following terms indicates the surgical removal of a portion of a lung?

   a. pneumothorax

   b. pleurocentesis

   c. pneumotomy

   d. lobectomy

7. If the surgeon places a drainage tube through the patient's chest cavity, it may be described as:

   a. pneumatic

   b. transthoracic

   c. intrapleural

   d. lobar

8. What word describes the normal location of pleural fluid?

   a. interpleural

   b. endotracheal

   c. contralateral

   d. circumoral

9. A patient who is breathing normally may be described as demonstrating:

   a. hyperpnea

   b. eupnea

   c. dyspnea

   d. tachypnea

10. An artificial opening in the neck that helps a person breathe is:

   a. a tracheostomy

   b. a tracheotomy

   c. a tracheotome

   d. none of these

11. Which of the following indicates a sense of urgency?

   a. CPAP

   b. CXR

   c. Stat

   d. R

12. Which of the following conditions involves infection?

    a. hemothorax

    b. empyema

    c. epistaxis

    d. hemoptysis

13. Which of the following involves abnormal tissue growths?

    a. nasal polyps

    b. histoplasmosis

    c. pneumoconiosis

    d. silicosis

14. Which of the following conditions involves birds?

    a. histoplasmosis

    b. asbestosis

    c. coryza

    d. legionellosis

15. Which of the following might cause a person to belch more frequently?

    a. bronchitis

    b. aerophagia

    c. coniosis

    d. dysphonia

16. Which of the following conditions is most likely to block a patient's airway?

    a. pneumonitis

    b. anthracosis

    c. epiglottic edema

    d. thoracentesis

17. All of the following involve the collection of a substance within the intrapleural space **except:**

    a. hemothorax

    b. pneumothorax

    c. empyema

    d. emphysema

18. Which of the following tests is most useful when the physician needs to evaluate circulation within the patient's lungs?

    a.   spirometry

    b.   pulmonary angiography

    c.   vital capacity

    d.   thoracentesis

19. Which of the following is done to cause the two membranes covering the lungs to adhere to one another?

    a.   oximetry

    b.   pleurodesis

    c.   angiography

    d.   sputum analysis

20. Which of the following is most useful in measuring the patient's lung capacity?

    a.   pulmonary function tests

    b.   Mantoux test

    c.   postural drainage

    d.   sputum analysis

DIGESTIVE SYSTEM

9

Chapter Outline

Structure and Function

The digestive system is also known as the **gastrointestinal (GI) system.** It includes all the structures of the alimentary canal, from the mouth to the anus, and the accessory organs. The digestive system has two key functions: digestion and excretion. The organs of the GI system break down food into usable nutrients and then eliminate bulk waste in the form of feces.

We will discuss the parts of the GI system in the same order in which food passes through the system. As we do this, please refer to Figure 9-1 to see the various parts of the GI system.

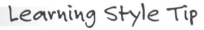 Learning Style Tip

After reading each paragraph, summarize the content and key points aloud before moving on to the next paragraph.

The first or most proximal part of the digestive system is the mouth, also known as the **oral** or **buccal cavity.** When we take a bite of food (**ingestion**) and begin chewing it, our tongue and teeth aid in the process of **mechanical digestion** as food is broken down into smaller and smaller parts. It is mixed and moistened with **saliva,** which is secreted from three different salivary glands. Saliva also contains ptyalin, a chemical that starts to break down starches. The **tongue** helps to form chewed food into a **bolus,** which is a rounded mass ready to be swallowed. The tongue also allows us to taste food. Specific areas on the tongue identify sweet, salty, sour, and bitter flavors (Fig. 9-2). Because taste can make

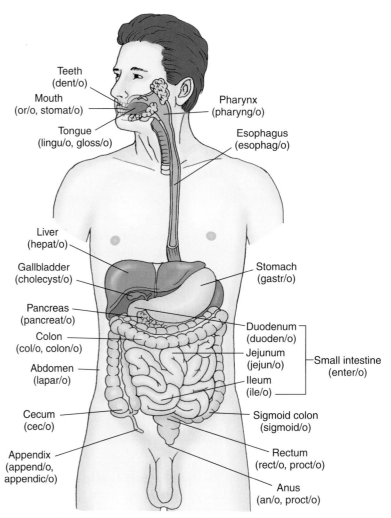

Teeth
(dent/o)

Mouth
(or/o, stomat/o)

Tongue
(lingu/o, gloss/o)

Pharynx
(pharyng/o)

Esophagus
(esophag/o)

Liver
(hepat/o)

Gallbladder
(cholecyst/o)

Stomach
(gastr/o)

Pancreas
(pancreat/o)

Colon
(col/o, colon/o)

Abdomen
(lapar/o)

Cecum
(cec/o)

Appendix
(append/o,
appendic/o)

Duodenum
(duoden/o)

Jejunum
(jejun/o)

Ileum
(ile/o)

Small intestine
(enter/o)

Sigmoid colon
(sigmoid/o)

Rectum
(rect/o, proct/o)

Anus
(an/o, proct/o)

FIGURE 9-1 **The gastrointestinal system.**

eating an enjoyable process, there are times when we may overeat. When we eat more calories than we burn through our daily activities or exercise, we gain weight (Box 9-1).

The **uvula** is a small, finger-shaped portion of soft tissue that hangs from the upper back of the mouth. It prevents food from entering the nasal cavity as we eat. At the back of the mouth is the **pharynx,** which is tissue that is shaped something like a funnel. The pharynx extends down to the **esophagus,** which is a long, tubelike structure that passes through the diaphragm and connects to the stomach. At the top of the esophagus is a small flap of cartilage covered with epithelial tissue; it is called the **epiglottis.** It acts to cover the trachea when we swallow, to keep food from entering the respiratory tract. Muscles in the esophageal wall contract intermittently and involuntarily, causing **peristalsis,** which moves the food bolus downward into the stomach. At the lower end of the esophagus is a muscular opening called the **lower esophageal sphincter (LES),** also called the cardiac sphincter because of its location near the heart. The LES acts as a doorway between the esophagus and the stomach and prevents backflow of gastric secretions.

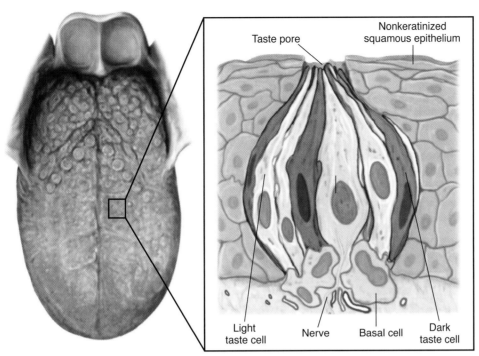

FIGURE 9-2 The tongue with structure of a taste bud and taste cells. (From Eagle, S., et al. [2009]. *The professional medical assistant.* Philadelphia, PA: F. A. Davis Company, p. 540; with permission)

Box 9-1 Obesity

Our bodies use the foods we eat for energy. When we eat more calories than our bodies burn through physical activity, the extra calories are stored as fat. Overeating and eating unhealthy foods are behaviors that can cause us to become overweight or even obese. In the United States, 1 in 3 adults and 1 in 6 children are obese. For these individuals, the chance of developing other conditions such as heart disease, diabetes, and cancer is greatly increased.

Our environment also plays a role in obesity. Low income families may not be able to afford healthier food choices. Our neighborhoods may not have sidewalks or crosswalks that enable us to exercise safely outdoors. Parks and community centers may be too far from our homes. While we are constantly told that we should eat healthier foods and get more exercise, we are often limited in our choices.

There are numerous online resources and free smartphone "apps" to help us lose weight or prevent us from gaining weight. If we don't have access to healthier type foods, these tools can help us to eat less of the unhealthier type. They can help us find ways to incorporate a little more exercise into our daily activities. The US Department of Agriculture (USDA) has an interactive website (*www.choosemyplate.gov*) that allows us to look up the nutritional value of more than 8000 foods and track what we are eating (*www.supertracker. usda.gov*). My Fitness Pal has an interactive website and a smartphone app with a nutrition and calorie database of more than 5 million foods. (*www.myfitnesspal.com*). Both of these resources can also track the type and amount of exercise we are getting every day. Being accountable for our food and exercise choices can help us reach our weight-related goals and decrease our risk for developing other chronic illnesses.

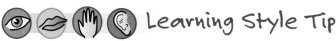 Learning Style Tip

Use inexpensive watercolor paints or colorful markers and sheets of paper to draw the GI system. Label anatomical parts and include the associated combining forms. Take pictures or make a video of your project so that you can "teach" yourself or your classmates in future study sessions.

The abdominal cavity holds the stomach, small intestine, large intestine, rectum, and anus. This cavity is lined with a membrane called the **peritoneum.** The inside of the stomach is lined with folds called **rugae** that allow the stomach to expand when we eat a large amount of food. The stomach is composed of three major areas: the **fundus** (upper portion), **body** (middle portion), and **pylorus** (lower portion). The fundus and body of the stomach are mostly holding areas for food; the majority of activity occurs in the pylorus. **Gastric secretions**—which are very acidic, with an average pH of 1.7—act on food to continue breaking it down and preparing it for absorption within the intestines. At this point, the food is now referred to as **chyme,** a more-liquid material made up of chewed food, saliva, and digestive juices. The **pyloric sphincter** lies between the pylorus and the small intestine. This sphincter acts as the stomach's exit way and releases chyme into the small intestine a little at a time.

The real digestive action occurs within the **small intestine.** It is small only in the sense that it is a relatively narrow tubelike structure; however, the small intestine is really quite long, around 20 feet in the average adult. Peristalsis continues to move the contents through the three parts of the small intestine: the **duodenum** (upper portion), **jejunum** (middle portion), and **ileum** (end portion). Here the majority of digestion is completed, and most nutrients are absorbed.

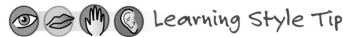 Learning Style Tip

Trace the GI system in Figure 9-1 with the tip of your finger as you recite the anatomical parts and the associated combining forms. Speak aloud and record your voice as you do this. Increase your available study time by listening to your recording while driving or doing household chores.

The small intestine is lined with **villi,** which are tiny, fingerlike structures surrounded by capillaries and lymphatic vessels. Villi increase the surface area of the small intestine, allowing greater absorption of water and nutrients into the blood (Fig. 9-3). All other products of digestion pass from the small intestine to the large intestine through the **ileocecal valve.** The first part of the large intestine is the **cecum.** A small tubelike structure called the **appendix** hangs from the cecum in the right lower quadrant (RLQ) of the abdomen. For years, the appendix was thought to serve no useful function. More recently, however, some experts have suggested that it may serve as a storage facility for normal bacteria, which may serve to repopulate the GI tract in the event that normal bacteria are eliminated (as can happen with certain GI disorders). Unfortunately, the appendix occasionally becomes clogged with intestinal matter and then becomes inflamed and infected. This condition is known as *appendicitis.* When this occurs, the appendix must be surgically removed by a procedure known as an *appendectomy.*

The **ascending colon** progresses upward from the cecum. It takes a 90-degree turn as it nears the top of the abdomen, beneath the liver, and becomes the **transverse colon** as it passes horizontally across the uppermost part of the

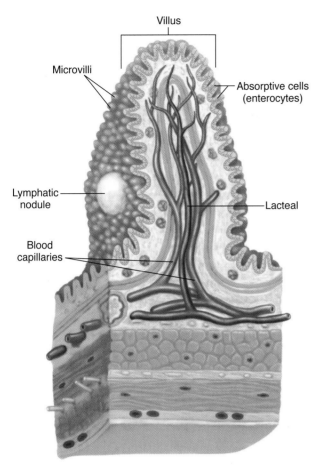

FIGURE 9-3 **Villi of the small intestine.** (From Eagle, S., et al. [2009]. *The professional medical assistant.* Philadelphia, PA: F. A. Davis Company, p. 540; with permission)

abdomen. It again takes a 90-degree turn, beneath the spleen, and heads down along the left side of the abdomen. This portion is known as the **descending colon.** The key function of the colon is absorption of water as the remaining waste products become less liquid and more solid. The colon then takes a gentle turn inward and becomes the **sigmoid colon,** which descends into the rectum and finally the anus. It is here that intestinal contents, now a waste product known as **feces,** are excreted in the process of **defecation.**

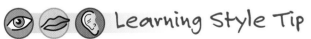 Learning Style Tip

Teach a classmate, friend, or family member about the GI tract. Beginning with the mouth and working all the way to the anus, say each anatomical part, its function, and its associated combining form.

Accessory Organs

There are several accessory organs that contribute to the process of digestion. These include the liver, gallbladder, and pancreas.

The **liver,** located in the upper right and center of the abdominal cavity, is the largest glandular organ of the body. Its many functions include digestion, absorption, storage, and excretion.

The **gallbladder** is a sac, 3 to 4 inches long, on the inner surface of the liver. It is connected to the common bile duct, which also connects to the duodenum. The gallbladder acts as a storage pouch for bile. When we eat fatty food, the gallbladder responds by secreting bile into the duodenum through the common bile duct to break down those fats for digestion and absorption.

The **pancreas** is a long, somewhat flat organ that lies just behind and beneath the stomach. Within the pancreas are specialized cells called the islets of Langerhans. The two types include alpha and beta cells. The pancreas is connected to the hepatic duct via the pancreatic duct at the duodenum. The pancreas secretes several substances into the duodenum through the pancreatic duct and directly into the bloodstream through capillaries of the islets of Langerhans. One of these substances is sodium bicarbonate, which acts to neutralize stomach acid. Others include the pancreatic enzymes trypsin, which breaks down proteins; lipase, which breaks down fats; and amylase, which breaks down carbohydrates.

The cells of the islets of Langerhans also secrete the hormones insulin and glucagon, which work together to regulate blood glucose levels. Insulin is secreted by beta cells in response to rising blood glucose levels after we eat. It binds to glucose molecules in the blood, which then allows them to diffuse into the tissues and enter cells to provide energy. Glucagon is secreted by alpha cells in response to dropping blood glucose levels. It stimulates the liver to release a storage form of glucose called glycogen. The liver then converts the glycogen into glucose for energy. This process will be discussed in more detail in Chapter 12.

Flashpoint

In type 1 diabetes, the body does not produce insulin. In type 2 diabetes, the body does not use insulin properly.

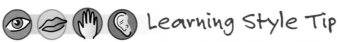 Learning Style Tip

In a group, take turns drawing individual parts of the GI system on a whiteboard or poster board. Begin with the mouth and work all the way to the anus. As each person draws their part, they should verbally explain it to the rest of the group.

Structure and Function Practice Exercises

Fill in the Blanks

Choose the term that matches the description.

Exercise 1

Oral Cavity
GI system
Oral or buccal cavity
Ingestion
Mechanical digestion
Saliva
Tongue
Bolus
Uvula
Pharynx
Esophagus
Epiglottis

Abdominal Cavity
Peritoneum
Rugae
Fundus, body, pyloris
Gastric secretions
Chyme
Pyloric sphincter
Intestines:
Small intestine
Duodenum, jejunum, ileum
Villi
Ileocecal valve

Colon:
Ascending colon
Transverse colon
Descending colon
Sigmoid colon
Feces
Defecation
Accessory Organs:
Liver
Gallbladder
Pancreas

Peristalsis   Cecum
Lower esophageal   Appendix
   sphincter (LES)

1. _____ Soft tissue that hangs from the upper back of the mouth that prevents food from entering the nasal cavity as we eat

2. _____ A structure that hangs from the cecum in which normal bacteria may be stored to repopulate the GI tract

3. _____ Fingerlike structures that increase the surface area of the small intestine

4. _____ An organ that secretes substances that neutralize stomach acids and break down proteins, fats, and carbohydrates

5. _____ A muscular opening between the esophagus and the stomach that prevents backflow of gastric secretions

6. _____ The portion of the colon found along the left side of the abdomen

7. _____ Upper, middle, and end portion of the small intestine

8. _____ A fluid secreted by the salivary glands that contains a chemical that starts to break down starches

9. _____ A long, tubelike structure that passes through the diaphragm and connects to the stomach

10. _____ A valve through which products of digestion pass from the small intestine to the large intestine

11. _____ Very acidic fluids that continue to break down food, preparing it for absorption within the intestines

12. _____ The waste product that is excreted through the process of defecation

13. _____ A rounded mass of chewed food that is ready to be swallowed

14. _____ The largest glandular organ of the body

15. _____ The portion of the colon that descends into the rectum

16. _____ Folds that line the stomach allowing it to expand when we eat a large amount of food

17. _____ All structures of the alimentary canal, from the mouth to the anus, and the accessory organs

18. _____ A more-liquid material made up of chewed food, saliva, and digestive juices

19. _____ The first part of the large intestine

20. _____ Muscular contractions that move the food bolus downward into the stomach and move chyme through the small intestine

21. _____ Taking a bite of food

22. _____ A very long, narrow, tubelike structure in which the majority of digestion is completed and most nutrients are absorbed

23. _____ The structure that progresses upward from the cecum

24. _____ The upper, middle, and lower portions of the stomach

25. _____ Releases chyme from the pylorus into the small intestine a little at a time

26. _____ A small flap of cartilage at the top of the esophagus that keeps food from entering the respiratory tract

27. _____ The mouth

28. _____ Funnel-shaped tissue at the back of the mouth that extends down to the esophagus

29. _____ A membrane that lines the abdominal cavity

30. _____ The process in which food is broken down into smaller parts by the teeth and the tongue

31. _____ A small sac found on the inner surface of the liver that acts as a storage pouch for bile

32. _____ The process in which products of digestion move through the colon, the rectum, and the anus to be excreted as feces

33. _____ The portion of the colon that passes horizontally across the uppermost part of the abdomen

34. _____ Allows us to taste food and helps to form chewed food into a bolus

Fill in the Blanks
Label Figure 9-4 with the appropriate anatomical terms and combining forms.

Exercise 2

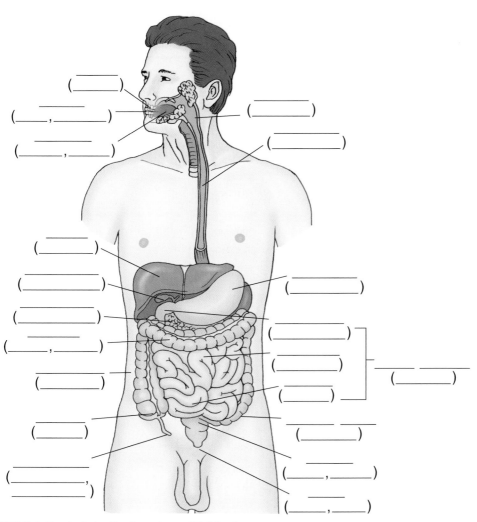

FIGURE 9-4 **Gastrointestinal system with blanks.**

Combining Forms and Abbreviations

Combining Forms

Table 9-1 contains combining forms that pertain to the digestive system, examples of medical terms that utilize the combining forms, and a pronunciation guide. Read aloud to yourself as you move from left to right across the table. Be sure to use the pronunciation guide so you can learn to say the terms correctly.

TABLE 9-1

COMBINING FORMS RELATED TO THE DIGESTIVE SYSTEM

Combining Form	Meaning	Example (Pronunciation)	Meaning of New Term
an/o	anus	anal (Ā-năl)	pertaining to the anus
append/o	appendix	appendectomy (ăp-ĕn-DĔK-tŏ-mē)	excision or surgical removal of the appendix
appendic/o		appendicitis (ă-pĕn-dĭ-SĪ-tĭs)	inflammation of the appendix
bil/i	bile	biliary (BĬL-ē-ār-ē)	pertaining to bile
bucc/o	cheek	buccogingival (bŭk-kō-JĬN-jĭ-văl)	pertaining to the cheek and gums
cec/o	cecum	cecectomy (sē-SĔK-tō-mē)	excision or surgical removal of the cecum
cheil/o	lip	cheiloplasty (KĪ-lō-plăs-tē)	surgical repair of the lip
labi/o		labiodental (lā-bē-ō-DĔN-tăl)	pertaining to the lips and teeth
chol/e	bile, gall	cholecystitis (kō-lē-sis-TĪ-tus)	inflammation of the gallbladder
cholangi/o	bile duct	cholangiography (kō-lăn-jē-ŎG-ră-fē)	process of recording a bile duct
cholecyst/o	gallbladder	cholecystectomy (kō-lē-sĭs-TĔK-tŏ-mē)	excision or surgical removal of the gallbladder
choledoch/o	common bile duct	choledocholith (kō-LĔD-ŏ-kō-lĭth)	stone of the common bile duct
col/o	colon	colectomy (kō-LĔK-tŏ-mē)	excision or surgical removal of the colon
colon/o		colonoscopy (kō-lŏn-ŎS-kō-pē)	visual examination of the colon
dent/o	teeth	dental (DĔN-tăl)	pertaining to the teeth
odont/o		odontodynia (ō-dŏn-tō-DĬN-ē-ă)	pain of the teeth
duoden/o	duodenum	duodenoscopy (dū-ŏd-ĕ-NŎS-kō-pē)	visual examination of the duodenum
enter/o	small intestine	enteritis (ĕn-tĕr-Ī-tĭs)	inflammation of the small intestine

TABLE 9-1

COMBINING FORMS RELATED TO THE DIGESTIVE SYSTEM—cont'd

Combining Form	Meaning	Example (Pronunciation)	Meaning of New Term
esophag/o	esophagus	esophagostenosis (ē-sŏf-ă-gō-stĕn-Ō-sĭs)	narrowing or stricture of the esophagus
gastr/o	stomach	gastralgia (găs-TRĂL-jē-ă)	pain of the stomach
gingiv/o	gums	gingivoglossitis (jĭn-jĭ-vō-glŏs-SĪ-tĭs)	inflammation of the gums and tongue
gloss/o	tongue	glossokinesthetic (glŏs-ō-kĭn-ĕs-THĔT-ĭk)	pertaining to tongue movement
lingu/o		sublingual (sŭb-LĬNG-gwăl)	pertaining to beneath the tongue
hepat/o	liver	hepatitis (hĕp-ă-TĪ-tĭs)	inflammation of the liver
ile/o	ileum	ileotomy (ĭl-ē-ŎT-ō-mē)	cutting into or incision of the ileum
jejun/o	jejunum	jejunostomy (jē-jū-NŎS-tō-mē)	mouthlike opening into the jejunum
lapar/o	abdomen, abdominal wall	laparoscope (LĂP-ă-rō-skōp)	instrument used to view inside the abdominal cavity
or/o	mouth	oral (ŌR-ăl)	pertaining to the mouth
pancreat/o	pancreas	pancreatitis (păn-krē-ă-TĪ-tĭs)	inflammation of the pancreas
pept/o	digestion	peptic (PĔP-tĭk)	pertaining to digestion
phag/o	eating, swallowing	phagocyte (FĂG-ō-sīt)	eating cell (specialized type of WBC)
pharyng/o	pharynx	pharyngeal (făr-ĬN-jē-ăl)	pertaining to the pharynx
proct/o	rectum, anus	proctoscopy (prŏk-TŎS-kō-pē)	visual examination of the rectum and/or anus
pylor/o	pylorus	pylorostenosis (pī-lōr-ō-stĕn-Ō-sĭs)	narrowing or stricture of the pylorus
rect/o	rectum	rectal (RĔK-tăl)	pertaining to the rectum
sial/o	saliva, salivary gland	sialolithiasis (sī-ă-lō-lĭ-THĪ-ă-sĭs)	pathological condition of a salivary-gland stone
sigmoid/o	sigmoid colon	sigmoidoscope (sĭg-MOY-dō-skōp)	viewing instrument for the sigmoid colon
steat/o	fat	steatorrhea (stē-ă-tō-RĒ-ă)	flow or discharge of fat (fatty stool)
stomat/o	mouth, mouthlike opening	stomatitis (stō-mă-TĪ-tĭs)	inflammation of the mouth

IN A FLASH!

It's time to print out all of the Combining Forms Flash Cards for Chapter 9 and run through them at least three times before you continue.

Abbreviations

Table 9-2 lists some of the most common abbreviations related to the GI system.

IN A FLASH!

It's time to print out all of the Abbreviations Flash Cards for Chapter 9 and run through them at least three times before you continue.

TABLE 9-2	
ABBREVIATIONS	
Abd	abdomen
BM	bowel movement
BRP	bathroom privileges
CA	cancer
EGD	esophagogastroduodenoscopy
ERCP	endoscopic retrograde cholangiopancreatography
GERD	gastroesophageal reflux disease
GI	gastrointestinal
IBD	inflammatory bowel disease
IBS	irritable bowel syndrome
LFT	liver function test
N&V	nausea and vomiting
NG	nasogastric
NPO	nothing by mouth
PO	by mouth
PR	per rectum
PUD	peptic ulcer disease
SBO	small bowel obstruction
UGI	upper GI x-ray

Combining Forms and Abbreviations Practice Exercises

Fill in the Blanks

Fill in the blanks below using Table 9-1.

Exercise 3

1. pertaining to the rectum _____

2. instrument used to view inside the abdominal cavity _____

3. pertaining to the mouth _____

4. pertaining to the pharynx _____

5. pertaining to the anus _____

6. narrowing or stricture of the esophagus _____

7. excision or surgical removal of the gallbladder _____

8. inflammation of the small intestine _____

9. mouthlike opening into the jejunum _____

10. visual examination of the colon _____

11. pertaining to beneath the tongue _____

12. visual examination of the duodenum _____

13. cutting into or incision of the ileum _____

14. inflammation of the mouth _____

15. pain of the stomach _____

16. inflammation of the liver _____

17. excision or surgical removal of the appendix _____

18. inflammation of the appendix _____

19. visual examination of the rectum and anus _____

20. excision or surgical removal of the colon _____

21. pertaining to the teeth _____

22. spasm of the tongue _____

23. inflammation of the pancreas _____

24. viewing instrument for the sigmoid colon _____

25. flow or discharge of fat (fatty stool) _____

26. pertaining to bile _____

27. pertaining to the cheeks and gums _____

28. stone of the common bile duct _____

29. pathological condition of a salivary-gland stone _____

30. excision or surgical removal of the cecum _____

31. process of recording a bile duct _____

32. surgical repair of the lip _____

33. pain of the teeth _____

34. pertaining to the lips and teeth _____

35. inflammation of the gums and tongue _____

36. pertaining to tongue movement _____

37. inflammation of the gallbladder _____

38. pertaining to digestion _____

39. eating cell (specialized type of WBC) _____

40. narrowing or stricture of the pylorus _____

Fill in the Blanks

Fill in the blanks below using Table 9-2.

Exercise 4

1. The abbreviation *ERCP* stands for _____

   _____ _____.

2. *Abdomen* may be abbreviated as _____.

3. The abbreviation *UGI* stands for _____

   _____.

4. The abbreviation *SBO* stands for _____

   _____ _____.

5. If a patient is not to eat or drink anything, the physician may write this

   order: _____.

6. If a medication is to be taken orally, the order will be

   _____.

7. A suppository medication that is given rectally may be ordered

   _____.

8. _____ is the abbreviation for *cancer.*

9. To allow the patient to have bathroom privileges, a physician might write

   "_____."

10. The physician dictates that the patient "c/o N&V." This means that the

    patient complains of _____ and

    _____

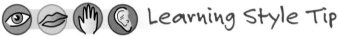 Learning Style Tip

Take short (5- to 10-minute) but frequent (every 30 to 60 minutes) study breaks and move your body. Exercise wakes you up, helps you feel better, and increases your ability to learn.

Pathologies, Procedures, and Pharmacology

Pathology Terms

Table 9-3 includes terms that relate to diseases or abnormalities of the digestive system. Use the pronunciation guide and say the terms aloud as you read them. This will help you get in the habit of saying the terms properly.

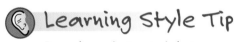 Learning Style Tip

Record your instructor's lectures, with his or her permission, and then play them back when you study. This allows you to hear information again later, as often as you wish. This technique will be especially helpful when your instructor discusses pathology terms and medical procedures.

IN A FLASH!

It's time to print out all of the Pathology Terms Flash Cards for Chapter 9 and run through them at least three times before you continue.

TABLE 9-3
PATHOLOGY TERMS

achalasia (ăk-ă-LĀ-zē-ă)	dilation and expansion of the lower esophagus, due to pressure from food accumulation

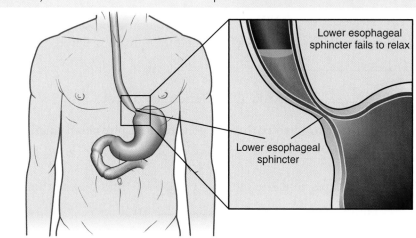

Achalasia.

anorexia nervosa (ăn-ō-RĔK-sē-ă nĕr-VŌ-să)	physical and psychiatric disorder that involves a combination of an intense fear of weight gain, distorted body image, and self-imposed starvation

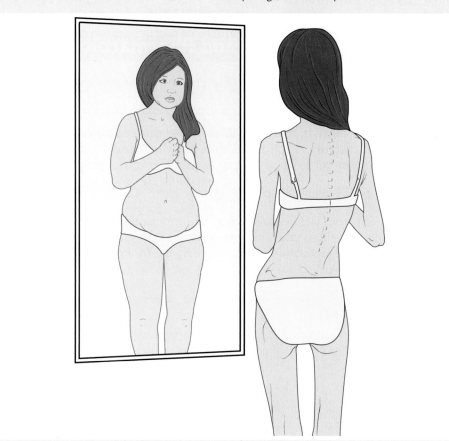

Anorexia.

TABLE 9-3
PATHOLOGY TERMS—cont'd

appendicitis (ă-pĕn-dĭ-SĪ-tĭs)	inflammation of the appendix

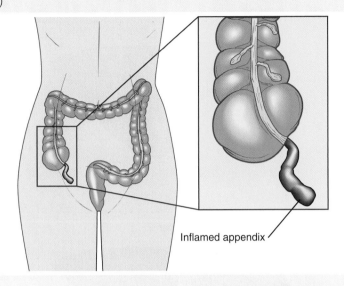

Inflamed appendix

Appendicitis.

ascites (ă-SĪ-tēz)	accumulation of serous fluid in the peritoneal (abdominal) cavity
bowel obstruction (BOW-ĕl ŏb-STRŬK-shŭn)	partial or complete blockage of the small or large intestine; common causes include volvulus, intussusception, tumors, and adhesions (scar tissue)
bulimia nervosa (bū-LĒ-mē-ă nĕr-VŌ-să)	physical and psychiatric disorder that involves a combination of obsessively eating huge quantities of food with purging behaviors
***Campylobacter* infection** (kăm-pĭ-lō-BĂK-tĕr ĭn-FĔK-shŭn)	infection with *Campylobacter* organisms via contaminated food or water, resulting in intestinal illness
celiac disease (SĒ-lē-ăk dĭ-ZĒZ)	disorder in which the lining of the small intestine is damaged due to dietary factors, resulting in impaired nutrient absorption
cholecystitis (kō-lē-sĭs-TĪ-tĭs)	inflammation of the gallbladder, usually secondary to the presence of gallstones
cholelithiasis (kō-lă-lĭ-THĪ-ăs-ĭs)	condition in which gallstones are present in the gallbladder, liver, or biliary ducts

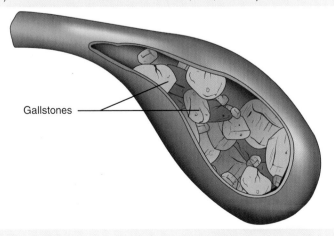

Gallstones

Cholelithiasis.

Continued

TABLE 9-3
PATHOLOGY TERMS—cont'd

cirrhosis (sĭ-RŌ-sĭs)	chronic liver disease characterized by scarring and loss of normal structure

Cirrhotic liver

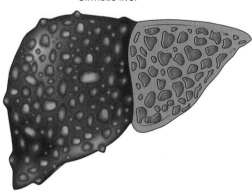

Normal liver

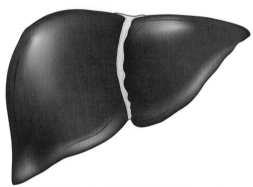

Cirrhosis.

Crohn's disease (krōn dĭ-ZĒZ)	disorder involving inflammation and edema deep into the layers of the lining of any part of the GI tract; also called *regional enteritis*
diverticulitis (dī-vĕr-tĭk-ū-LĪ-tĭs)	inflammation of one or more diverticula (tiny pouches in the intestinal wall)

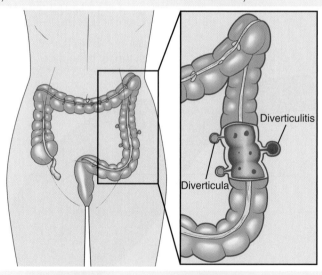

Diverticulitis

Diverticula

Diverticulitis.

TABLE 9-3
PATHOLOGY TERMS—cont'd

diverticulosis
(dĭ-vĕr-tĭk-ū-LŌ-sĭs)

condition in which diverticula form in the intestinal wall due to increased pressure

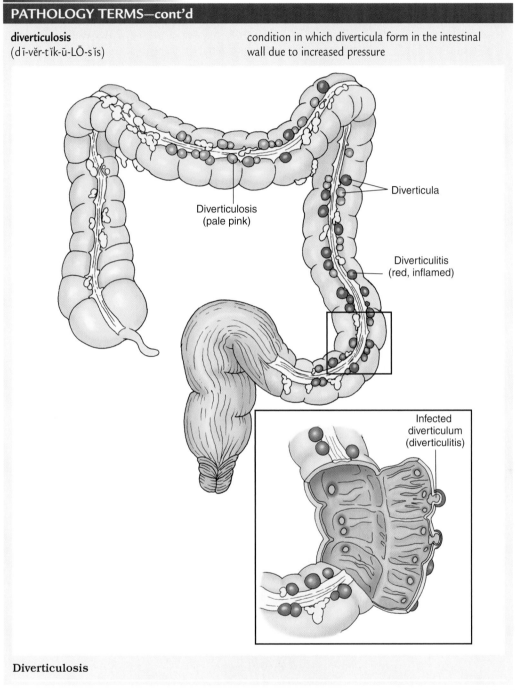

Diverticula

Diverticulosis
(pale pink)

Diverticulitis
(red, inflamed)

Infected
diverticulum
(diverticulitis)

Diverticulosis

Continued

TABLE 9-3
PATHOLOGY TERMS—cont'd

E. coli O157:H7 infection (ē KŌ-lī ĭn-FĔK-shŭn)	dangerous strain of _Escherichia coli_ that produces toxins that can severely damage the intestinal lining, resulting in bloody diarrhea
emesis (ĔM-ĕ-sĭs)	vomiting
esophageal varices (ē-sŏf-ă-JĒ-ăl VĂR-ĭ-sēz)	varicose veins of the distal end of the esophagus

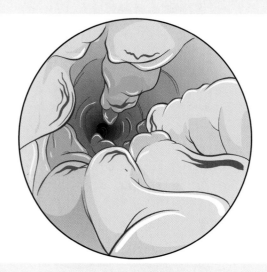

Esophageal varices.

esophagitis (ē-sŏf-ă-JĪ-tĭs)	inflammation of the esophageal lining

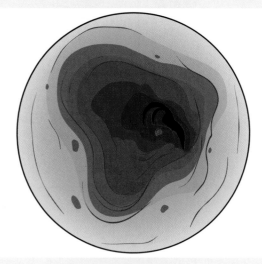

Esophagitis.

food poisoning (fūd POY-zun-ing)	common term for a number of illnesses caused by eating food contaminated with bacterial or toxic organisms; sometimes called _dysentery_

TABLE 9-3
PATHOLOGY TERMS—cont'd

gastritis (găs-TRĪ-tĭs)	inflammation of the stomach's mucosal lining

Gastritis.

gastroenteritis (găs-trō-ĕn-tĕr-Ī-tĭs)	inflammation of the stomach and intestines; often referred to as the *stomach flu* (although influenza is not the cause)
gastroesophageal reflux disease (GERD) (găs-trō-ĕ-sŏf-ă-JĒ-ăl RĒ-flŭks dĭ-ZĒZ)	backflow of acidic gastric contents into the esophagus, causing esophagitis

Esophageal sphincter

Esophagus

Stomach acid

Gastroesophageal reflux.

Continued

TABLE 9-3
PATHOLOGY TERMS—cont'd

hemorrhoids (HĔM-ō-roydz)	internal or external varicose veins of the anal area

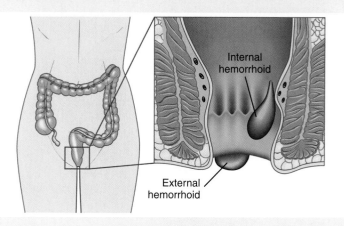

Internal hemorrhoid

External hemorrhoid

Hemorrhoids.

hepatitis (hĕp-ă-TĪ-tĭs)	chronic inflammation of the liver, caused by one of several viruses (types A, B, C, D, or E)
hernia (HĔR-nē-ă)	protrusion of a structure through the wall that normally contains it

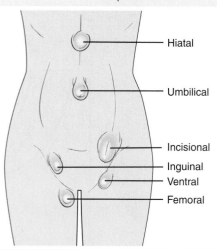

Hiatal

Umbilical

Incisional

Inguinal

Ventral

Femoral

Hernia.

TABLE 9-3

PATHOLOGY TERMS—cont'd

hiatal hernia (hī-Ā-tăl HĔR-nē-ă)	protrusion of a portion of the stomach through the diaphragm into the chest cavity; also called *hiatus hernia*

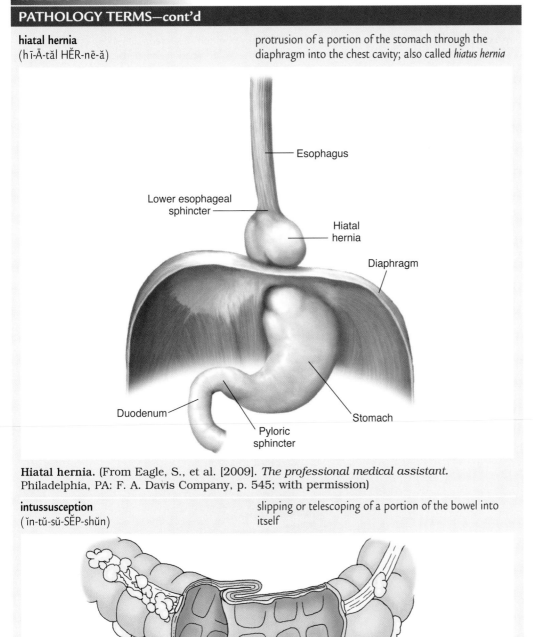

Esophagus

Lower esophageal sphincter

Hiatal hernia

Diaphragm

Duodenum

Pyloric sphincter

Stomach

Hiatal hernia. (From Eagle, S., et al. [2009]. *The professional medical assistant.* Philadelphia, PA: F. A. Davis Company, p. 545; with permission)

intussusception (ĭn-tŭ-sŭ-SĔP-shŭn)	slipping or telescoping of a portion of the bowel into itself

Intussusception.

Continued

TABLE 9-3
PATHOLOGY TERMS—cont'd

irritable bowel syndrome (ĬR-ĭt-ă-bul BOW-ĕl SĬN-drōm)	chronic condition characterized by alternating episodes of constipation and diarrhea
jaundice (JAWN-dĭs)	condition marked by yellow staining of body tissues and fluids as a result of excessive levels of bilirubin in the blood
malabsorption syndrome (măl-ăb-SŌRP-shŭn SĬN-drōm)	inadequate absorption of nutrients from the intestinal tract, especially the small intestine
malnutrition (măl-nū-TRĬ-shŭn)	nutritional deficiency due to inadequate intake or absorption of protein, vitamins, minerals, or other vital nutrients
oral herpes (OR-ăl HĔR-pēz)	vesicular eruption in or on the mouth caused by herpesvirus; also called *herpes labialis* or *cold sore*

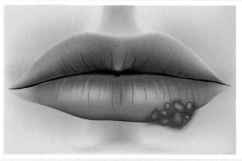

Oral herpes.

oral thrush (OR-ăl thrŭsh)	infection of the skin or mucous membrane with any species of candida, but mainly *Candida albicans;* also called *candidiasis*

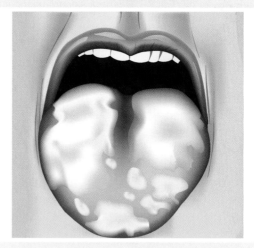

Oral thrush.

TABLE 9-3
PATHOLOGY TERMS—cont'd

pancreatitis (păn-krē-ă-TĪ-tĭs)	acute or chronic inflammation of the pancreas
peptic ulcer (PĔP-tĭk ŬL-sĕr)	inflamed lesion in the gastric or duodenal lining

Peptic ulcer. (From Eagle, S., et al. [2009]. *The professional medical assistant.* Philadelphia, PA: F. A. Davis Company, p. 547; with permission)

peritonitis (pĕr-ĭ-tō-NĪ-tĭs)	inflammation of the organs and structures within the peritoneal cavity
pseudomembranous enterocolitis (soo-dō-MĔM-brān-ŭs ĕn-tĕr-ō-kō-LĪ-tĭs)	inflammatory condition of both small and large bowels that results in severe watery diarrhea; also commonly called C. *diff. colitis*
salmonellosis (săl-mō-nĕ-LŌ-sĭs)	intestinal infection caused by various types of salmonella organisms
short bowel syndrome (shōrt BOW-ĕl SĬN-drōm)	malabsorption and malnutrition disorder created by the loss of a significant portion of functioning bowel

Continued

TABLE 9-3

PATHOLOGY TERMS—cont'd

small bowel obstruction (SBO) (smăl BOW-ĕl ŏb-STRŬK-shŭn)	blockage of normal passage of intestinal contents
ulcerative colitis (ŬL-sĕr-ā-tĭv kō-LĪ-tĭs)	chronic inflammatory disease of the lining of the colon and rectum marked by up to 20 liquid, bloody stools per day
volvulus (VŎL-vū-lŭs)	twisting of the bowel upon itself, causing obstruction

Large intestine

Small intestine

Twisted portion of small intestine

Volvulus.

Common Diagnostic Tests and Procedures

Barium enema: Enema containing a substance that shows up clearly under x-ray and fluoroscopic examination

Barium swallow: X-ray examination of the esophagus after the patient has swallowed a liquid that contains barium

Computed tomography (CT) scan: Computerized collection and translation of multiple x-rays into a three-dimensional picture, creating a more-detailed and accurate image than traditional x-rays (Fig. 9-5)

Endoscopic retrograde cholangiopancreatography (ERCP): Radiographic examination through a fiber-optic endoscope of vessels that connect the liver, gallbladder, and pancreas to the duodenum after injection of a radiopaque material

Fecal occult blood test (Hemoccult): Test of fecal specimen for presence of hidden blood

Gastroccult: Test of gastric contents for pH level and presence of blood

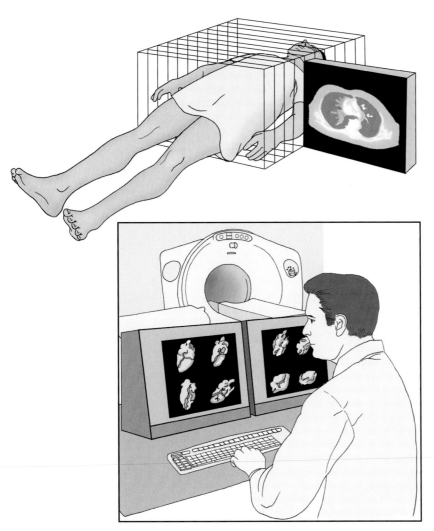

FIGURE 9-5 Computed tomography scan.

***Helicobacter pylori* test:** Test that detects the presence of antibodies to *Helicobacter pylori (H. pylori)*, the most common cause of gastric ulcers

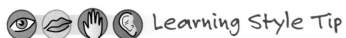 Learning Style Tip

Visit a medical clinic to obtain patient-education pamphlets about some (or all) of these diagnostic tests and procedures; then read them aloud.

Laparoscopy: Exploration of abdominal contents with a laparoscope

Liver function tests (LFTs): Tests, including aspartate aminotransferase (AST) and alanine aminotransferase (ALT), that determine the liver's ability to perform its many complex functions

Lower endoscopy: Visual examination of the GI tract from the rectum to cecum; variations include the colonoscopy, sigmoidoscopy, and proctoscopy (Fig. 9-6)

Lower GI x-ray: X-ray of the large intestine after rectal instillation of barium sulfate

Stool culture: Examination of a fecal specimen for abnormal bacteria and other microorganisms

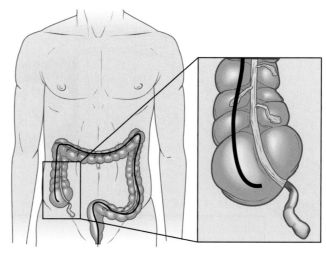

FIGURE 9-6   Lower endoscopy.

Ultrasound: Test in which ultrahigh-frequency sound waves are used to outline the shapes of various body structures

Upper endoscopy: Visual examination of the GI tract, from the esophagus to duodenum (Fig. 9-7)

Upper GI x-ray (UGI): X-ray that involves the use of a contrast medium to help visualize abdominal organs, including the stomach and esophagus

Pharmacology

Table 9-4 provides a list of common digestive system medications used to treat constipation, diarrhea, nausea and vomiting, gastroesophageal reflux disease (GERD), and ulcers.

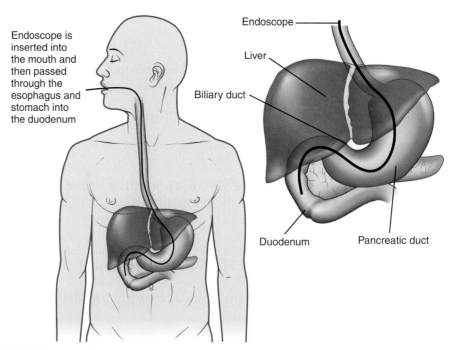

Endoscope is inserted into the mouth and then passed through the esophagus and stomach into the duodenum

Endoscope

Liver

Biliary duct

Duodenum

Pancreatic duct

FIGURE 9-7   Upper endoscopy.

TABLE 9-4

PHARMACOLOGY

Therapeutic Classification	Generic Name	Brand Name	Common Use
Anti-diarrheal	bismuth	Pepto-Bismol	Reduce diarrhea by slowing forward propulsion of intestinal contents
	kaolin and pectin	Kaopectate	
	loperamide	Imodium	
Anti-emetic	dimenhydrinate	Dramamine	Prevent or treat nausea and vomiting
	diphenhydramine	Benadryl	
	meclizine	Antivert	
	phosphorated carbohydrate solution	Emetrol	
	promethazine	Phenergan	
Histamine 2 blocker	cimetidine	Tagamet	Block histamine to reduce stomach acidity
	famotidine	Pepcid	
	ranitidine	Zantac	
Osmotic-type laxative	docusate	Colace	Increase water in the intestinal tract to soften or increase number of bowel movements
	polyethylene glycol	Miralax	
	psyllium	Metamucil	
Proton pump inhibitor	esomeprazole	Nexium	Decrease amount of acid in the stomach
	lansoprazole	Prevacid	
	omeprazole	Prilosec	
	rabeprazole	Aciphex	

   Learning Style Tip

Go to *www.youtube.com* to find videos that match the information in this chapter. Enter *gastrointestinal system* or *digestive system* into the YouTube search bar. Send a couple of your favorite videos to your classmates by clicking on "share." You can copy and paste the highlighted link into an e-mail, upload it onto a class discussion board, or post it on a social media site.

Pathologies, Procedures, and Pharmacology Practice Exercises

Deciphering Terms

Write the correct meaning of these medical terms.

Exercise 5

1. cholecystectomy _____

2. enteritis _____

3. proctoscopy _____

4. gastroscope _____

5. laparoscopy _____

6. jejunoplasty _____

7. pancreatolith _____

8. sublingual _____

9. pharyngitis _____

10. gastroenterologist _____

11. microgastric _____

12. dyskinesia _____

13. diarrhea _____

14. gastroparesis _____

15. dysphoria _____

Fill in the Blanks

Fill in the blanks below using Table 9-3.

Exercise 6

1. _____ is the accumulation of serous fluid in the peritoneal cavity.

2. A condition in which tiny pouches form in the intestinal wall is _____.

3. When the condition in the previous question includes inflammation, it is known as _____.

4. Another term for *vomiting* is _____.

5. A chronic disease of the colon marked by inflammation and frequent bloody diarrhea is _____ _____.

6. When a portion of the bowel slips inside of itself, it is called _____.

7. Excessive levels of bilirubin in the blood may result in a yellow staining of body tissues, known as _____.

8. _____ _____

    _____ is a chronic condition characterized by alternating episodes of constipation and diarrhea.

9. Internal or external varicose veins of the anal area are known as

    _____.

10. The term for a condition in which gallstones are present in the gallbladder, liver, or biliary ducts is _____.

Multiple Choice

Select the one best answer to the following multiple-choice questions.

Exercise 7

1. Mr. Green is a 63-year-old man with heartburn (GERD). When it flares up, he experiences:
    a. gastromegaly
    b. esophagostenosis
    c. esophagodynia
    d. gastromalacia

2. Mr. Smith, a 36-year-old man, has come to the clinic complaining of symptoms that are consistent with heartburn (GERD). Which of the following will accurately diagnose this condition?
    a. laparoscopy
    b. upper endoscopy
    c. esophagectomy
    d. enteropathy

3. Ms. Diaz is a 47-year-old woman with a bowel obstruction caused by a portion of her bowel twisting upon itself. This condition is known as:
    a. intussusception
    b. ulcerative colitis
    c. volvulus
    d. cirrhosis

4. Which of the following terms is **not** related to a part of the small intestine?

   a. duoden/o

   b. jujen/o

   c. colon/o

   d. ile/o

5. To obtain multiple three-dimensional images of a body structure, the physician will order:

   a. a barium swallow

   b. a CT scan

   c. an ERCP

   d. a UGI

Fill in the Blanks

Using Table 9-4, write the common use of the generic or brand name medication.

Exercise 8

1. dimenhydrinate _____

2. Zantac _____

3. Kaolin and pectin _____

4. ketamucil _____

5. Nexium _____

6. famotidine _____

7. loperamide _____

8. diphenhydramine _____

9. Colace _____

10. Prevacid _____

CASE STUDY

Read the case study and answer the questions that follow. Most of the terms are included in this chapter. Refer to the glossaries or to your medical dictionary for the other terms.

Ulcerative Colitis

Cynthia Summers is a 34-year-old married woman with two small children. She was seen by a physician at Valley Clinic this morning for an exacerbation of her ulcerative colitis. Her chief complaints were three to five episodes of bloody diarrhea per day, cramping abdominal pain, and fatigue. Mrs. Summers is thin and pale. She appears anxious and is reluctant to go to the hospital, stating that she needs to go home to take care of her family.

The physician prescribed prednisone and gave her the following dietary recommendations: Eat high-calorie foods, avoid strong spices and caffeine, and drink plenty of fluids. She is to return in 3 days for a follow-up visit or sooner if her condition worsens. If her condition cannot be controlled with medications and dietary changes, hospitalization and possibly surgery will be considered.

Ulcerative colitis is characterized by chronic inflammation of the large intestine, primarily the rectum and sigmoid colon. Onset is usually in a patient's early 20s. Lesions form in the mucosal layer, causing very tiny hemorrhages that may, in time, develop abscesses. The lesions may become necrotic and may ulcerate. The primary symptom of ulcerative colitis is bloody diarrhea accompanied by cramping abdominal pain. Episodes of diarrhea may vary from once or twice a day to as many as 30 to 40 times a day in very severe cases. As a result, anorexia, anemia, and fatigue are common. The disease usually has periods of exacerbation and remissions. Treatment includes steroid medication such as prednisone, which has a powerful anti-inflammatory effect, and dietary modifications. Severe cases may require partial or complete colectomy. People with ulcerative colitis are at increased risk for developing colon cancer.

Case Study Questions

Exercise 9

1. Ulcerative colitis usually affects which part of the intestine?
   a. ileum
   b. jejunum
   c. proximal colon
   d. distal colon

2. The medication the physician prescribed should help Mrs. Summers because:
   a. It is an analgesic, which reduces pain.
   b. It is an antibiotic, which promotes healing.
   c. It will reduce inflammation in her colon.
   d. It reduces pain by reducing acids in the intestine.

3. The age of onset of ulcerative colitis is usually:
   a. childhood
   b. the early 20s
   c. the 40s
   d. after 60

4. Lesions may become abscessed, which means that they:
   a. become infected
   b. bleed
   c. swell
   d. contain dead tissue

5. The lesions may eventually become necrotic, which means that they:
   a. heal
   b. contain dead tissue
   c. swell
   d. bleed

6. In severe cases of ulcerative colitis, the patient experiences:
   a. weight gain
   b. constipation
   c. frequent nausea
   d. loss of appetite

7. Ulcerative colitis is characterized by:
   a. Periods of improvement alternating with periods of worsening
   b. Sudden, acute onset; short duration; and total healing
   c. Gradual onset, lengthy illness, and eventual complete healing
   d. Gradual onset, chronic disability, and eventual death

8. Describe how the common symptoms of ulcerative colitis could impact a person's activities of daily living (ADLs).

9. Create a list of foods and beverages that should, and should not, be consumed to help relieve the symptoms of ulcerative colitis.

End-of-Chapter Practice Exercises

Word Building

Using **only** *the word parts in the lists provided, create medical terms with the indicated meanings.*

Exercise 10

Prefixes	Combining Forms	Suffixes
circum-	an/o	-al
hyper-	append/o	-ectomy
hypo-	appendic/o	-emesis
peri-	chol/e	-ic
	cholecyst/o	-itis
	colon/o	-lith
	dent/o	-megaly
	esophag/o	-oma
	gastr/o	-pathy
	hepat/o	-scopy
	ile/o	-stomy
	jejun/o	-tomy
	or/o	

1. disease of the liver _____

2. inflammation of the esophagus _____

3. visual examination of the esophagus and stomach _____

4. pertaining to around the mouth _____

5. excision or surgical removal of the gallbladder _____

6. enlargement of the stomach _____

7. pertaining to excessive colon _____

8. pertaining to near the anus _____

9. instrument used in examining the pharynx ————————————

10. tumor of the liver ————————————

11. inflammation of the appendix ————————————

12. excision or surgical removal of the appendix ————————————

13. cutting into or incision of the ileum ————————————

14. excessive vomiting ————————————

15. pertaining to the teeth ————————————

16. inflammation of the gallbladder ————————————

17. pertaining to below or beneath the stomach ————————————

18. visual examination of the colon ————————————

19. bile stone ————————————

20. disease of the colon ————————————

True or False

Decide whether the following statements are true or false.

Exercise 11

1. True   False   The abbreviation **BRP** stands for *bathroom prohibited.*

2. True   False   The abbreviation **NPO** means *no eating or drinking.*

3. True   False   **Crohn's disease** is a chronic inflammatory disease of the lining of the colon, marked by up to 20 liquid, bloody stools per day.

4. True   False   The abbreviation **LFT** stands for *liver function test.*

5. True   False   **Irritable bowel syndrome** is a chronic condition characterized by alternating episodes of constipation and diarrhea.

6. True   False   The abbreviation **PUD** stands for *peptic ulcer disease.*

7. True   False   An **EGD** is a procedure that involves examination of the liver.

8. True   False   The abbreviation **BM** stands for *basal metabolic rate.*

9. True   False   An accumulation of fluid in the peritoneal cavity is known as **cirrhosis.**

10. True   False   The abbreviation **GI** stands for *gastrointestinal.*

Deciphering Terms

Write the correct meaning of these medical terms.

Exercise 12

1. atrophy _____

2. gingivostomatitis _____

3. proctology _____

4. glossospasm _____

5. lithotripsy _____

6. phagophobia _____

7. dyspepsia _____

8. labionasal _____

9. odontectomy _____

10. cecectomy _____

Multiple Choice

Select the one best answer to the following multiple-choice questions.

Exercise 13

1. Mr. Washington, a 27-year-old man, has a sore throat caused by inflammation. Which of the following is the correct medical term for this condition?

   a.   pharyngitis

   b.   pharyngopathy

   c.   colitis

   d.   stomatitis

2. Which of the following terms means *bad, difficult, or painful swallowing?*

   a.   dyspepsia

   b.   dysphagia

   c.   dysphasia

   d.   dyspnea

3. Which of the following tests most accurately detects the cause of gastric ulcers?

   a. Gastroccult

   b. *H. pylori* test

   c. laparoscopy

   d. ultrasound

4. To detect gastrointestinal bleeding, the physician may order which of the following?

   a. barium enema

   b. lower endoscopy

   c. stool culture

   d. fecal occult blood test

5. Which of the following abbreviations refers to measurement of the patient's pulse, respiratory rate, blood pressure, and temperature?

   a. VS

   b. N&V

   c. CA

   d. LFT

6. Which of the following abbreviations involves the pancreas?

   a. GERD

   b. BRP

   c. ERCP

   d. EGD

7. Which of the following abbreviations refers to a procedure?

   a. IBS

   b. IBD

   c. PUD

   d. UGI

8. Which of the following indicates a route of medication administration?

   a. PO

   b. c/o

   c. GI

   d. Q

9. Which of the following disorders involves dilation and expansion of the lower esophagus due to pressure from food accumulation?

    a. cholelithiasis

    b. achalasia

    c. esophageal varices

    d. ascites

10. The definition of *pseudomembranous enterocolitis* is:

    a. accumulation of serous fluid in the peritoneal (abdominal) cavity

    b. inflammatory condition of both small and large bowels that results in severe watery diarrhea

    c. disorder of inflammation and edema deep into the layers of the lining of any part of the GI tract

    d. chronic condition characterized by alternating episodes of constipation and diarrhea

11. Which of the following is **not** a common cause of bowel obstruction?

    a. volvulus

    b. intussusception

    c. adhesions

    d. hernia

12. All of the following disorders involve the large intestine **except:**

    a. celiac disease

    b. pseudomembranous enterocolitis

    c. ulcerative colitis

    d. diverticulosis

13. The term *enterobiliary* means:

    a. abnormal condition of the cheek and esophagus

    b. pertaining to the small intestine and bile

    c. disease of the bowel

    d. within the small intestine

14. The term *gingivostomatitis* means:

    a. inflammation of the tongue and mouth

    b. inflammation of the teeth and gums

    c. inflammation of the gums and mouth

    d. inflammation of the cheek and throat

15. The term *glossolabial* means:

    a. pertaining to the gums and teeth

    b. pertaining to the gallbladder and liver

    c. pertaining to the cheek and tongue

    d. pertaining to the tongue and lips

16. Which of the following terms means *inflammation of the salivary gland?*

    a. steatitis

    b. sialadenitis

    c. stomatitis

    d. lymphadenitis

17. Which of the following terms means *enlargement of the liver and spleen?*

    a. hepatosplenomegaly

    b. splenolaparotomy

    c. splenonephric

    d. microlipolysis

18. Which of the following terms means *suturing of the rectum?*

    a. proctorrhaphy

    b. rectostenosis

    c. rectoplasty

    d. sigmoid surgery

19. Which of the following terms means *cutting instrument for the pharynx?*

    a. pharyngoscopy

    b. pharyngoscope

    c. pharyngotome

    d. pharyngotomy

20. Which of the following terms means *cutting into or incision of the abdomen and spleen?*

    a. pylorogastrectomy

    b. laparosplenotomy

    c. splenomalacia

    d. hepatopexy

10 URINARY SYSTEM

Chapter Outline

Structure and Function

The **urinary system** consists of the kidneys, ureters, bladder, and urethra. Each structure is uniquely designed and suited to its purpose. The urinary system's main functions are to filter and excrete waste products from the body, help regulate blood pressure, and maintain an optimal level of fluid and electrolytes within the body (Fig. 10-1).

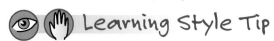 Learning Style Tip

If you are highly kinesthetic, be sure to take notes in class even if the instructor does not require it. Embellish your notes with your own diagrams, illustrations, or flowcharts. If you are a visual learner, you will get more out of this if you use colored pens or highlighters to jazz up your notes.

The key organs of the urinary system are the **kidneys,** which are located in the back of the abdominal cavity in the **retroperitoneal space,** to either side of the vertebral column. The right kidney is slightly lower than the left. Each one is surrounded by a renal capsule, made up of connective tissue and a thick layer of fat. This provides protection by acting as a cushion and a shock absorber. The renal artery, vein, nerves, and ureter exit the kidneys on the medial (inner) side.

Both kidneys are highly vascular organs made up of an outer cortex and an inner medulla. In fact, over 20% of the blood pumped by the heart each minute passes through the kidneys. The vascular nature of the kidneys lends itself to their function, which is to filter blood for the elimination of wastes and excess fluid and to regulate **electrolytes** (the ions in bodily fluids). Major electrolytes include sodium (Na), potassium (K), magnesium (Mg), and calcium (Ca).

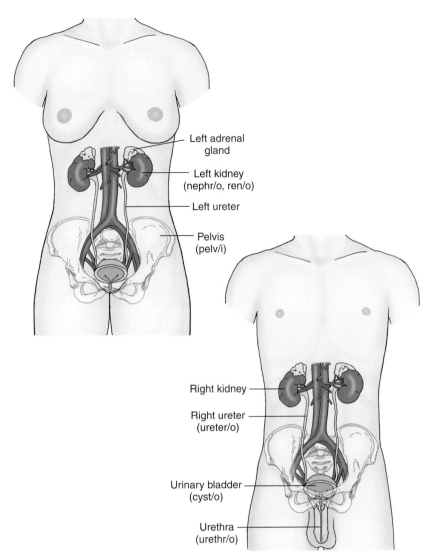

Left adrenal
gland

Left kidney
(nephr/o, ren/o)

Left ureter

Pelvis
(pelv/i)

Right kidney

Right ureter
(ureter/o)

Urinary bladder
(cyst/o)

Urethra
(urethr/o)

FIGURE 10-1 **The urinary system.**

Located primarily within the outer cortex of the kidneys are microscopic structures called **nephrons** (Fig. 10-2). There are more than one million nephrons in each kidney. Each nephron is composed of an arteriole, venule, Bowman's capsule, **glomerulus** (capillary cluster within the Bowman's capsule), proximal tubule, Henle's loop, distal tubule, and capillary bed. The nephron has long been called the functional unit of the kidney, because it is where most of the action takes place. To begin the filtration process, blood passes from a tiny arteriole into the glomerulus. The walls of the glomerulus and Bowman's capsule are designed to permit filtration of water, electrolytes, urea, and other small molecules. A large amount of this fluid (approximately 180 liters), called **filtrate,** is created each day. However, as it moves on through the proximal tubule, Henle's loop, and distal tubule, nearly all of the water and useful solutes (99%) are reabsorbed, and additional wastes are excreted. After the kidneys make final adjustments in the composition of the leftover fluid, it is called **urine.** The kidneys produce and excrete an average of 1 to 2 liters of urine each day.

Flashpoint

One in nine adults have kidney disease and millions more are at risk for getting it. The National Kidney Foundation (NKF) provides information on awareness, prevention, and treatment of this disease. Visit their website at *www.kidney.org.*

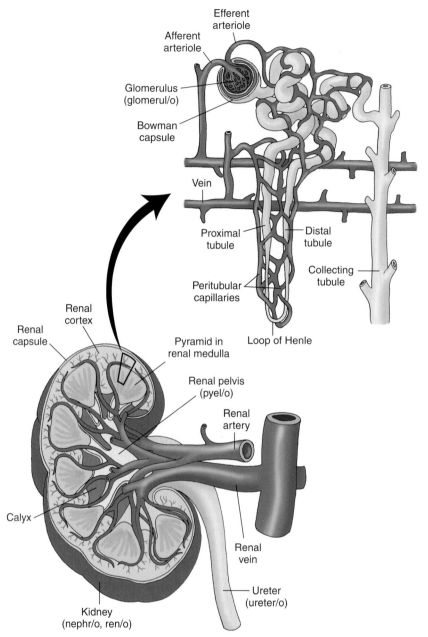

FIGURE 10-2 **The kidney and the nephron.**

Within the kidney's **medulla,** the innermost part, are several oval-shaped renal pyramids, which point inward. Cupping each one is a calyx (plural *calyces*). The area where all of the calyces join is called the **renal pelvis.** As the renal pelvis narrows, it joins the uppermost part of the ureter. When urine is formed, it drains into the calyces, which funnel the urine inward through the renal pelvis and into the ureter, which in turn drains urine from the kidney downward to the urinary bladder.

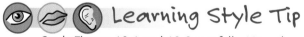 Learning Style Tip

Study Figures 10-1 and 10-2 carefully. Now close your eyes and visualize the urinary system. Note each structure in the order of urine creation and flow. As you do so, visualize it, say it aloud, and name the associated combining forms.

In addition to filtering fluid and wastes from the body, the kidneys play active roles in maintaining blood pressure and **blood pH** (acidity or alkalinity). They help regulate blood pressure by retaining or excreting more fluid and electrolytes (especially sodium). They help maintain a healthy acid-base balance by retaining or excreting buffers and acids as needed. Acid-base level is measured according to the **pH scale,** which ranges from 0 to 14 (Fig. 10-3). The pH level of human blood must remain slightly alkaline, within the very narrow range of 7.35 to 7.45. Even minor fluctuations in this balance will result in illness or even death.

The **ureters** are long, narrow tubes that drain urine from the renal pelvis to the urinary bladder. The **bladder** is a flexible, muscular container for urine; its lining is uniquely designed to stretch to accommodate varying amounts of fluid. Urine accumulates here until the volume reaches a level that stimulates stretch receptors and initiates the **micturition reflex,** which is the urge to urinate. We may temporarily ignore this urge; however, eventually, the increased urine volume stimulates the stretch receptors again, and our urge to urinate will be even stronger. At the base of the bladder is the exit into the urethra, a tube that varies in length depending on the patient's gender. The male urethra is approximately 20 cm (just under 8 inches) long, and the female urethra is approximately 4 cm (just over 1 ½ inches) long. The **urethra** functions as a passageway for final urine elimination and emptying of the bladder. *Urinary incontinence (UI)* is the involuntary leakage of urine. There are different types of UI as well as a variety of treatment options (Box 10-1).

Flashpoint
The kidneys play an important role in maintaining the body's acid-base balance.

Flashpoint
Kegel exercises can help manage the type of UI known as stress incontinence. These exercises are performed by repeatedly contracting and relaxing the muscles of the pelvic floor, as if you were starting and stopping the flow of urine.

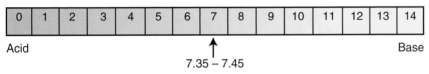

0	1	2	3	4	5	6	7	8	9	10	11	12	13	14

Acid   ↑   Base
                          7.35 – 7.45

FIGURE 10-3 **The pH scale.**

Box 10-1 Urinary Incontinence

Urinary incontinence (UI) affects millions of Americans. It is most common in older adults but it occurs in all age groups. For some people, it is slightly bothersome; for others, it is totally debilitating. Many individuals living with UI have such a strong fear of embarrassment that they stop going out in public and may even isolate themselves from friends and family. Some take unhealthy measures such as decreasing their liquid intake to avoid episodes of involuntary urine leakage.

There are different types of UI. *Stress incontinence* is a leakage of urine that occurs with coughing, sneezing, heavy lifting, or other movements that put pressure on the bladder. This type of incontinence is especially common in women because the pelvic floor muscles that support the bladder may weaken during pregnancy, childbirth, or menopause. *Urge incontinence* does not involve any particular movement or activity. A strong urge to urinate is immediately followed by an involuntary contraction, or spasm, of the bladder muscles that causes a leakage of urine. Damage to the nerves that control bladder function may cause this type of UI.

Anybody who has urine leakage should see a doctor to find out the cause. There are various treatment options including special exercises, medications, bladder retraining techniques, and surgery. UI affects people of all ages but it does not have to affect their quality of life.

Occasionally, a person may experience kidney failure, also known as **renal failure** or **end-stage renal disease (ESRD).** The most common causes of renal failure are high blood pressure and type 2 diabetes. Diabetes is a disorder in which the pancreas does not produce enough insulin or the body is resistant to the insulin that is produced. This results in abnormal metabolism of **glucose** (sugar) and fat. (This disorder is discussed more thoroughly in Chapter 12, Endocrine System.)

In some cases, when a person experiences renal failure, he or she is able to receive a kidney transplant. You may have heard of situations in which one person donates a kidney to another person. This illustrates two important points: One is that most people can live a long and normal life with only one healthy kidney; the other is that it is very difficult to lead a long and normal life without any kidneys at all.

If the person is not able to receive a transplant, he or she may live for months or even years by having regular **hemodialysis.** This is a process in which the blood is filtered through a special membrane in a dialysis machine to remove excess fluid and wastes (Fig. 10-4). Another type of dialysis, in which the patient is not hooked up to a machine, is **peritoneal dialysis.** In this case, the patient's own peritoneal membrane (in the abdominal cavity) is used as a filter. Dialysis fluid enters the peritoneal cavity through a catheter in the abdomen then is drained and replaced a few hours later (Fig. 10-5).

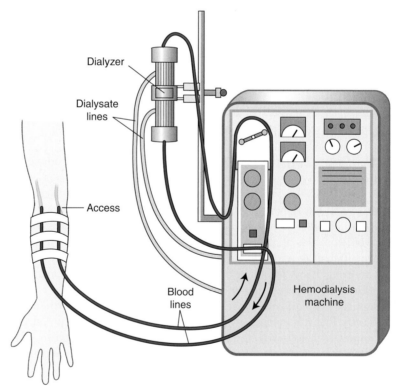

FIGURE 10-4 **Hemodialysis.**

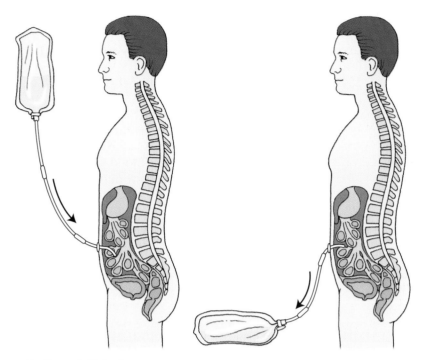

FIGURE 10-5 Peritoneal dialysis.

Structure and Function Practice Exercises

Fill in the Blanks

Choose the term that matches the description.

Exercise 1

Kidneys	Urine	Micturition reflex
Retroperitoneal space	Medulla	Urethra
Electrolytes	Blood pH	Renal failure
Nephrons	pH scale	Glucose
Filtrate	Ureters	Hemodialysis
Glomerulus	Bladder	Peritoneal dialysis
Renal pelvis	Urinary system	

1. _____ Passageway for final urine elimination and emptying of the bladder

2. _____ Microscopic structures located primarily within the outer cortex of the kidneys

3. _____ Capillary cluster within the Bowman's capsule

4. _____ The area where all of the calyces join

5. _____ The urge to urinate

6. _____ The key organs of the urinary system

7. _____ A flexible, muscular container for urine

8. _____ The acidity or alkalinity in the blood

9. _____ The innermost part of the kidney

10. _____ Long, narrow tubes that drain urine from the renal pelvis to the urinary bladder

11. _____ A process by which blood is filtered through a special membrane in a machine to remove excess fluid and wastes

12. _____ The kidneys produce an average of 1 to 2 liters of this each day

13. _____ The kidneys, ureters, bladder, and urethra

14. _____ Sugar

15. _____ A process by which blood is filtered through the patient's own membrane in the abdominal cavity to remove excess fluid and wastes

16. _____ High blood pressure and type 2 diabetes are the most common cause

17. _____ Fluid that has been filtered by the walls of the glomerulus and Bowman capsule

18. _____ Used to measure the acid-base that ranges from 0–14

19. _____ The ions in bodily fluids

20. _____ Location in the back of the abdominal cavity

Short Answer

Exercise 2

Consider all of the things you do in a typical day. Describe how having urinary incontinence would affect your activities of daily living (ADLs). Ask your class-mates or family members how it might affect their ADLs. Label Figures 10-6 and 10-7 with the appropriate anatomical terms and combining forms.

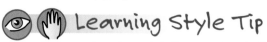 Learning Style Tip

Make copies of your labeling exercises before you fill in the blanks. This will enable you to practice labeling multiple times.

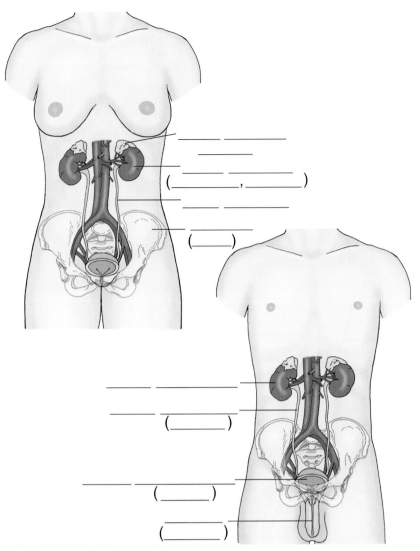

FIGURE 10-6 **Urinary system with blanks.**

Combining Forms and Abbreviations

Combining Forms

Table 10-1 contains combining forms that pertain to the urinary system, examples of terms that utilize the combining forms, and a pronunciation guide. Read aloud to yourself as you move from left to right across the table. Be sure to use the pronunciation guide so that you can learn to say the terms correctly.

IN A FLASH!

It's time to print out all of the Combining Form Flash Cards for Chapter 10 and run through them at least three times before you continue.

Flashpoint

Many of the combining forms in Table 10-1 are paired with the commonly used suffix *-uria* to describe abnormalities of urine.

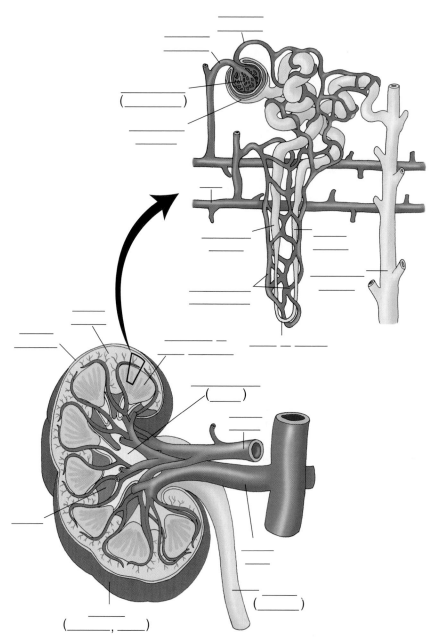

FIGURE 10-7 Kidney and nephron with blanks.

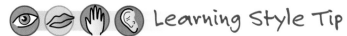 Learning Style Tip

You will get more out of class if you remain awake and alert. Therefore, if you sometimes find yourself feeling sleepy during a lecture, try adjusting your posture to sitting up straight and tall.

Abbreviations

Table 10-2 lists some of the most common abbreviations related to the urinary system, as well as others often used in medical documentation.

TABLE 10-1

COMBINING FORMS RELATED TO THE URINARY SYSTEM

Combining Form	Meaning	Example (Pronunciation)	Meaning of New Term
azot/o	nitrogenous compounds	azoturia (Ăz-ō-TŪ-rē-Ă)	nitrogenous compounds in the urine
bacteri/o	bacteria	bacteriuria (BĂK-tē-rē-Ū-rē-Ă)	bacteria in the urine
cyst/o	bladder	cystitis (sĭs-TĪ-tĭs)	inflammation of the bladder
		cystoscopy (sĭs-TŎS-kō-pē)	visual examination of the bladder
glomerul/o	glomerulus	glomerulopathy (glō-mĕr-Ū-LŎP-Ă-thē)	disease of the glomerulus
gluc/o	glucose, sugar, sweet	glucogenesis (gloo-kō-JĔN-ĕ-sĭs)	creation of glucose
glucos/o		glucosuria (gloo-kō-SŪR-ē-Ă)	sugar in the urine
glyc/o		glycemia (glī-SĒ-mē-Ă)	sugar in the blood
glycos/o		glycosuria (glī-kō-SŪ-rē-Ă)	sugar in the urine
keton/o	ketone bodies (acids and acetones)	ketonuria (kē-tō-NŪ-rē-Ă)	ketone bodies in the urine
lith/o	stone	nephrolithiasis (nĕf-rō-lĭth-Ī-Ă-sĭs)	pathological condition of kidney stones
meat/o	meatus, opening	meatotome (mē-ĂT-ŏ-tōm)	cutting (enlarging) instrument for a meatus
nephr/o	kidney	nephritis (nĕ-FRĪ-tĭs)	inflammation of the kidney
		nephropathy (nĕ-FRŎP-Ă-thē)	disease of the kidney
noct/o	night	nocturia (nŏk-TŪ-rē-Ă)	urination at night
olig/o	deficiency	oliguria (ōl-ĭ-GŪR-ē-Ă)	deficiency of urine
peritone/o	peritoneum	peritoneal (pĕr-ĭ-tō-NĒ-Ăl)	pertaining to the peritoneum
py/o	pus	pyuria (pī-ŪR-ē-Ă)	pus in the urine
pyel/o	renal pelvis	pyelonephritis (pī-ĕ-lō-nĕ-FRĪ-tĭs)	inflammation of the renal pelvis and kidney
pelv/i	pelvis	pelvic	pertaining to the pelvis
ren/o	kidney	renal (RĒ-nĂl)	pertaining to the kidneys
ur/o	urine	urology (Ū-RŎL-ō-jē)	study of disorders of the urinary tract
urin/o		urinometer (Ū-rĭ-NŎM-ĕ-tĕr)	measuring instrument for urine

Continued

TABLE 10-1
COMBINING FORMS RELATED TO THE URINARY SYSTEM—cont'd

Combining Form	Meaning	Example (Pronunciation)	Meaning of New Term
ureter/o	ureter	ureterostenosis (Ū-rē-tĕr-ō-stĕ-NŌ-sĭs)	narrowing or stricture of the ureter
urethr/o	urethra	urethropexy (Ū-RĒ-thrō-pĕk-sē)	surgical fixation of the urethra
vesic/o	bladder	vesicocele (VĔS-ĭ-kō-sēl)	hernia of the bladder
		vesicoscopy (VĔS-ĭ-kō-skō-pē)	visual examination of the bladder

TABLE 10-2
ABBREVIATIONS

AGN	acute glomerulonephritis
ARF	acute renal failure
ATN	acute tubular necrosis
BNO	bladder neck obstruction
BPH	benign prostatic hypertrophy (benign prostatic hyperplasia)
BUN	blood urea nitrogen
C&S	culture and sensitivity
Cath	catheterization, catheter
CRF	chronic renal failure
Cysto	cystoscopy
ESRD	end-stage renal disease
HD	hemodialysis
H_2O	water
I&O	intake and output
IVP	intravenous pyelogram
KUB	kidney, ureter, and bladder
PKD	polycystic kidney disease
RP	retrograde pyelogram
SG, sp. gr.	specific gravity
TURP	transurethral resection of the prostate
UA	urinalysis
UI	urinary incontinence
UC	urine culture
UTI	urinary tract infection
VCUG	voiding cystourethrography
VUR	vesicoureteral reflux

IN A FLASH!

It's time to print out all of the Abbreviations Flash Cards for Chapter 10 and run through them at least three times before you continue.

Combining Forms and Abbreviations Practice Exercises

Fill in the Blanks

Fill in the blanks below using Table 10-1.

Exercise 3

1. pertaining to the peritoneum _____

2. urination at night _____

3. hernia of the bladder _____

4. sugar in the blood _____

5. surgical fixation of the urethra _____

6. inflammation of the renal pelvis and kidney _____

7. disease of the kidney _____

8. visual examination of the bladder _____

9. nitrogenous compounds in the urine _____

10. specialist in the study of the kidneys _____

11. narrowing or stricture of the ureter _____

12. study of disorders of the urinary tract _____

13. measuring instrument for urine _____

14. sugar in the urine _____

15. ketone bodies in the urine _____

16. abnormal condition of kidney stones _____

17. inflammation of the kidney _____

18. pus in the urine _____

19. pertaining to the kidneys _____

20. cutting (enlarging) instrument for a meatus _____

21. creation of glucose _____

22. bacteria in the urine _____

23. deficiency of urine _____

24. disease of the glomerulus _____

25. inflammation of the bladder _____

Fill in the Blanks

Say the pronunciation of the term and then write the term and the abbreviation correctly. Use Table 10-2 to check your work.

Exercise 4

1. Ū-rǐ-nār-ē trĂkt ǐn-FĔK-shŭn _____

2. pŏl-ē-SĬS-tǐk KĬD-nē dǐ-ZĒZ _____

3. Ă-KYÜT glō-mĕr-Ū-lō-nĕ-FRĪ-tǐs _____

4. VĔS-ǐ-kō-ū-RĒ-tĕr-ăl RĒ-fluks _____

5. TŪ-bŪ-lĂr nĕ-KRŌ-sǐs _____

6. KRÄN-ik RĒ-nĂl FĂL-yĕr _____

7. Ū-rǐ-nār-ē ǐn-KŎNT-ǐn-ĕns _____

8. ǐn-tră-vē' nŭs pī-ĕ-lō-gr_m _____

Pathologies, Procedures, and Pharmacology

Pathology Terms

Table 10-3 includes terms that relate to diseases or abnormalities of the urinary system. Use the pronunciation guide and say the terms aloud as you read them. This will help you get in the habit of saying them properly.

TABLE 10-3

PATHOLOGY TERMS

acute glomerulonephritis (Ă-KYŪT glō-měr-Ū-lō-ně-FRĪ-tĭs)	type of nephritis (kidney infection) in which the glomeruli are the key structures affected; also called *acute nephritic syndrome*
bacterial cystitis (bak-TIR-ē-ul sĭs-TĪ-tĭs)	inflammation of the bladder caused by bacterial infection, commonly coexisting with bacterial urethritis, both of which together constitute a *UTI*, sometimes referred to as a *bladder infection*
chronic glomerulonephritis (KRÄN-ik glō-měr-Ū-lō-ně-FRĪ-tĭs)	condition in which the glomeruli suffer gradual, progressive, destructive changes, with resulting loss of kidney function; also called *chronic nephritis*
diabetic nephropathy (dī-Ă-BĚT-ĭk ně-FRŎP-Ă-thē)	kidney disease associated with diabetes that results in inflammation, degeneration, and sclerosis of the kidneys
diuresis (dī-Ū-RĒ-sĭs)	abnormal secretion of large amounts of urine
end-stage renal disease (ESRD) (END-stāj RĒ-năl dĭ-ZĒZ)	final phase of kidney disease
enuresis (ěn-Ū-RĒ-sĭs)	involuntary urination during sleep; also called *bedwetting*
frequency (FRĒ-kwun-sē)	need to urinate more often than normal
glucosuria, glycosuria (gloo-kō-SŪ-rē-Ă, glī-kō-SŪ-rē-Ă)	sugar in the urine
hydronephrosis (hī-drō-něf-RŌ-sĭs)	condition in which the renal pelvis and calyces become distended and dilated and begin to atrophy due to urine outflow obstruction

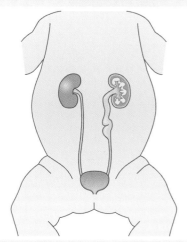

Hydronephrosis.

interstitial cystitis (ĭn-těr-STĬSH-Ăl sĭs-TĪ-tĭs)	chronic inflammatory condition of the bladder lining not caused by infection or other identified pathology
interstitial nephritis (ĭn-těr-STĬSH-Ăl něf-RĪ-tĭs)	pathological changes in renal tissue that destroy nephrons and impair kidney function
nephrotic syndrome (ně-FRŎT-ĭk SĬN-drōm)	uncommon disorder marked by massive proteinuria, edema, hypoalbuminemia (low blood albumin), hyperlipidemia (high blood lipids), and hypercoagulability (high tendency to form blood clots)

Continued

TABLE 10-3
PATHOLOGY TERMS—cont'd

neurogenic bladder (nŪ-rō-JĔN-ĭk BLĂD-ĕr)	bladder dysfunction (retention, incontinence, or altered capacity) due to disease or injury of the central nervous system or certain peripheral nerves
phimosis (fī-MŌ-sĭs)	narrowing or stricture of the foreskin opening of the penis

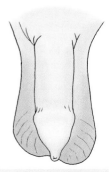

Phimosis.

polycystic kidney disease (PKD) (pŏl-ē-SĬS-tĭk KĬD-nē dĭ-ZĒZ)	group of hereditary, progressive disorders in which cysts (small sacs of fluid) form in the kidneys, eventually destroying them
pyelonephritis (pī-ĕ-lō-nĕ-FRĪ-tĭs)	inflammation and infection caused by bacterial growth in the renal pelvis and kidney
renal calculus (RĒ-nĂl KĂL-kŪ-lŭs)	small stone, composed of mineral salts, that may obstruct portions of the kidneys or a ureter; also called *kidney stone*

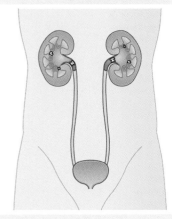

Renal calculus.

renal colic (RĒ-nĂl KĂL-ik)	severe, intermittent pain caused by spasms of the ureter
renal failure (RĒ-nĂl FĀL-yĕr)	acute or chronic failure of the kidneys to effectively eliminate fluids or wastes from the body
tubular necrosis (TŪ-bŪ-lĂr nĕ-KRŌ-sĭs)	renal failure caused by acute injury to the renal tubules
uremia (Ū-RĒ-mĕ-Ă)	increased level of urea or other wastes in the blood
urgency (UR-jĭn-sē)	need to urinate immediately

TABLE 10-3
PATHOLOGY TERMS—cont'd

urinary incontinence (UI) (Ū-rĭ-nār-ē ĭn-KŎNT-ĭn-ĕns)	involuntary urine leakage upon physical stress, such as a cough or sneeze (stress incontinence), after failing to reach a toilet in time (functional incontinence), or directly following the strong urge to urinate (urge incontinence)

Stress incontinence.

urinary retention (Ū-rĭ-nār-ē rĭ-TĚN-shŭn)	inability to urinate
urinary tract infection (UTI) (Ū-rĭ-nār-ē trĂkt ĭn-FĔK-shŭn)	inflammation and infection caused by bacterial growth in the urinary tract, usually the bladder
vesicoureteral reflux (VUR) (VĚS-ĭ-kō-ū-RĒ-tĕr-ăl RĒ-fluks)	abnormal flow of urine from the bladder back into the ureter
Wilms' tumor (vĭlmz TŪ-mor)	rapidly growing type of kidney cancer that most commonly affects children; also known as *nephroblastoma* or *malignant neoplasm of kidney*

IN A FLASH!
It's time to print out all of the Pathology Terms Flash Cards for Chapter 10 and run through them at least three times before you continue.

Common Diagnostic Tests and Procedures

24-hour urine specimen: Total urine excreted over 24 hours, collected for analysis

Bladder ultrasound (bladder scan): Noninvasive use of a portable ultrasound device to measure the amount of retained urine

Blood urea nitrogen (BUN): Lab value used to measure kidney function, based on nitrogen levels in the blood

Culture and sensitivity (C&S): Process of growing microorganisms and then exposing them to antimicrobial drugs to determine which ones kill them most effectively

Cystoscopy: Visual examination of the bladder lining with a cystoscope (Fig. 10-8)

Extracorporeal shock wave lithotripsy: Procedure in which shock waves or sound waves crush stones in the kidneys or urinary tract (Fig. 10-9)

Flashpoint
Remember the differences in the meanings of the following terms by using the associations shown below:
Diuresis happens in the **d**aytime (usually) in response to **d**rugs.
Enuresis occurs "en" (in) bed while you sleep.
Nocturia **n**udges you from bed (wakes you) at **n**ight.

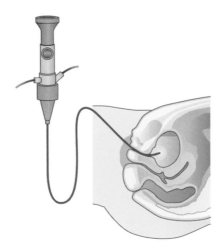

FIGURE 10-8 Cystoscopy.

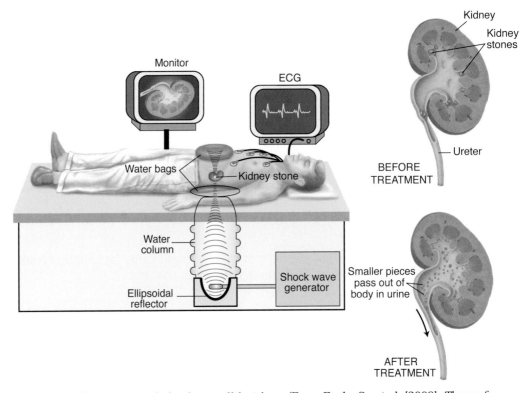

FIGURE 10-9 **Extracorporeal shock wave lithotripsy.** (From Eagle, S., et al. [2009]. *The professional medical assistant*. Philadelphia, PA: F. A. Davis Company, p. 581; used with permission)

Hemodialysis: Filtration of wastes and fluid from blood as it passes through selectively permeable membranes; also called *dialysis* (Fig. 10-4)

Intravenous pyelogram (IVP): X-ray examination of the kidneys, ureters, and bladder after injection of a contrast medium

KUB: Radiological imaging (x-ray) of the abdomen, specifically the kidneys, ureters, and bladder

Peritoneal dialysis: Filtration of fluid and wastes from the blood using the lining of the patient's peritoneal cavity as a dialyzing membrane (Fig. 10-5)

Serum creatinine: Lab value used to measure kidney function that is more specific than BUN

Urinalysis (UA): Visual and microscopic analysis of a urine specimen (Table 10-4)

Urinary catheterization: Insertion of a tube into the bladder via the urethra to drain urine, obtain a urine specimen, or instill medication (Fig. 10-10). Foley is a type of urinary catheter commonly used with hospital inpatients. A small balloon keeps the catheter in place. The urine is collected in a bag, which is usually kept hanging low, on the side of the patient's bed (Fig. 10-11).

Voiding cystourethrography (VCUG): Radiological examination of the bladder and urethra during urination

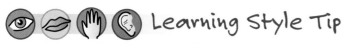 Learning Style Tip

After reading aloud the brief definition of each test or procedure from this book, look up each one in a medical dictionary and read the expanded definition found there. Then reread aloud the brief definition in this book.

Pharmacology

The most common medications for the urinary system include diuretics, electrolyte supplements, and antispasmodics (Table 10-5). Diuretics help to rid the body of excessive amounts of fluid by increasing urine output. They are used in

TABLE 10-4

NORMAL VALUES OF A URINALYSIS

Chem Stick		Microscope	
Color	Light yellow or straw	Epithelial cells	3-4
Appearance	Clear	WBCs	0-1
SG	1.010–1.030	RBCs	0
pH	5-8	Bacteria	0
Protein	Neg		
Glucose	Neg		
Ketones	Neg		
Bilirubin	Neg		
Blood	Neg		
Nitrites	Neg		

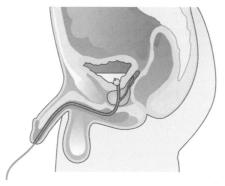

FIGURE 10-10 Urinary catheterization.

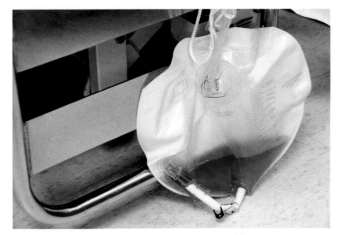

FIGURE 10-11 **Foley catheter bag.** (Photograph © Thinkstock)

TABLE 10-5			
PHARMACOLOGY			
Therapeutic Classification	**Generic Name**	**Brand Name**	**Common Use**
Antispasmodic	fesoterodine	Toviaz	Prevent uncontrollable bladder contractions
	oxybutynin	Ditropan, Oxytrol	
	solifenacin	Vesicare	
	tolterodine	Detrol	
Diuretic (loop, thiazide, or potassium sparing)	bumetanide	Bumex	Increase urine flow
	furosemide	Lasix	
	hydrochlorothiazide	Microzide, Hydrodiuril	
	spironolactone	Aldactone	
Mineral supplement	potassium chloride	Klor-Con, Micro-K	Prevent low potassium levels

Flashpoint

Muscle spasms are sudden, involuntary muscle contractions that can happen to any muscle in the body. You may have called a strong, painful, muscle spasm a "cramp."

the treatment of pathologies such as high blood pressure, congestive heart failure, kidney failure, liver failure, and edema. Some diuretics can cause low levels of the electrolyte potassium (hypokalemia). Electrolyte supplements can help to maintain, or restore, appropriate potassium levels. Antispasmodics relieve, or prevent, muscle spasms. Since the bladder is a muscular container for urine, antispasmodics are used in the treatment of overactive bladder and urinary incontinence.

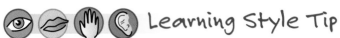 Learning Style Tip

Arrange to meet regularly with study partners. If you cannot get together in person, use a camera to have virtual study sessions. This way you are able to engage your visual and kinesthetic senses along with your verbal and auditory senses.

Pathologies, Procedures, and Pharmacology Practice Exercises

Fill in the Blanks

Fill in the blanks below.

Exercise 5

1. The term that refers to involuntary urination during sleep is

   _____.

2. The term _____ means *narrowing or stricture of the foreskin opening.*

3. The term _____ refers to an increased level of urea or other waste in the blood.

4. The term _____ refers to an abnormal secretion of large amounts of urine.

5. The term that indicates a chronic condition of inflammation of the bladder lining is _____ _____.

6. A condition in which the glomeruli suffer gradual, progressive, destructive changes, with a resulting loss of kidney function, is

   _____ _____.

7. The term _____ refers to inflammation and infection caused by bacterial growth in the renal pelvis and kidney.

8. When a person is unable to urinate or completely empty the bladder, the condition is known as _____ _____.

9. Leakage of urine when one coughs or sneezes is known as

   _____ _____.

10. The term _____ _____ refers to pathological changes in renal tissue that destroy nephrons and impair kidney function.

Multiple Choice

Select the one best answer to the following multiple-choice questions.

Exercise 6

1. During her annual health check with her nurse practitioner, Mrs. Tran states that she has recently been experiencing involuntary leakage of urine when she laughs, coughs, or sneezes. Her symptoms are most consistent with which of the following disorders?

   a. enuresis

   b. polyuria

   c. stress incontinence

   d. nocturia

2. Mrs. Fernandez tells her physician that she has been having pain in her abdomen and lower pelvic area. To gather further information, the physician orders a KUB, an x-ray procedure that specifically looks at the:

   a. kidney, uterus, and bowel

   b. kidney stones, urine, and blood

   c. kyphosis, uremia, and bones

   d. kidney, ureter, and bladder

3. Ms. Johansen has had chronic complaints of frequency, urgency, dysuria, and intermittent low-back and pelvic pain. She was initially treated with antibiotics for a presumed urinary tract infection (UTI), without any relief. A cystoscopy reveals that she has chronic inflammation of her bladder lining. This is most consistent with which of the following diagnoses?

   a. urinary retention

   b. interstitial cystitis

   c. interstitial nephritis

   d. uremia

4. Which of the following terms means *involuntary urination during sleep?*

   a. enuresis

   b. diuresis

   c. glycosuria

   d. uremia

5. A patient with which of the following conditions will typically complain of pain?

   a. neurogenic bladder

   b. renal colic

   c. diuresis

   d. enuresis

6. Which of the following conditions involves inflammation or infection?

    a. bacterial cystitis

    b. pyelonephritis

    c. glomerulonephritis

    d. all of these

7. Which of the following conditions involves a disruption in urine flow?

    a. glomerulonephritis

    b. phimosis

    c. hydronephrosis

    d. Wilms' tumor

8. Which of the following procedures involves microscopic examination of the urine?

    a. acute glomerulonephritis (AGN)

    b. urinalysis (UA)

    c. TURP

    d. polycystic kidney disease (PKD)

9. A patient with kidney stones may benefit from which of the following tests or procedures?

    a. culture and sensitivity

    b. extracorporeal shock wave lithotripsy

    c. urinary catheterization

    d. voiding cystourethrography

10. Which of the following tests will most accurately help with the diagnosis of urinary retention?

    a. bladder ultrasound

    b. blood urea nitrogen

    c. hemodialysis

    d. intravenous pyelogram

Fill in the Blanks

Using Table 10-5, write the common use of the medication next to each generic or brand name.

Exercise 7

1. spironolactone _____

2. potassium chloride _____

3. Lasix _____

4. fesoterodine _____

5. Detrol _____

6. hydrochlorothiazide _____

7. solifenacin _____

8. Vesicare _____

9. Klor-Con _____

10. Toviaz _____

CASE STUDY

Read the case study and answer the questions that follow. Most of the terms are included in this chapter. Refer to the glossaries or to your medical dictionary for the other terms.

Interstitial Cystitis

Lisa Galerno is a 32-year-old woman who came to her nurse practitioner 2 months ago with complaints of frequency, urgency, dysuria, and low-back and pelvic pain. A urine specimen was collected and analyzed. The findings were normal except for a small number of red blood cells (RBCs). Because of her symptoms, Ms. Galerno was treated for a possible UTI and was put on a course of antibiotics. She returned a week later with her symptoms unchanged. A second urine specimen was tested and showed the same results as the first. Next, Ms. Galerno was put on a different antibiotic. When she returned a week later, with still no improvement in symptoms, she was referred to a urologist for further evaluation.

After an initial consultation with the urologist, a cystoscopy was done under general anesthesia and tissue collected for a biopsy. The cytology report revealed that the specimen was benign; however, visual inspection during the cystoscopy confirmed the presence of hemorrhagic lesions and ulcerations, as well as smaller-than-normal bladder capacity. Based on these findings, a diagnosis of interstitial cystitis was confirmed. A bladder distention was performed at that time.

Interstitial cystitis (IC) is a disorder of the bladder lining that affects approximately one million people in the United States, mostly women. The cause has not been clearly identified, although severe stress appears to be a contributor. There is also some speculation that it may be autoimmune in nature. There is no known cure, and treatments are few and provide variable results.

People with IC manage their disease most effectively by noticing what seems to trigger or worsen their symptoms and what brings relief. It is essentially a process of trial and error; the results are not the same for everyone. Dietary triggers may include caffeine, alcohol, chocolate, or acidic foods such as citrus fruits; therefore, the usual remedy of drinking cranberry juice for a bladder infection is *not* helpful and may exacerbate symptoms. Some interventions that may bring relief include taking Elmiron (the only medication approved so far for IC), taking NSAIDs such as ibuprofen or naproxen, and applying heat. People with IC generally notice wide fluctuations in symptoms and will have good days and bad days. They may need to adopt lifestyle modifications and avoid activities that seem to increase their pain.

Common symptoms of IC include low-back and pelvic pain, **frequency** (the need to urinate often, caused by bladder irritation), **urgency** (the need to urinate *now*), and **dysuria** (pain or burning on urination). The symptoms are extremely variable in duration and intensity and may fluctuate dramatically throughout any given day.

Definitive diagnosis is concluded via cystoscopy, which may be performed under general anesthesia if bladder distention is planned. In this procedure, the bladder is filled with sterile saline to stretch it and increase its capacity.

Flashpoint

During cystoscopy, the physician closely examines the inner bladder wall.

Case Study Questions

Exercise 8

1. Both times that a urinalysis was performed, the findings confirmed the presence of:
   a. pus
   b. bacteria
   c. blood
   d. protein

2. Ms. Galerno was referred to a physician who specializes in the treatment of:
   a. female disorders
   b. urinary-tract disorders
   c. colorectal disorders
   d. endocrine disorders

3. The urologist performed which of the following procedures?
   a. surgical removal of the bladder
   b. surgical incision into the bladder
   c. visual examination of the bladder
   d. surgical fixation of the bladder

4. Which of the following abnormal findings were noted during the cystoscopy?
   a. small cracks and sores that bleed
   b. presence of cancerous lesions
   c. presence of an infection
   d. large bladder capacity

5. During the cystoscopy, the urologist also:
   a. injected antibiotics into the bladder
   b. used sterile salt water to stretch the bladder
   c. applied medication to the bladder lining
   d. cauterized the lesions to stop the bleeding

6. Which of the following statements is **not** true about IC?
   a. It affects women more often than men.
   b. All people with IC experience the same symptoms.
   c. There is no known cure.
   d. Each person with IC must learn by trial and error what makes symptoms better or worse.

7. Describe how the common symptoms of IC could impact a person's ADLs.

8. Create a list of foods and beverages that could worsen the symptoms of IC.

End-of-Chapter Practice Exercises

Word Building

*Using **only** the word parts in the lists provided, create medical terms with the indicated meanings.*

Exercise 9

Prefixes	Combining Forms	Suffixes
an-	azot/o	-al
dys-	bacteri/o	-algia
poly-	cyst/o	-ary
	glomerul/o	-dynia
	hemat/o	-ectomy
	lith/o	-gram
	nephr/o	-iasis
	noct/o	-ic
	olig/o	-itis
	py/o	-lith
	pyel/o	-logist
	ren/o	-plasty
	ureter/o	-scopy
	urethr/o	-uria
	ur/o	
	urin/o	
	vesic/o	

1. absence of urination _____

2. much urination _____

3. pus in the urine _____

4. bad, painful, or difficult urination _____

5. pertaining to deficient urination _____

6. pain of the urethra _____

7. visual examination of the bladder _____

8. blood in the urine _____

9. condition of a kidney stone _____

10. urination at night _____

11. bacteria in the urine _____

12. excision or surgical removal of a ureter _____

13. abnormal movement of urine from the bladder into the ureters _____

14. record of the urethra and bladder _____

15. pertaining to urine _____

16. surgical repair of the bladder _____

17. pertaining to the kidneys _____

18. inflammation of the glomerulus and kidney _____

19. nitrogenous compounds in the urine _____

20. specialist in the study and treatment of urinary disorders _____

Deciphering Terms

Write the correct meaning of these medical terms.

Exercise 10

1. retroperitoneal _____

2. meatorrhaphy _____

3. cystourethropexy _____

4. lithotripsy _____

5. urogenic _____

6. urostasis _____

7. polyuresis _____

8. ureterospasm _____

9. cystocele _____

10. nephromegaly _____

11. renopathy _____

12. urethropexy _____

13. periurethral _____

14. cystectomy _____

15. nephrotomy _____

16. ureterostomy _____

17. glomerulonephritis _____

18. polydipsia _____

19. nephrectomy _____

20. nocturia _____

21. bacteriuria _____

22. hematuria _____

23. nephrolith _____

24. anuric _____

25. cystomegaly _____

Multiple Choice

Select the one best answer to the following multiple-choice questions.

Exercise 11

1. All of the following abbreviations indicate a urinary-tract disorder **except:**

    a. ATN

    b. BUN

    c. VUR

    d. UTI

2. Which of the following terms means *blood in the urine?*

    a. bacteriuria

    b. hematuria

    c. pyuria

    d. oliguria

3. Which of the following terms means *sugar in the blood?*

    a. glycosuria

    b. glucogenesis

    c. glucosuria

    d. glycemia

4. Which of the following terms indicates absence of urination?

    a. oliguria

    b. anuria

    c. polyuria

    d. nocturia

5. Which of the following terms means pertaining to the bladder and urethra?

    a. cystoureteral

    b. vesicourethral

    c. cholecystic

    d. none of these

6. All of the following combining forms indicate sugar **except:**

    a. gluc/o

    b. glyc/o

    c. glomerul/o

    d. glycos/o

7. Which of the following combining forms refers to pus?

    a. pyel/o

    b. peritone/o

    c. py/o

    d. none of these

8. Which of the following combining forms means *stone?*

    a. lith/o

    b. azot/o

    c. cyst/o

    d. none of these

9. Which of the following combining forms means *deficiency?*

    a. nephr/o

    b. vesic/o

    c. pyel/o

    d. olig/o

10. The term *urostasis* means:

     a.   absence of urination

     b.   cessation or stopping of urine

     c.   movement of urine

     d.   resembling urine

11. The term *ureteroscope* means:

     a.   visualization of the urethra

     b.   viewing instrument for the ureter

     c.   mouthlike opening into the ureter

     d.   none of these

12. The term *nephrocentesis* means:

     a.   surgical puncture of the kidney

     b.   hernia of the kidney

     c.   behind the kidney

     d.   none of these

REPRODUCTIVE SYSTEM 11

Chapter Outline

Structure and Function

The major function of the male and female reproductive systems is procreation. The two systems work together in a complementary fashion to join a sperm and an egg at the moment of conception to create a new human being.

> *Flashpoint*
> There are approximately 20 million sperm in a normal sample amount; however, only one sperm is needed for conception, or fertilization of the egg, to occur.

Male Reproductive System

The male reproductive system shares some structures with other body systems: The penis and urethra are shared by the urinary system, and the testes are shared by the endocrine system. Other structures within the male reproductive system include the prostate gland, the scrotum, and a series of ducts and glands (Fig. 11-1).

 Learning Style Tip

If you are a strong auditory learner, you may notice that you take incomplete lecture notes because you focus more energy on listening than on writing. If this is the case, ask for your instructor's permission to record lectures to play back at a later time, with the purpose of filling in the gaps in your own notes.

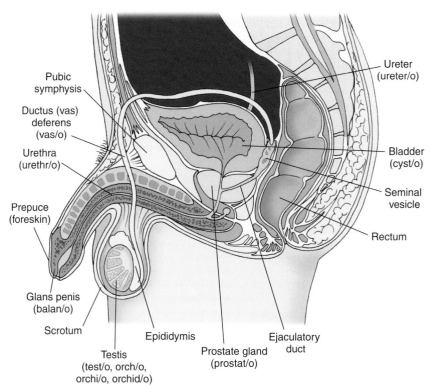

FIGURE 11-1 **The male reproductive system.**

The **testes** are located within the scrotum. They are oval-shaped structures composed of an outer capsule, made of thick, white connective tissue, and an inner part divided into 200 to 300 lobules, which contain the seminiferous tubules. **Spermatogenesis** (creation of sperm cells) occurs in the seminiferous tubules. **Spermatocytes** are the male reproductive cells, which carry half of the genetic material needed to form a new human being. These cells are sensitive to heat and must live within an environment that is slightly below normal body temperature.

Therefore, prior to birth, the testes in the male fetus normally descend from the lower abdomen into the scrotum. The **scrotum** is composed of two internal compartments surrounded by loose connective tissue and a smooth muscle layer. A second muscle group, called the **cremasters,** extends from the abdomen into the scrotum. The structures of the scrotum are designed to maintain an optimal temperature for spermatogenesis. In a cold environment, the smooth muscle of the scrotum and the cremaster muscles contract, bringing the scrotum and testes closer to the body to keep them warmer. In a warm environment, the same muscles relax and allow the scrotum and testes to descend away from the body to keep them cooler.

When spermatocytes have reached a sufficient stage of maturity, they exit the testes through a series of ducts beginning with the seminiferous tubules, then the rete testis, efferent ductules, **epididymis, vas deferens,** and finally the **ejaculatory duct,** which joins with the urethra. From there, they exit the body during ejaculation.

The penis is composed of three sections of erectile tissue and a distal, rounded end, which is the **glans penis.** A fold of skin commonly called the **foreskin** covers the glans penis. In many cultures, a procedure called circumcision is commonly practiced, in which part or all of the foreskin is removed.

Flashpoint

Male circumcision is usually performed for cultural, religious, or social reasons. Many people feel that it is an unnecessary and risky surgical procedure. Recently, the American Academy of Pediatrics (AAP) concluded that health benefits associated with circumcision outweigh the risks of the procedure.

The **urethra** serves a dual purpose, as the exit passageway for both urine and semen; however, both do not exit at the same time. During sexual activity, the **internal urinary sphincter** contracts to keep semen from entering the bladder and to keep urine from exiting the bladder.

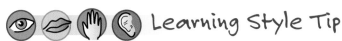 Learning Style Tip

Search for free "apps" for your mobile device. They provide a fun way to practice your new medical terminology while appealing to your learning style.

During arousal, the erectile tissue of the penis becomes engorged with blood, and the penis becomes firm and erect, to facilitate sexual intercourse and ejaculation. The state of erection ends with expulsion of semen or seminal fluid from the urethra, known as ejaculation, or when sexual arousal diminishes.

Secretions from a variety of sources contribute to the seminal fluid. Mucous secretions from the **bulbourethral glands** and the inner urethral wall lubricate the urethra and neutralize its normally acidic environment. **Seminal vesicles** secrete fructose and other nutrients for sperm cells. They also secrete a substance called **prostaglandin,** which stimulates smooth muscle contractions in the female reproductive tract. This is thought to help move sperm through that environment. The **prostate gland** secretes prostatic fluid that flows through a number of ducts to the urethra and helps to create a more alkaline environment, which is important to sperm motility.

Flashpoint

Motility is the ability of the sperm to "swim" to its destination.

Female Reproductive System

The female reproductive system is made of internal and external structures. The primary function of the female reproductive system is to bear offspring, or produce another human being. The internal and external organs and structures of the female reproductive system all function toward achieving this ultimate goal. The female reproductive system also manufactures **hormones** (chemicals secreted into the bloodstream that cause bodily reactions) that are necessary for the development and functioning of reproductive organs.

Internal organs and structures of the female reproductive system include the ovaries, fallopian tubes, uterus, cervix, and vagina (Fig. 11-2).

The **ovaries** are oval-shaped structures located on each side of the uterus in the lower abdominal cavity, attached to the broad ligament. They are the primary sex organs in females. They contain **graafian follicles,** in which are immature ova, or eggs. Approximately every 28 days, one of the ovaries produces a **mature ovum,** which contains one-half of the necessary components of a new life. The ovaries also produce the two female hormones estrogen and progesterone. **Estrogen** acts to develop the female reproductive organs during puberty, produces secondary sexual characteristics such as breasts and pubic hair, and prepares the uterus for a fertilized egg. **Progesterone** is responsible for the changes in the endometrium (uterine lining) in preparation for implantation of a developing embryo.

Flashpoint

The ovaries and the testes are somewhat round in shape, like the letter O. Terms associated with the ovaries and testes usually have lots of Os in them: *ovari/o, oophor/o, orch/o, orchi/o, orchid/o,* and so on.

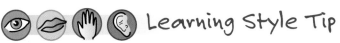 Learning Style Tip

Study Figures 11-1 and 11-2 and then draw them as accurately as you can from memory. Try speaking aloud as you do so. Add anatomical labels and related combining forms. Next, check your work against the book illustrations and make any needed corrections.

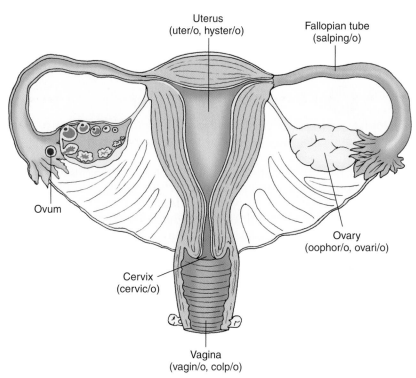

FIGURE 11-2 **The female reproductive system.**

The two **fallopian tubes** extend approximately 4 inches from the sides of the uterus toward the ovaries. Although the fallopian tubes do not connect to the ovaries directly, they are attached to the broad ligament for stability. Each fallopian tube ends with structures called fimbriae. They move in a wavelike fashion to help direct the ovum into the tube through which it travels on its way to the uterus. As the ovum travels down the fallopian tube, the ovary secretes estrogen and progesterone, which act to change the endometrial lining of the uterus to become more receptive to implantation.

The uterus is a thick-walled, muscular organ located behind the urinary bladder and in front of the rectum. It consists of the fundus, the rounded upper portion; the corpus, the body of the uterus; and the cervix, the narrowed section that opens into the vagina. The cavity of the uterus is triangular in shape; the innermost lining is called the endometrium. The myometrium, or muscular wall of the uterus, consists of muscle fibers that run in many directions, including circular, longitudinal, and diagonal. During pregnancy, the cervix and **uterus** house and protect the developing fetus. The muscular tissue of the uterus is able to expand during pregnancy to accommodate the growing fetus. The **cervix** dilates during the birth process to allow delivery of the fetus. The multidirectional muscles of the myometrium also enable forceful contraction of the uterus during the birth process. The **vagina** connects the cervix with the external surface. It acts as the passageway for the penis during sexual intercourse and as the birth canal during the birth process.

The external structures of the female reproductive system, also called the **vulva,** include the clitoris, urethral meatus, labia, mons pubis, and Bartholin's glands (Fig. 11-3). This area in men and women is also called the perineum.

The **clitoris,** made up of elongated erectile tissue, is located beneath the anterior portion of the labia. It responds to stimulation, causing orgasm. The

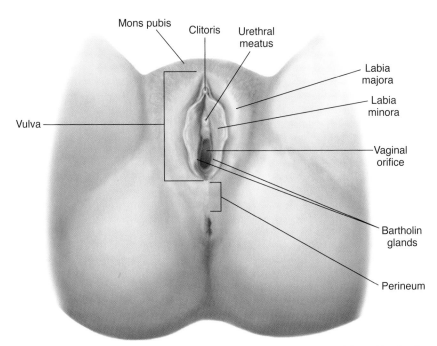

Mons pubis   Clitoris   Urethral meatus

Labia majora

Labia minora

Vulva

Vaginal orifice

Bartholin glands

Perineum

FIGURE 11-3 External structures of the female reproductive system. (From Eagle, S., et al. [2009]. *The professional medical assistant.* Philadelphia, PA: F. A. Davis Company, p. 602; with permission)

urethral meatus, located posterior to the clitoris and anterior to the vaginal opening, is the opening to the urinary bladder. The **labia** consist of two layers, covering and protecting the clitoris, urethral meatus, and vaginal opening. The inner labia minora extends from the anterior clitoris to the posterior aspect of the vaginal opening. The outer labia majora forms the lateral borders of the vulva. The labia majora and mons pubis, the pad of fatty tissue that covers the pubic symphysis (or pubic bone), are covered in coarse hair.

During puberty, increased secretion of estrogen causes breast development (Fig. 11-4). The center surface of each breast has a region of pigmented tissue called the **areola.** At the center of the areola is the **nipple.** Inside each breast are 15 to 20 lobes of glandular tissue, including mammary glands, which are milk-producing glands in a female. This glandular tissue is surrounded by connective tissue, which provides support, and adipose tissue, which provides insulation. The amount and distribution of adipose tissue determine the size and shape of the breasts. The role of the breasts in reproduction is nourishing the neonate, or newborn baby, with the mother's breast milk, a process called **lactation.**

The mammary glands of the breasts produce milk in response to the later part of pregnancy and after giving birth. During pregnancy, the breasts respond to four different hormones: Estrogen increases breast size, progesterone stimulates the development of the duct system (for lactation), prolactin stimulates milk production, and oxytocin promotes the flow of milk from the glands.

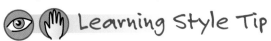 Learning Style Tip

Use social media with classmates to write "test" questions. Challenge each other every day and don't make the questions too easy! For variety, include multiple-choice, true-false, and fill-in-the-blank questions.

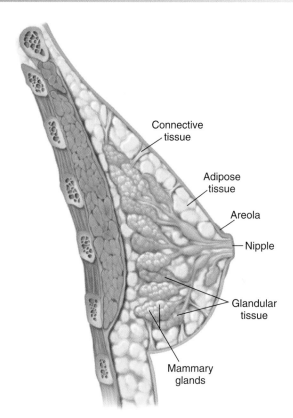

FIGURE 11-4 **Female breast.** (From Eagle, S., et al. [2009]. *The professional medical assistant.* Philadelphia, PA: F. A. Davis Company, p. 602; with permission)

Female Reproductive Cycle

The female reproductive system follows a cycle that parallels the life span. The cycle includes menarche, menstruation, pregnancy and childbirth (for some women), and menopause.

Menarche (onset of menstruation) varies widely in adolescent females, with the average age of onset being 13 years. Menstruation, also called the menstrual cycle or menses, occurs approximately every 28 days, but this timing varies. During **menstruation,** the uterus sheds the layer of endometrial tissue that develops each month in preparation for pregnancy. Phases of the 28-day cycle include the follicular, luteal, and menstrual phases.

During the **follicular phase,** the hypothalamus of the brain secretes gonadotropin-releasing hormone (GnRH), which stimulates the anterior pituitary gland to secrete follicle-stimulating hormone (FSH) and luteinizing hormone (LH). These hormones act on the graafian follicles within the ovaries to secrete estrogen, which stimulates the growth and thickening of the endometrium. Between day 9 and day 14, the ripened graafian follicle ruptures out of the ovarian wall and begins to secrete the hormone progesterone. Some women know when they are ovulating because they experience mild to moderately sharp pain on the side of the ovulating ovary. The next month, they may notice similar pain on their other side.

During the **luteal phase,** the ovum (egg cell) is propelled toward the fallopian tube by the wavelike action of the fimbriae. During this phase, progesterone produced by the **corpus luteum,** the remainder of the follicle after a woman

Flashpoint

Premenstrual syndrome (PMS) can affect women during the late stages of the menstrual cycle. Regular exercise, regular sleep, stress management, and dietary changes can help lessen the emotional and physical symptoms that may interfere with normal activities. A more severe form of PMS called premenstrual dysphoric disorder (PMDD) may require prescription medications.

ovulates, continues to cause extensive growth of the functional layer of the endometrium. If fertilization of the ovum, also called **conception,** occurs, the corpus luteum will secrete human chorionic gonadotropin (HCG) hormone. If no conception occurs, the corpus luteum does not secrete HCG but instead atrophies into a mass of fibrous tissue called the **corpus albicans.** In the absence of HCG and with decreasing progesterone levels, the endometrium begins to deteriorate, and menstruation begins.

The third and final phase of the menstrual cycle is the **menstrual phase.** In this phase, the uterus sheds the unneeded endometrial lining. The menstrual phase lasts between 5 and 7 days, after which the follicular phase begins again (Fig. 11-5).

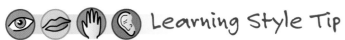 Learning Style Tip

Gather a group of two or more classmates. Use the bold terms from the Structure and Function section of this chapter to make additional flash cards. Then draw large outlines of Figures 11-1 through 11-3. Shuffle your stack of cards and take turns choosing a card from the top of the stack. Depending on the term on the card, either "label" your drawings by placing the card on the appropriate area or state the definition of the term.

Pregnancy

Fertilization occurs when one sperm penetrates an egg and forms a zygote (Box 11-1). The resulting **zygote** has 23 chromosomes from the ovum and 23 chromosomes from the sperm. The zygote immediately begins growing and multiplying as it travels down the fallopian tube. When it reaches the uterus in 4 to 6 days, it implants into the uterine wall. Implantation of the zygote causes

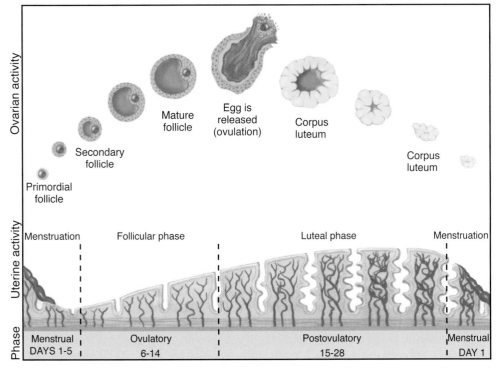

FIGURE 11-5 **Phases of the menstrual cycle.** (From Eagle, S., et al. [2009]. *The professional medical assistant.* Philadelphia, PA: F. A. Davis Company, p. 605; with permission)

Box 11-1 Twins

Fraternal twins develop when two separate eggs are fertilized by two separate sperm. They are *dizygotic*. They are not always the same sex and do not always have the same blood type. Fraternal twins may be difficult to tell apart, such as the famous Mary-Kate and Ashley Olsen, or they may not look any more alike than siblings born at separate times. Approximately two-thirds of twin pregnancies result in fraternal twins.

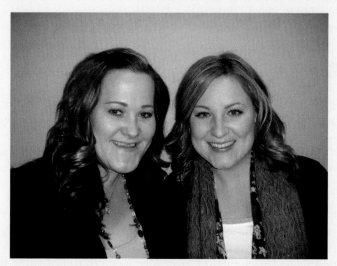

Fraternal twins.

Identical twins develop when a single egg is fertilized by a single sperm and then splits into two identical halves. They are *monozygotic*. They are always the same sex, always have the same blood type, and essentially have the same DNA. They are not clones, however, and environmental factors contribute to differences between them.

Hyperovulation, or releasing more than one egg during an ovulation cycle, is the most common reason for twin pregnancy. Several factors can increase the likelihood that hyperovulation will occur: if the mother is nearing the end of her reproductive years (i.e., 35 to 39 years old), if she is using fertility treatments, or if she has inherited a gene for hyperovulation.

a change in the menstrual cycle: The ovaries respond to implantation by releasing high levels of estrogen and progesterone, which increases the endometrium's receptivity to implantation. The corpus luteum secretes a substance called inhibin. As its name implies, inhibin acts to inhibit secretion of FSH in the anterior pituitary gland. It also causes the secretion of relaxin, which prevents uterine contraction, increasing the likelihood of successful zygote implantation. The resulting low level of FSH, along with low levels of LH, prevent stimulation of a new follicle and disrupt the 28-day menstrual cycle. After implantation, the **placenta,** the organ of nutrition for the growing zygote, forms within the wall of the uterus.

As the zygote develops into an embryo and then a fetus, the placenta also grows to provide nourishment and oxygen. The placenta begins forming early after conception and is completely formed by 12 weeks. The mature, disk-shaped placenta is approximately 7 inches in diameter. It adheres to the wall of the uterus and connects to the developing fetus through the umbilical cord. The **umbilical cord** contains two arteries and one vein; the arteries supply oxygen and nutrients to the fetus, while the vein removes carbon dioxide and wastes.

The corpus luteum secretes HCG, a hormone that stimulates the maternal ovary so that it will continue to secrete estrogen and progesterone. As the placenta increases in size, it secretes estrogen and progesterone itself, and HCG levels in the bloodstream drop. Estrogen prevents the secretion of FSH and LH (in the anterior pituitary gland); without these hormones, the menstrual cycle ceases. Progesterone prevents contractions of the uterus that could result in a miscarriage.

Pregnancy, also called **gestation,** is broken into three equal time periods called **trimesters.** The first trimester lasts 12 weeks. During this period, the zygote becomes an **embryo** and develops all its tissues and organs. At 9 weeks, the embryo is called a **fetus.** Symptoms commonly experienced by the pregnant woman during the first trimester include fatigue, nausea, vomiting, breast tenderness, urinary frequency, constipation, and insomnia.

The second trimester begins around week 13. At 15 to 28 weeks, the uterus expands to above the umbilicus, and the expectant mother can feel the first fetal movements. By 20 weeks, the fetus can open its eyes, and by 24 weeks it can hear sounds made outside the uterus. As the second trimester progresses, fetal movements become more vigorous, and the mother may be aware of when the fetus is sleeping or awake. This is a time of rapid growth, during which the fetus develops eyelashes, eyebrows, and subcutaneous fat deposits. Even so, the fetus still weighs less than 2 pounds and is not yet ready for birth.

During the third trimester, the fetus adds more subcutaneous fat, the lungs grow toward full development, and the testes descend in males. Maternal weight gain can be in excess of 1 pound per week. During this trimester, the mother may experience low back pain and fatigue because of increasing fetal size and quantity of amniotic fluid. By the end of the seventh month, or 28 weeks, the fetus has typically moved into the head-down position in anticipation of birth. At full term, 38 to 40 weeks, average fetal weight is approximately 3400 grams (7 1/2 pounds) (Fig. 11-6).

Flashpoint
Even though we refer to it as 9 months, pregnancy lasts about 40 weeks. An average newborn infant typically weighs about 7 pounds and is about 20 inches long.

Birth Process

Toward the end of gestation, the placental secretion of progesterone decreases, while the levels of estrogen remain high. The uterus begins to gently contract at irregular intervals. These early **Braxton Hicks contractions** are sometimes called *false labor.* The beginning of labor and delivery is usually signaled by the expulsion of the mucous plug that develops in the cervix to protect the fetus from organisms in the vagina. After expulsion of the mucous plug, amniotic fluid may begin to leak slowly or may flow quickly. The uterus begins more rhythmic contractions because of the drop in the secretion of progesterone from the placenta.

The first stage of active labor begins with **dilation** (expansion or opening) and **effacement** (thinning) of the cervix. The degree of cervical dilation is measured in centimeters, from 1 to 10 centimeters. At 10 centimeters, the cervix is large enough to accommodate delivery. Uterine contractions increase in frequency and intensity in this stage, which can last from 1 to 24 hours.

The second stage of labor involves delivery of the infant. In this stage, the posterior pituitary gland secretes oxytocin, a powerful hormone that causes even more forceful contraction of the uterus. During these contractions, the woman typically feels the need to "push," or bear down. Eventually the top of the infant's head appears at the cervical opening, a process called **crowning.** As soon as the infant's head delivers, it rotates to the side, and then the shoulders are delivered, followed by the rest of the body.

Period of dividing zygote, implantation, and bilaminar embryo (in weeks)

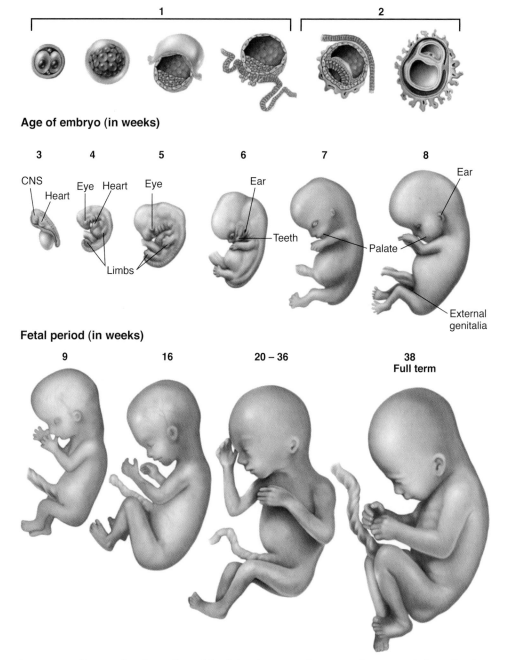

Age of embryo (in weeks)

Fetal period (in weeks)

FIGURE 11-6 **Stages of embryonic and fetal development.** (From Eagle, S., et al. [2009]. *The professional medical assistant.* Philadelphia, PA: F. A. Davis Company, p. 606; with permission)

In the third stage of labor, the placenta detaches from the uterine wall and is expelled from the body, usually with a few more uterine contractions. The uterus continues to contract after delivery, to constrict blood vessels and control bleeding.

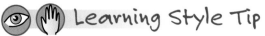 Learning Style Tip

Identify whether there are museums in your area with anatomical displays. One that allows you to touch the displays would be especially useful. Visit and study the models.

Menopause

The menstrual cycle continues throughout a woman's life until a period called **menopause,** the normal cessation of menses. Menopause occurs naturally in most women approximately 40 years after menarche. Menses may stop suddenly, or the flow and frequency of menses may decrease gradually.

Symptoms of menopause begin soon after the ovaries stop functioning, vary widely in severity, and may last from a few months to several years. Common signs and symptoms of menopause include hot flashes, chills, night sweats, mood swings, and insomnia. Treatment of menopausal symptoms may include hormone replacement therapy (HRT). However, because there are some associated risks, each woman should consult with her health-care provider to determine whether or not HRT is a viable option for her.

Flashpoint
Postmenopausal women have an increased risk of developing osteoporosis because of decreased levels of the hormone estrogen.

Structure and Function Practice Exercises

Fill in the Blanks

Choose the male or female reproductive system term that matches the description.

Exercise 1

Testes
Spermatogenesis
Spermatocytes
Scrotum
Cremasters
Epididymis, vas deferens, and ejaculatory duct
Glans penis
Foreskin
Urethra
Internal urinary sphincter

Bulbourethral glands
Seminal vesicles
Prostaglandin
Prostate gland
Hormones
Ovaries
Graafian follicles
Mature ovum
Estrogen
Progesterone

Fallopian tubes
Uterus
Cervix
Vagina
Vulva
Clitoris
Labia
Areola
Nipple
Lactation

1. _____ Lubricate the urethra and neutralize its acidic environment

2. _____ Acts as the passageway for the penis during sexual intercourse and as the birth canal during the birth process

3. _____ The distal, rounded end of the penis

4. _____ Chemicals secreted into the bloodstream that cause bodily reactions

5. _____ Contains one-half of the necessary components of a new life and is produced by the ovaries every 28 days

6. _____ Composed of two internal compartments and structures designed to maintain an optimal temperature for spermatogenesis

7. _____ Two of these extend approximately 4 inches from the sides of the uterus toward the ovaries

8. _____ The narrowed section of the uterus that dilates during the birth process to allow delivery of the fetus

9. _____ The exit passageway for both urine and semen

10. _____ Two layers of tissue that cover and protect the clitoris, the urethral meatus, and the vaginal opening

11. _____ A region of pigmented tissue at the center surface of each breast

12. _____ Secrete fructose, prostaglandin, and other nutrients for sperm cells

13. _____ The production of breast milk to nourish the newborn baby

14. _____ Located within the scrotum and contain the seminiferous tubules

15. _____ Houses and protects the developing fetus; its muscular tissue is able to expand as the fetus grows

16. _____ Stimulates smooth muscle contractions in the female reproductive tract to help move sperm

17. _____ The oval-shaped structures on each side of the uterus that are the primary sex organs in females

18. _____ Spermatocytes will exit the testes through these ducts that join with the urethra

19. _____ A hormone that is responsible for changes in the uterine lining in preparation for implantation of a developing embryo

20. _____ Male reproductive cells

21. _____ Are found within the ovaries and contain the immature ova, or eggs

22. _____ Secretes fluid that helps to create a more alkaline environment in the urethra

23. _____ A muscle group that extends from the abdomen into the scrotum

24. _____ The center of the areola

25. _____ A hormone that prepares the uterus for a fertilized egg

26. _____ Creation of sperm cells

27. _____ Elongated erectile tissue located beneath the anterior portion of the labia

28. _____ Contracts to keep semen from entering the bladder and to keep urine from exiting the bladder

29. _____ The external structures of the female reproductive system

30. _____ A fold of skin that covers the penis

Fill in the Blanks

Choose the reproductive cycle, pregnancy, birth process, or menopause term that matches the description.

Exercise 2

Menarche	Menstrual phase	Embryo
Menstruation	Fertilization	Fetus
Follicular phase	Zygote	Braxton Hicks contractions
Luteal phase	Placenta	Dilation
Corpus luteum	Umbilical cord	Effacement
Conception	Gestation	Crowning
Corpus albicans	Trimesters	Menopause

1. _____ Organ of nutrition that begins forming early after conception and connects to the developing fetus through the umbilical cord

2. _____ Fertilization of the ovum

3. _____ The zygote becomes this as all of the tissues and organs develop during the first nine weeks

4. _____ A term for pregnancy

5. _____ The second phase of the menstrual cycle in which the ovum is propelled toward the fallopian tube and conception may occur

6. _____ A term for expansion or opening of the cervix

7. _____ When one sperm penetrates an egg and forms a zygote

8. _____ The top of the infant's head appears at the cervical opening

9. _____ Approximately every 28 days, the uterus sheds the layer of endometrial tissue that develops each month in preparation for pregnancy

10. _____ The normal cessation of menses that occurs approximately 40 years after menarche

11. _____ Three equal time periods in a pregnancy

12. _____ The corpus luteum atrophies into this mass of fibrous tissue if conception does not occur

13. _____ At nine weeks, the embryo is called this

14. _____ The first phase of the menstrual cycle in which a woman is ovulating

15. _____ A term for thinning of the cervix

16. _____ Contains 23 chromosomes from the ovum and 23 chromosomes from the sperm and will develop into an embryo and then a fetus

17. _____ Gentle contractions of the uterus at irregular intervals also known as false labor

18. _____ The remainder of the graafian follicle after ovulation

19. _____ Contains two arteries, which supply oxygen and nutrients to the fetus, and one vein that removes carbon dioxide and wastes

20. _____ The third phase of the menstrual cycle in which the uterus sheds the unneeded endometrial lining

21. _____ Onset of menstruation

Fill in the Blanks

Label Figure 11-7 with the appropriate anatomical terms and combining forms.

Exercise 3

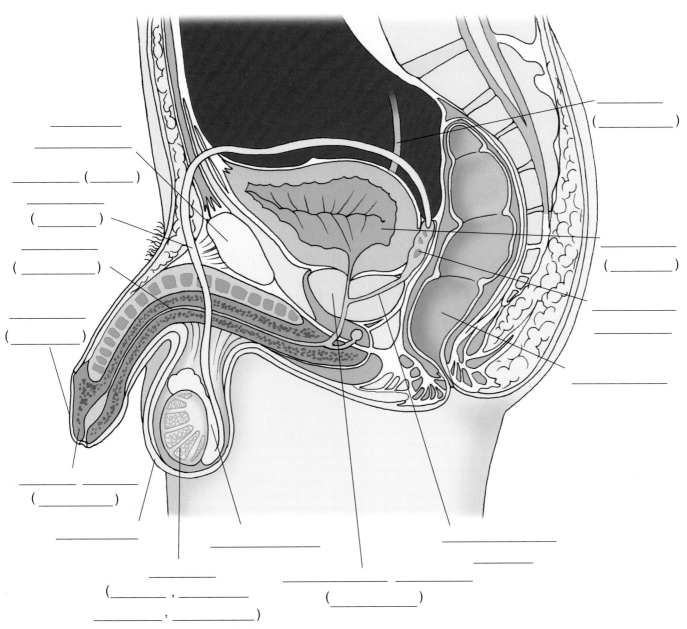

FIGURE 11-7 **Male reproductive system with blanks.**

Fill in the Blanks

Label Figure 11-8 with the appropriate anatomical terms and combining forms.

Exercise 4

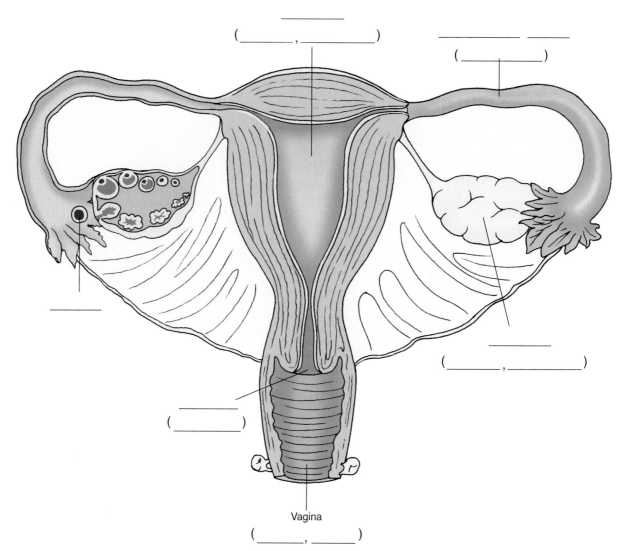

FIGURE 11-8 **Female reproductive system with blanks.**

Combining Forms and Abbreviations

Combining Forms

Tables 11-1 and 11-2 contain combining forms that pertain to the male and female reproductive systems, respectively, along with examples of terms that utilize the combining forms, and a pronunciation guide. Read aloud to yourself as you move from left to right across the table. Be sure to use the pronunciation guide so that you can learn to say the terms correctly.

IN A FLASH!

It's time to print out all of the Combining Form Flash Cards for Chapter 11 and run through them at least three times before you continue.

TABLE 11-1

COMBINING FORMS RELATED TO THE MALE REPRODUCTIVE SYSTEM

Combining Form	Meaning	Example (Pronunciation)	Meaning of New Term
andr/o	male	androgynous (ăn-DRŎJ-ĭ-nŭs)	pertaining to male and female
balan/o	glans penis	balanitis (băl-ă-NĪ-tĭs)	inflammation of the glans penis
crypt/o	hidden	cryptorchidism (krĭpt-OR-kĭd-ĭ-zum)	condition of hidden testes
epididym/o	epididymis	epididymitis (ĕp-ĭ-dĭd-ĭ-MĪ-tĭs)	inflammation of the epididymis
orch/o	testis	orchiopathy (ōr-kē-OP-ă-thē)	disease of a testis
orchi/o		orchiectomy (ŏr-kē-ĔK-tō-mē)	surgical removal of a testis
orchid/o		orchidopexy (ŎR-kĭ-dō-pĕk-sē)	surgical fixation of a testis
testicul/o		testicular (tĕs-TĬK-ū-lăr)	pertaining to the testes
phall/i	penis	phalloid (FĀL-oyd)	resembling a penis
prostat/o	prostate	prostatectomy (PRŎS-tă-tĔK-tō-mē)	surgical removal of part or all of the prostate gland
semin/o	sperm	seminuria (sē-mĭn-Ū-rē-ă)	semen in the urine
sperm/o		aspermia (ă-SPĔR-mē-ă)	failure to form semen or to ejaculate
spermat/o		spermatogenesis (spĕr-măt-ō-JĔN-ĕ-sĭs)	production of sperm
vas/o	vessel	vasotomy (văs-ŎT-ō-mē)	incision of the vas deferens

TABLE 11-2

COMBINING FORMS RELATED TO THE FEMALE REPRODUCTIVE SYSTEM

Combining Form	Meaning	Example (Pronunciation)	Meaning of New Term
amni/o	amnion (amniotic sac), amniotic fluid	amniocentesis (ăm-nē-ō-sěn-TĒ-sĭs)	surgical puncture of the amnion
cervic/o	cervix	cervical (SĚR-vĭ-kăl)	pertaining to the cervix
colp/o	vagina	colposcopy (kŏl-PŎS-kō-pē)	visual examination of the vagina
vagin/o		vaginopexy (VĂJ-ĭn-ō-pěk-sē)	surgical fixation of the vagina
embry/o	embryo	embryonic (ěm-brē-ŎN-ĭk)	pertaining to an embryo
episi/o	vulva	episiotomy (ě-pĭz-ē-ŎT-ō-mē)	cutting into or incision of the vulva (perineum)
vulv/o		vulvodynia (vŭl-vō-DĬN-ē-ă)	pain of the vulva
fet/o	fetus	fetotoxic (fē-tō-TŎK-sĭk)	poisonous to a fetus
galact/o	milk	galactorrhea (gă-lăk-tō-RĒ-ă)	flow or discharge of milk
lact/o		lactotherapy (lăk-tō-THĚR-ă-pē)	milk therapy
gonad/o	gonads	gonadectomy (gŏn-ă-DĚK-tō-mē)	surgical removal of a gonad
gynec/o	woman, female	gynecology (gī-ně-KŎL-ō-jē)	study of female (disorders)
hyster/o	uterus	hysterotomy (hĭs-těr-ŎT-ō-mē)	cutting into or incision of the uterus
metr/o		metrocarcinoma (MET-ro-kärs-ă-nō-mă)	cancerous tumor of the uterus
uter/o		uterocervical (ū-těr-ō-SĚR-vĭ-kăl)	pertaining to the uterus and cervix
lapar/o	abdomen, abdominal wall	laparoscopy (lăp-ăr-ŎS-kō-pē)	visual examination of the abdomen
mamm/o	breast	mammoplasty (MĂM-ō-plăs-tē)	surgical repair of a breast
mast/o		mastectomy (măs-TĚK-tō-mē)	surgical removal of a breast
men/o	menses	dysmenorrhea (dĭs-měn-ō-RĒ-ă)	bad, painful, or difficult menstrual flow
nat/o	birth	natal (NĀ-tăl)	pertaining to birth
oophor/o	ovary	oophorectomy (ō-ŏf-ō-RĚK-tō-mē)	surgical removal of an ovary
ovari/o		ovariocele (ō-vă-rē-ō-sēl)	tumor or hernia of the ovary
ov/o	ovum	ovogenesis (ō-vō-JĚN-ě-sĭs)	creation of an ovum

TABLE 11-2

COMBINING FORMS RELATED TO THE FEMALE REPRODUCTIVE SYSTEM—cont'd

Combining Form	Meaning	Example (Pronunciation)	Meaning of New Term
perine/o	perineum	perineoplasty (pĕr-ĭ-NĒ-ō-plăs-tē)	surgical repair of the perineum
placent/o	placenta	placental (plă-SĔN-tăl)	pertaining to the placenta
salping/o	tube (fallopian or eustachian)	salpingitis (săl-pĭn-JĪ-tĭs)	inflammation of a fallopian tube
son/o	sound	sonorous (sun-ŌR-ŭs)	full and loud in sound
vagin/a	vagina	vaginapexy (vă-JĪ-nă-pexē)	surgical fixation of the vagina

Abbreviations

Table 11-3 lists some of the most-common abbreviations related to the reproductive system, as well as others often used in medical documentation.

IN A FLASH!
It's time to print out all of the Abbreviation Flash Cards for Chapter 11 and run through them at least three times before you continue.

TABLE 11-3

ABBREVIATIONS

Female Reproductive System

♀	female
AB	abortion
BSE	breast self-examination
C-section	cesarean section
D&C	dilation and curettage
EDC	estimated date of confinement (due date)
ERT, HRT	estrogen replacement therapy, hormone replacement therapy
FHR	fetal heart rate
GYN	gynecology
IUD	intrauterine device
IVF	in vitro fertilization
L&D	labor and delivery
LMP	last menstrual period

Continued

TABLE 11-3	
ABBREVIATIONS—cont'd	
OB-GYN	obstetrics and gynecology
OC	oral contraceptive
Pap	Papanicolaou smear
PID	pelvic inflammatory disease
PMS	premenstrual syndrome
TAH	total abdominal hysterectomy
TAH-BSO	total abdominal hysterectomy, bilateral salpingo-oophorectomy
TSS	toxic shock syndrome

Male Reproductive System

♂	male
BPH	benign prostatic hypertrophy; also called *benign prostatic hyperplasia*
CIRC, circum	circumcision
DRE	digital rectal examination
ED	erectile dysfunction
PSA	prostate-specific antigen
TSE	testicular self-examination
TURP	transurethral resection of the prostate

Male and Female Reproductive Systems

GC	gonorrhea
GU	genitourinary
HPV	human papilloma virus
STD, STI	sexually transmitted disease, sexually transmitted infection
Trich	trichomoniasis
VD	venereal disease; sexually transmitted disease

Combining Forms and Abbreviations Practice Exercises

Fill in the Blanks

Fill in the blanks below using Table 11-1.

Exercise 5

1. resembling a penis _____

2. surgical removal of a testis _____

3. cutting into or incision of a vessel _____

4. pertaining to male and female _____

5. inflammation of the glans penis _____

6. production of sperm _____

7. condition of hidden testes _____

8. surgical fixation of a testis _____

9. inflammation of the epididymis _____

10. enlargement of a testis _____

11. disease of a testis _____

12. surgical repair of the prostate _____

13. pertaining to the penis and scrotum _____

14. condition of no sperm _____

15. pertaining to the testes _____

16. semen in the urine _____

Fill in the Blanks

Fill in the blanks below using Table 11-2.

Exercise 6

1. surgical puncture of the amnion _____

2. prolapse of the ovary _____

3. pertaining to the embryo _____

4. pertaining to the cervix _____

5. poisonous to the fetus _____

6. surgical removal of an ovary _____

7. flow or discharge of milk _____

8. pertaining to the uterus _____

9. milk therapy _____

10. visual examination of the vagina _____

11. surgical removal of a gonad _____

12. surgical repair of a breast _____

13. cancerous tumor of the uterus _____

14. bad, painful, or difficult menstrual flow _____

15. pertaining to the uterus and cervix _____

16. cutting into or incision of the vulva (perineum) _____

17. creation of an ovum _____

18. pain of the vulva _____

19. drooping of the ovary _____

20. cutting into or incision of the uterus _____

21. surgical repair of the perineum _____

22. visual examination of the abdomen _____

23. pertaining to the placenta _____

24. inflammation of a fallopian tube _____

25. surgical removal of a breast _____

Fill in the Blanks

Fill in the blanks below using Table 11-3.

Exercise 7

1. The abbreviation *Gyn* stands for _____.

2. *STI* stands for _____ _____

   _____.

3. The abbreviation *TAH-BSO* stands for _____

_____ _____

_____ _____

_____.

4. Marcella will see her OB-GYN physician every week during her 9th month of pregnancy. *OB-GYN* stands for _____

_____ _____.

5. The abbreviation for oral contraceptive is _____.

6. Danielle's nurse practitioner recommends that she have a Pap test once a year. *Pap* is an abbreviation that stands for _____.

7. Carla and her husband have tried unsuccessfully for 4 years to have a baby. They are now considering IVF, which is _____

_____ _____.

8. Nicholas is a 65-year-old man with BPH, or _____

_____ _____.

9. The inability of a man to achieve or maintain erection is known as

_____.

10. Nicholas will undergo a procedure known as a TURP, or

_____ _____

_____ _____

_____.

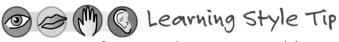 Learning Style Tip

Trace your finger across the terms as you read them, and the definitions, aloud. Then close your eyes, visualize each term, and say it and its corresponding definition aloud again.

Pathologies, Procedures, and Pharmacology

Pathology Terms

Table 11-4 includes terms that relate to diseases or abnormalities of the reproductive system. Use the pronunciation guide and say the terms aloud as you read them. This will help you get in the habit of saying them properly.

TABLE 11-4	
PATHOLOGY TERMS	
Female Reproductive System	
amenorrhea (ă-měn-ō-RĒ-ă)	absence of menses in a woman between the ages of 16 and 40
Bartholin's gland cyst (BĂR-tō-lĭnz glănd sĭst)	blockage of one or both of the Bartholin's glands, causing inflammation and tenderness

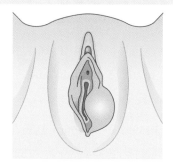

Bartholin's gland cyst.

candidiasis (kăn-dĭ-DĪ-ă-sĭs)	vaginal fungal infection caused by *Candida albicans,* with key symptoms including itching, burning, and a thick, curdy discharge; also known as a vaginal *yeast infection*

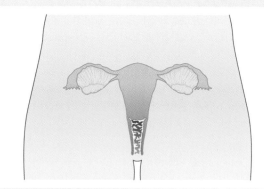

Candida albicans (vaginal yeast infection).

dysmenorrhea (dĭs-měn-ō-RĒ-ă)	pain in the lower abdominopelvic area and other discomfort associated with menses

TABLE 11-4

PATHOLOGY TERMS—cont'd

ectopic pregnancy (ĕk-TŎ-pĭk PRĔG-năn-sē)	implantation of a fertilized ovum outside of the uterus, often in the fallopian tube; also called *tubal pregnancy*

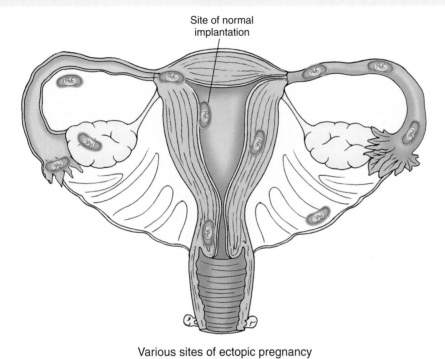

Various sites of ectopic pregnancy

Ectopic pregnancy.

endometriosis (ĕn-dō-mē-trē-Ŏ-sĭs)	growth of endometrial tissue in abnormal sites in the lower abdominopelvic area

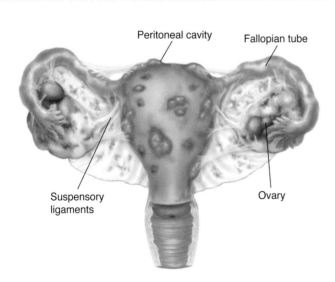

Endometriosis. (From Eagle, S., et al. [2009]. *The professional medical assistant.* Philadelphia, PA: F. A. Davis Company, p. 616; with permission)

Continued

TABLE 11-4

PATHOLOGY TERMS—cont'd

fibrocystic breast disease (fī-brō-SĬS-tĭk brĕst dĭ-ZĒZ)	presence of multiple lumps in the breast, consisting of fibrous tumors or fluid-filled cysts

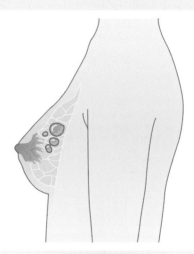

Fibrocystic breast disease.

infertility (ĭn-fĕr-TIL-ĭ-tē)	inability to achieve pregnancy after trying to conceive for a period of 1 year or more; may be primary, which is an inability to conceive a first child, or secondary, which is infertility in a woman who has previously conceived
ovarian cyst (ō-VĂ-rē-ăn sĭst)	sac of fluid or semisolid mass that grows within the ovary

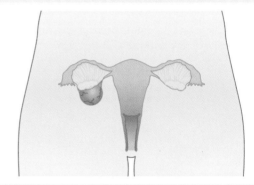

Ovarian cyst.

pelvic inflammatory disease (PID) (PĔL-vĭk ĭn-FLĂ-mă-tōrē dĭ-ZĒZ)	any acute or chronic infection of the female reproductive system, including the uterus, fallopian tubes, and ovaries
premenstrual syndrome (prē-MĔN-stroo-ăl SĬN-drōm)	range of symptoms occurring 7 to 14 days before menstruation, including fluid retention, bloating, temporary weight gain, breast tenderness, headaches, depression, irritability, diarrhea, constipation, and appetite changes
toxic shock syndrome (TSS) (TŎKS-ĭk shŏk SĬN-drōm)	rare disorder caused by bacterial exotoxins; most commonly occurs in young women who use tampons

TABLE 11-4

PATHOLOGY TERMS—cont'd

uterine fibroids (Ŭ-tĕr-ĭn FĪ-broyds)	benign, smooth tumors made of muscle and fat; also called *leiomyomas*

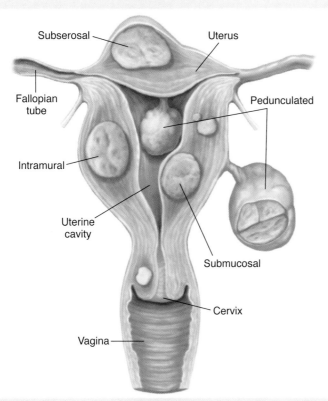

Uterine fibroids. (From Eagle, S., et al. [2009]. *The professional medical assistant.* Philadelphia, PA: F. A. Davis Company, p. 617; with permission)

uterine prolapse (Ŭ-tĕr-ĭn PRŌ-lăps)	downward protrusion of the uterus into the vaginal opening

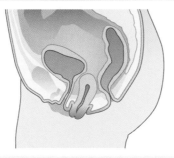

Uterine prolapse.

Complications of Pregnancy

abortion (ă-BOR-shŭn)	spontaneous or therapeutic loss of a pregnancy at less than 20 weeks; also called *miscarriage*

Continued

TABLE 11-4
PATHOLOGY TERMS—cont'd

abruptio placentae (ă-BRŬP-shē-ō plă-SĔN-tă)	sudden, premature detachment of the placenta from the uterine wall

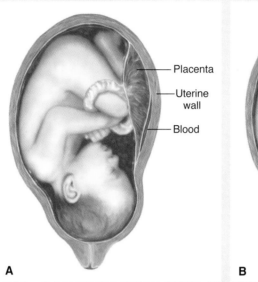
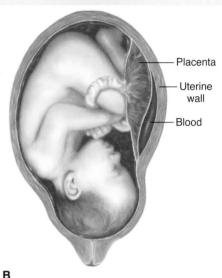

A

B

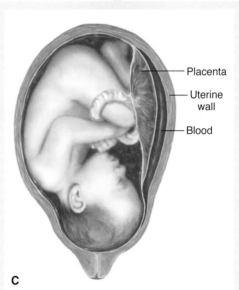

C

Abruptio placentae: (A) grade 1, (B) grade 2, (C) grade 3. (From Eagle, S., et al. [2009]. *The professional medical assistant.* Philadelphia, PA: F. A. Davis Company, p. 620; with permission)

eclampsia (ĕ-KLĂMP-sē-ă)	complication of pregnancy characterized by severe hypertension, seizures, and possible coma
gestational diabetes (jĕs-TĀ-shŭn-ăl dī-ă-BĒ-tēz)	development of type 2 diabetes mellitus in a pregnant woman who did not have diabetes before becoming pregnant

TABLE 11-4

PATHOLOGY TERMS—cont'd

placenta previa (plă-SĔN-tă PRĒ-vē-ă)	implantation of the placenta in the lower uterine segment rather than the central or upper portion of the uterine wall, which may cause maternal hemorrhage during labor

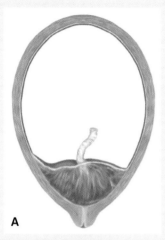 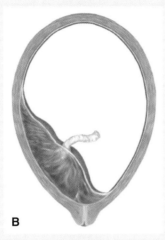 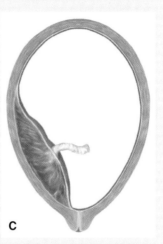

A B C

Placenta previa: (A) centralis, (B) marginalis, (C) lateralis. (From Eagle, S., et al. [2009]. *The professional medical assistant.* Philadelphia, PA: F. A. Davis Company, p. 620; with permission)

Male Reproductive System

balanoposthitis (băl-ă-nō-pŏs-THĪ-tĭs)	inflammation of the glans penis and foreskin covering the glans penis; also called *balanitis*
benign prostatic hypertrophy (BPH) (bē-NĬN prŏs-TĀT-ĭc hī-PĔR-trŏ-fē)	noncancerous enlargement of the prostate gland, common in elderly men

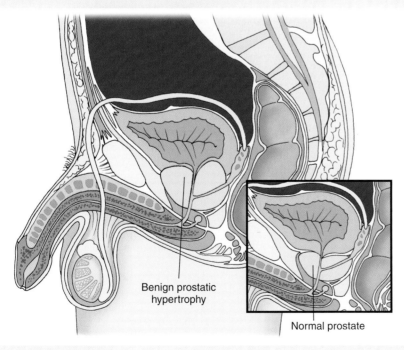

Benign prostatic hypertrophy. / Normal prostate

Benign prostatic hypertrophy.

Continued

TABLE 11-4
PATHOLOGY TERMS—cont'd

cryptorchidism (krĭpt-ŎR-kĭd-ĭ-zum)	failure of one or both testes to descend into the scrotum
epididymitis (ĕp-ĭ-dĭd-ĭ-MĪ-tĭs)	acute or chronic inflammation or infection of the epididymis, a tubular structure on the posterior surface of the testicle
erectile dysfunction (ED) (ĕ-RĔK-tĭl dĭs-FŬNK-shŭn)	general term that describes a number of disorders, all of which impact the ability of a man to attain an erection adequate to achieve a satisfactory sexual experience; also called *impotence*
impotence (ĬM-pŏ-tĕns)	inability of a male to achieve or maintain an erection
orchitis (or-KĪ-tĭs)	acute or chronic condition of inflammation of one or both testicles, caused by (usually viral) infection
prostatitis (prŏs-tă-TĪ-tĭs)	acute or chronic inflammation of the prostate gland
testicular torsion (tĕs-TĬK-ū-lăr TŎR-shŭn)	condition in which the testicles become twisted and the spermatic cord, blood vessels, nerves, and vas deferens become strangled

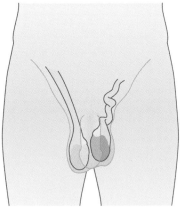

Testicular torsion.

varicocele (VĂR-ĭ-kō-sēl)	enlargement and dilation or herniation of the veins of the spermatic cord that drain the testis

Male and Female Reproductive Systems

chlamydia (klă-MĬD-ē-ă)	the most common STI, a bacterial infection caused by *Chlamydia trachomatis*
gonorrhea (gŏn-ō-RĒ-ă)	STI caused by *Neisseria gonorrhoeae* that results in inflammation of mucous membranes

TABLE 11-4

PATHOLOGY TERMS—cont'd

herpes genitalis (HĔRP-ēs jĕn-ĭ-TĀL-ĭs)	STI caused by herpes simplex virus type 2 that results in painful vesicles; commonly called *genital herpes*

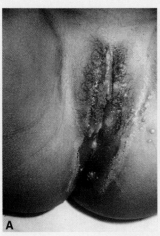 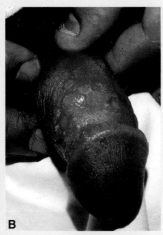

A   B

Herpes genitalis as manifested in female (A) and male (B) patients. (From Dillon, P.M. (2008). *Nursing health assessment.* Philadelphia, PA: F. A. Davis Company, pp. 543 and 577; with permission)

human papillomavirus (HŪ-măn păp-ĭ-LŌ-mă VĪ-rŭs)	STI caused by human papillomavirus that results in painless, cauliflower-like warts; a cause of cervical cancer in women
sterility (stĕr-ĬL-ĭ-tē)	inability to produce offspring
syphilis (SĬF-ĭ-lĭs)	multistage STI caused by the spirochete *Treponema pallidum*, with key symptoms including skin lesions; eventually fatal unless treated
trichomoniasis (trĭk-ō-mō-NĪ-ă-sĭs)	STI infestation with *Trichomonas vaginalis* parasites; key symptoms include vaginitis, urethritis, and cystitis

IN A FLASH!

It's time to print out all of the Pathology Terms Flash Cards for Chapter 11 and run through them at least three times before you continue.

Common Diagnostic Tests and Procedures

Cryosurgery: Destruction of abnormal tissue by freezing

Dilation and curettage (D&C): Dilation of the cervix followed by scraping of the endometrial lining

Needle biopsy: Aspiration of tissue or fluid through a large-gauge needle for analysis (Fig. 11-9)

Papanicolaou smear: Removal of tissue cells from the cervix for analysis

Pelvic sonography: Ultrasound imaging of the structures in the female pelvis

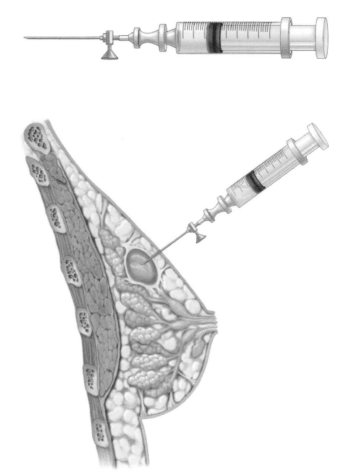

FIGURE 11-9 Needle biopsy. (From Eagle, S., et al. [2009]. *The professional medical assistant*. Philadelphia, PA: F. A. Davis Company, p. 387; with permission)

Prostate-specific antigen (PSA): Blood test used to screen for prostate cancer

Transurethral resection of the prostate (TURP): Removal of tissue from the prostate gland with an endoscope, via the urethra

Tubal ligation: Sterilization procedure in which fallopian tubes are cut and ligated (Fig. 11-10)

Uterine ablation: Procedure that destroys the entire surface of the endometrium and superficial myometrium

Vasectomy: Sterilization procedure in which a small section of the vas deferens is removed (Fig. 11-11)

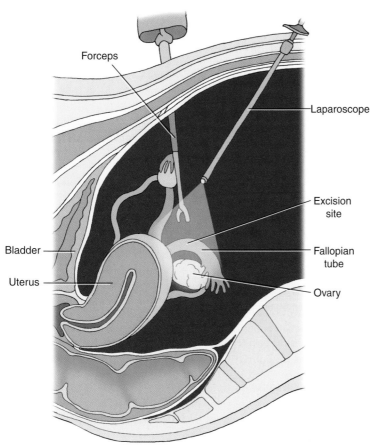

FIGURE 11-10 **Tubal ligation.**

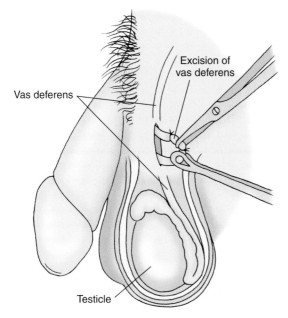

FIGURE 11-11 **Vasectomy.**

Pharmacology

Table 11-5 provides a list of common reproductive system medications.

TABLE 11-5

PHARMACOLOGY

Therapeutic Classification	Generic Name	Brand Name	Common Use
Contraceptives	ethinyl estradiol/drospirenone	Beyaz, Yasmine, Yaz	Prevent ovulation
	ethinyl estradiol/levonorgestrel	Alesse, Aviane, Lutera, Seasonique	
	ethinyl estradiol/norgestimate	Ortho Tri-Cyclen, Sprintec, TriNessa	
	medroxyprogesterone	Depo-Provera, Provera	
Gonadotropins	human chorionic gonadotropin (HCG)	Chorex, Novarel, Ovidrel, Profasi, Pregnyl	Stimulate ovulation
	menotropins	Menopur, Repronex	
	urofollitropin	Bravelle, Fertinex, Metrodin	
Impotence agents	alprostadil	Caverject, Edex, Muse	Cause vasodilation and increase blood flow to penis to cause an erection
	sildenafil	Viagra	
	tadalafil	Cialis	
	vardenafil	Levitra	
Synthetic ovulation stimulants	clomiphene citrate	Clomid, Serophene	Stimulate ovulation
Uterine relaxants	magnesium sulfate		Inhibit uterine muscle contractions
	terbutaline	Brethine	
Uterine stimulants	carboprost	Hemabate	Stimulate uterine muscle contractions
	dinoprostone	Cervidil	
	oxytocin	Pitocin, Syntocinon	

Pathologies, Procedures, and Pharmacology Practice Exercises

Fill in the Blanks

Write the correct meaning of these medical terms.

Exercise 8

1. Uterine fibroids are _____.

2. Ectopic pregnancy occurs when _____.

3. Endometriosis occurs when _____.

4. *Trichomoniasis* is a(n) _____.

5. The term *orchidoptosis* means _____.

6. The term *salpingo-oophorectomy* means _____.

7. The term *balanoplasty* means _____.

8. The term *dysplasia* means _____.

9. The term *neoplastic* means _____.

10. The term *laparoscopy* means _____.

Fill in the Blanks

Fill in the blanks below.

Exercise 9

1. When a fertilized ovum is implanted outside of the uterus, it is called an

   _____ pregnancy.

2. Lacey has dysmenorrhea due to endometrial tissue growth in her

   abdominopelvic area. This condition is known as _____.

3. _____ is an STI that is eventually fatal if not treated.

4. _____ is an STI infestation caused by a parasite.

5. _____ is the inability to produce offspring.

6. The term *seminuria* means _____.

7. The term *galactorrhea* means _____.

8. The term *phalloid* means ————————————.

9. The definition of *cryptorchidism* is ————————————.

10. The term *sonorous* means ————————————.

Multiple Choice

Select the one best answer to the following multiple-choice questions.

Exercise 10

1. Ms. Andretti came to the clinic today complaining of severe menstrual pain and cramping. Which of the following medical terms best describes her complaint?

   a. menostasis

   b. vaginodynia

   c. dysmenorrhea

   d. cervicitis

2. Mrs. Ramirez had a painful ovarian cyst on her left side. The ovary and the cyst were surgically removed through her lower abdomen with a small endoscope. The proper name for this procedure is a:

   a. laparoscopic oophorectomy

   b. colposcopic oophoretomy

   c. vaginoscopic salpingo-oophorectomy

   d. laparoscopic hysterectomy

3. Mr. Smyth had to be circumcised as a result of chronic balanitis. He had:

   a. a continual prostate infection

   b. constant inflammation of his testes

   c. constant inflammation of his glans penis

   d. continual pain of his vas deferens

4. Mrs. Brown is 6 months pregnant and sees her physician each month for care. This type of care is known as:

   a. prenatal care

   b. perinatal care

   c. postnatal care

   d. circumnatal care

5. Which of the following combining forms does **not** mean testis?

   a. test/o

   b. orchi/o

   c. orchid/o

   d. oophor/o

Fill in the Blanks

Using Table 11-5, write the therapeutic classification of the medication next to each generic or brand name.

Exercise 11

1. Seasonique _____

2. Clomid _____

3. carboprost _____

4. vardenafil _____

5. Novarel _____

6. sildenafil _____

7. oxytocin _____

8. Yasmine _____

9. Brethine _____

10. clomiphene citrate _____

CASE STUDY

Read the case study and answer the questions that follow. Most of the terms are included in this chapter. Refer to your medical dictionary for the other terms.

Endometriosis

Susan Brownlee is a 32-year-old woman with a history of dysmenorrhea since the age of 13. Her primary symptoms include pelvic pain and cramping prior to and during her menses. The severity of her symptoms caused her to occasionally miss 1 or 2 days of school each month when she was young. Over time, her symptoms have slowly worsened, currently causing her to miss an average of 2 or 3 days of work each month. Treatment with acetaminophen and NSAIDs provided only partial relief, so she was eventually started on hormonal therapy.

Mrs. Brownlee has been married for 8 years and has been trying to get pregnant for the past 5 years. During evaluation and treatment for infertility, a laparoscopy was performed and a diagnosis of endometriosis confirmed. Surgical treatment was performed at the same time, in which endometrial implants and cysts were removed from the outer surface of her ovaries and fallopian tubes. She was informed that this procedure might reduce her dysmenorrhea symptoms and increase the chance of a successful pregnancy but that the only definitive treatment for endometriosis is a total hysterosalpingo-oophorectomy. Mrs. Brownlee stated that she understood this but wanted to postpone that decision because of her wish to have children.

Endometriosis occurs in 10% to 15% of all women of reproductive age and in 50% of infertile women. The cause is not clearly understood, but there seems to be a genetic predisposition. One theory involves the implantation of endometrial cells from menstrual flow, which moves up the fallopian tubes and into the pelvic cavity. Another theory involves the spread of endometrial cells through blood and lymphatic vessels. Other theories list possible immunological factors. A presumptive diagnosis is made based on history and symptoms, but a definitive diagnosis is made by the performance of a laparoscopy, which allows direct visualization of the reproductive organs and surrounding structures. Treatment depends on the severity of the symptoms; options include analgesics, hormone therapy, and surgery.

Case Study Questions

Exercise 12

1. Since the age of 13, Mrs. Brownlee has experienced:
   a. painful or difficult menstrual flow
   b. absence of menses
   c. excessive menstrual flow
   d. fear of menses

2. Treatment for her dysmenorrhea has included:
   a. cystoscopy with bladder distention
   b. steroids
   c. nonsteroidal anti-inflammatory drugs
   d. hysterectomy

3. The diagnosis of endometriosis was confirmed by:
   a. visual examination of the bladder
   b. incision into the abdomen
   c. visual examination of the abdomen
   d. visual examination of the vagina and cervix

4. What was removed from Mrs. Brownlee's abdomen during her laparoscopy?
   a. her uterus
   b. her fallopian tubes
   c. cancerous growths
   d. endometrial tissue

5. As a result of the surgical procedure, Mrs. Brownlee understands that:
   a. Her endometriosis is probably cured.
   b. Her symptoms of dysmenorrhea will likely worsen.
   c. Her chances of becoming pregnant have increased.
   d. The only reliable cure for her endometriosis is surgical removal of her fallopian tubes.

6. Which of the following statements is true regarding endometriosis?
   a. It is common among women.
   b. There is no relationship to infertility.
   c. Severity of symptoms tends to remain constant over time.
   d. Endometrial tissue proliferates in abnormal areas.

7. Which of the following statements is true regarding endometriosis?
   a. The most effective permanent treatment is complete removal of the uterus, fallopian tubes, and ovaries.
   b. A definite diagnosis can be made based on history and current symptoms.
   c. Standard treatment for endometriosis involves the use of steroids.
   d. Symptoms tend to improve as the woman ages.

8. Describe how Susan's symptoms may have affected her activities of daily living (ADLs) both when she was young and when she was an adult.

9. Examine the impact of Susan missing school and work on a regular basis and how it may also affect others.

End-of-Chapter Practice Exercises

Word Building

*Using **only** the word parts in the lists provided, create medical terms with the indicated meanings.*

Exercise 13

Prefixes	**Combining Forms**	**Suffixes**
an-	balan/o	-al
dys-	cervic/o	-algia
neo-	colp/o	-dynia
oligo-	episi/o	-ectomy
peri-	gynec/o	-esthesia
retro-	hyster/o	-gram
	lapar/o	-ia
	mamm/o	-ism
	mast/o	-itis
	men/o	-logist
	nat/o	-pause
	orchid/o	-pexy
	prostat/o	-plasia
	sperm/o	-plasm
	vagin/o	-rrhaphy
	vas/o	-scope
		-stenosis
		-tomy

1. inflammation of the glans penis _____

2. cutting into or incision of the vulva (perineum) _____

3. condition of absent testes _____

4. surgical fixation of a testis _____

 5. condition of deficient sperm _____

 6. pertaining to near (the time of) birth _____

 7. bad, painful, or difficult formation or growth _____

 8. new formation or growth _____

 9. pertaining to behind the vagina _____

10. absence of sensation _____

11. narrowing or stricture of a vessel _____

12. pain of the prostate _____

13. inflammation of the cervix _____

14. suturing of the vagina _____

15. specialist in the study of female (disorders) _____

16. viewing instrument for the abdomen _____

17. excision or surgical removal of the uterus _____

18. record (x-ray) of a breast _____

19. surgical fixation of a breast _____

20. cessation or stopping of menses _____

True or False

Decide whether the following statements are true or false.

Exercise 14

1. True   False   **Herpes genitalis** is caused by herpes simplex virus type 2.

2. True   False   The abbreviation **PID** stands for *pelvic invasive disorder.*

3. True   False   The key symptoms of **candidiasis** are itching, burning, and a thick curdy discharge.

4. True   False   The abbreviation **IUD** stands for *interurinary disorder.*

5. True   False   **Uterine prolapse** is a herniation of the vaginal wall.

6. True   False   **VD** and **STD** are the same thing.

7. True   False   The symbol for male is ♂.

8. True   False   The symbol for female is ♀.

9. True   False   The abbreviation **GU** stands for *gonorrhea.*

10. True   False   **Cryptorchidism** is the absence of testes.

Deciphering Terms

Write the correct meaning of these medical terms.

Exercise 15

1. orchidorrhaphy _____

2. cervicocolpitis _____

3. multigravida _____

4. gynecomastia _____

5. menopause _____

6. phallodynia _____

7. hyperplasia _____

8. spermolytic _____

9. prostatocele _____

10. cryptomenorrhea _____

Multiple Choice

Select the one best answer to the following multiple-choice questions.

Exercise 16

1. The term *android* means:

    a.   resembling female

    b.   resembling amnion

    c.   resembling male

    d.   none of these

2. The term *salpingolysis* means:

   a.   process of recording sound

   b.   pertaining to the destruction of sperm

   c.   destruction of a tube

   d.   none of these

3. The term *uteropexy* means:

   a.   surgical fixation of the uterus

   b.   suturing of the uterus

   c.   slight or partial paralysis of the uterus

   d.   none of these

4. The term *balanic* means:

   a.   condition of the penis

   b.   pertaining to the glans penis

   c.   disease of the prostate

   d.   none of these

5. The term *sonography* means:

   a.   process of recording sound

   b.   record of sound

   c.   instrument used to record sound

   d.   none of these

6. All of the following abbreviations indicate a type of sexually transmitted infection **except:**

   a.   HPV

   b.   GC

   c.   Trich

   d.   TSS

7. All of the following are matched with the correct definition **except:**

   a.   ♀ : male

   b.   PMS: premenstrual syndrome

   c.   TSS: toxic shock syndrome

   d.   ED: erectile dysfunction

8. Which of the following statements is true?

   a.   The abbreviations *STI* and *STD* mean the same thing.

   b.   EDC is a type of contraceptive device.

   c.   The abbreviation *OC* stands for ovarian cyst.

   d.   The abbreviation *FHR* stands for female hormone.

9. Which of the following abbreviations pertains to the male reproductive system?

   a.   TSE

   b.   BSE

   c.   D&C

   d.   PID

10. Which of the following abbreviations pertains to the female reproductive system?

   a.   PSA

   b.   HRT

   c.   DRE

   d.   TURP

11. All of the following abbreviations indicate a type of procedure **except:**

   a.   AB

   b.   TAH

   c.   GU

   d.   DRE

12. All of the following abbreviations indicate a type of disease or disorder **except:**

   a.   PID

   b.   BPH

   c.   STI

   d.   OC

13. All of the following terms are matched with the correct definition **except:**

   a.   endometriosis: tissue growth in abnormal sites in lower abdominopelvic area

   b.   eclampsia: condition marked by severe hypertension, seizures, and possible coma

   c.   abruptio placentae: implantation of the placenta in the lower uterine segment rather than the central or upper portion of the uterine wall

   d.   uterine fibroids: benign, smooth tumors made of muscle and fat

14. All of the following terms are matched with the correct definition **except:**

    a.   cryptorchidism: failure of one or both testes to descend into the scrotum

    b.   impotence: inability to produce offspring

    c.   varicocele: enlargement and dilation of veins of the spermatic cord

    d.   testicular torsion: condition in which the testicles become twisted and the spermatic cord, blood vessels, nerves, and vas deferens become strangled

15. Balanoposthitis is:

    a.   inflammation caused by blockage of one or both of the Bartholin's glands

    b.   protrusion of the uterus through the vaginal opening

    c.   inflammation of the glans penis and foreskin

    d.   pain in the lower abdominal and pelvic area, associated with menses

16. Which of the following procedures destroys the entire surface of the endometrium and superficial myometrium?

    a.   cryosurgery

    b.   ablation

    c.   dilation and curettage

    d.   none of these

17. Which of the following procedures involves freezing of tissue?

    a.   cryosurgery

    b.   needle biopsy

    c.   ablation

    d.   prostate-specific antigen

18. Which of the following combining forms means *sound?*

    a.   salping/o

    b.   son/o

    c.   semin/o

    d.   none of these

19. Which of the following combining forms means *vulva?*

    a.   andr/o

    b.   episi/o

    c.   colp/o

    d.   none of these

20. The combining form *phall/i* means:

   a.　hidden

   b.　amnion

   c.　fetus

   d.　none of these

12 ENDOCRINE SYSTEM

Chapter Outline

Structure and Function

The endocrine system is made up of all the major glands, which act to regulate hormones in the body (Fig. 12-1). Various endocrine organs produce and secrete these hormones in order to maintain **homeostasis,** which is defined as the state of dynamic equilibrium. In other words, the hormones act together to keep the body's internal environment healthy. Some hormones act directly on target organs; others stimulate certain glands to secrete yet different hormones.

Hormone levels in the blood may vary according to bodily functions. **Hormones** usually work in pairs to maintain a healthy balance, with one acting to raise levels of other substances when needed and the other acting to lower levels when needed. For example, the hormones calcitonin and parathyroid hormone function in an opposite, yet complementary, fashion to maintain a healthy level of calcium in the blood.

Endocrine glands are responsible for the sexual maturation of individuals from childhood to adolescence and into adulthood. Endocrine glands also play a role in the body's ability to metabolize food and store energy.

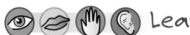 Learning Style Tip

Study Figure 12-1 and then create a fun and colorful 3-D model that similarly illustrates the pituitary gland, the hormones it produces, and the target organs the hormones affect. An example might be a hanging mobile with the pituitary gland at the top and labeled "hormone" strings, each of which dangles its respective target organ(s). Once you've completed it, show and explain your model to one or more classmates.

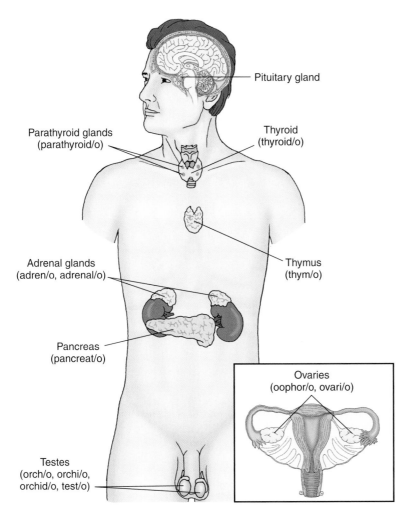

FIGURE 12-1 **The endocrine system.**

The **pituitary gland** is a small, round, pea-sized structure attached to the lower surface of the hypothalamus in the brain. It is commonly called the master gland because it controls all of the other glands in the body. (Even so, the pituitary is actually controlled by the hypothalamus.) The pituitary gland is divided into an anterior lobe and a posterior lobe. These two parts function separately to produce many different hormones (Fig. 12-2). The **anterior lobe** secretes the following six hormones:

- **Growth hormone (GH)** promotes the growth of body structures, such as bones.
- **Thyroid-stimulating hormone (TSH)** affects the growth and functioning of the thyroid gland.
- **Follicle-stimulating hormone (FSH)** and **luteinizing hormone (LH)** are referred to as gonadotropins because they act on the gonads—the ovaries in the female, to produce an ovum, and the testes in the male, to produce sperm.
- **Prolactin** acts on the mammary glands to produce milk.
- **Adrenocorticotropic hormone (ACTH)** acts on the adrenal glands to secrete glucocorticoids, including cortisol.

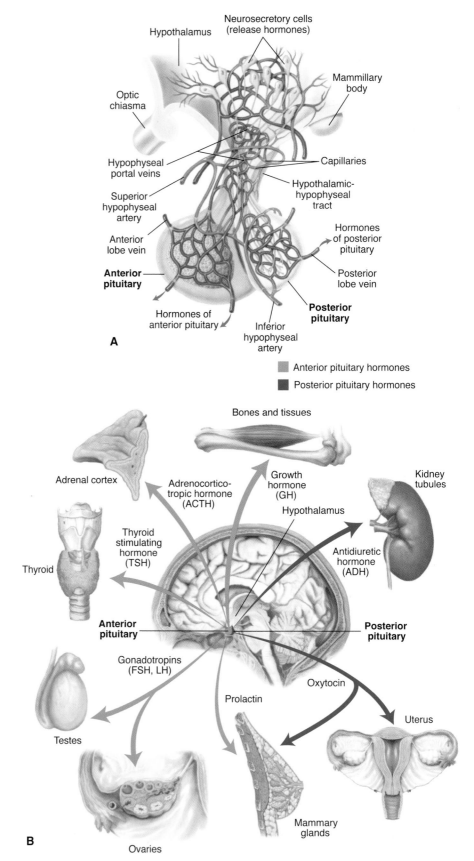

FIGURE 12-2 Pituitary gland: (A) anterior and posterior view (B) hormones and target glands. (From Eagle, S., et al. [2009]. *The professional medical assistant.* Philadelphia, PA: F. A. Davis Company, p. 523; with permission)

The **posterior lobe** of the pituitary gland secretes the following two hormones:

- **Oxytocin** acts on the uterus to promote contractions during labor and delivery.
- **Antidiuretic hormone (ADH)** acts on the kidneys to increase the absorption of water.

The tiny **pineal gland** is sometimes referred to as the pineal body. It is shaped like a pinecone and is located in the brain, above and behind the thalamus. The pineal gland produces the hormone **melatonin,** which influences the body's natural **circadian rhythm,** or sleep-wake cycle.

The **thyroid gland** is one of the largest endocrine glands; it is highly vascular and is located in the base of the neck. It is shaped similarly to the letter H and has two lobes, one located on each side of the trachea, which are connected by a narrow band. It produces the two thyroid hormones, **triiodothyronine (T3)** and **thyroxine (T4),** which are responsible for growth throughout childhood and regulation of body metabolism. For the thyroid gland to function properly, iodine must be obtained in the diet. The thyroid gland also secretes the hormone **calcitonin,** which is responsible for regulating calcium and phosphorus levels in the blood.

Four tiny **parathyroid glands** lie on the posterior surface of the thyroid gland, within its connective tissue. They secrete **parathormone (PTH),** also called parathyroid hormone, which also helps regulate calcium and phosphorus levels in the blood.

The two triangular-shaped **adrenal glands** are located on top of each kidney, within the retroperitoneal cavity (behind the abdomen). They are made up of an outer layer called the *adrenal cortex* and an inner part called the *adrenal medulla.* The adrenal glands secrete several hormones:

- **Epinephrine,** also known as *adrenaline,* is released during the fight-or-flight response, which increases your ability to cope with stress or trauma. Epinephrine enables the body to respond to stressful situations by converting glycogen into glucose for quick energy, dilating the pupils, opening the airways, and decreasing peristalsis.
- **Aldosterone** plays a role in regulating and maintaining the body's water, sodium, and electrolyte balance.
- **Cortisol** is the body's natural steroid and works to decrease inflammation.
- **Androgens** are responsible for secondary sexual characteristics in females and males.

The **pancreas** is a long, somewhat flat organ located in the upper-left quadrant of the abdomen. It plays an active role in the digestive system as well as the endocrine system. The endocrine portion of the pancreas includes the pancreatic islets, also called the *islets of Langerhans.* The beta cells of the pancreas secrete **insulin** after food is eaten, to metabolize carbohydrates and break them down into glucose. Insulin also stimulates cells to take up glucose from the blood so that it can be delivered to tissue cells for energy. As a result, blood glucose levels decrease. The alpha cells of the pancreas secrete **glucagon,** which acts on the liver to convert glycogen into glucose. (Glycogen is also stored in the muscles.) Glycogen is converted into glucose to meet energy needs, such as during exercise or prolonged periods without meals.

Normally, pancreatic hormones work cooperatively to maintain healthy blood glucose levels. However, when dysregulation occurs, as with **diabetes mellitus,** blood glucose levels may widely fluctuate, resulting in **hyperglycemia** (high blood sugar) or **hypoglycemia** (low blood sugar). The classic signs of new onset of undiagnosed diabetes are the three "polys": *polydipsia* (much thirst), *polyphagia* (much eating, which indicates an increased appetite), and *polyuria*

Flashpoint

If you feel threatened or frightened, your body reacts by triggering a survival mechanism called the fight-or-flight response. Your adrenal glands secrete cortisol and epinephrine (adrenaline), which causes changes that include increasing your heart rate and your respiratory rate, dilating your pupils, and shunting blood away from your digestive tract, toward your muscles, to provide extra energy for fighting or for running away.

(much urination). In spite of eating more, an undiagnosed diabetic may lose weight because of faulty carbohydrate metabolism; in spite of drinking more, an undiagnosed diabetic may become dehydrated because of polyuria. In severe cases, as these symptoms worsen and blood glucose levels rise, lethargy may progress to loss of consciousness. This is called **_diabetic ketoacidosis (DKA),_** otherwise known as a _diabetic coma._ Treatment includes admission to the hospital for fluid rehydration and insulin therapy.

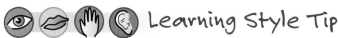 Learning Style Tip

As you read the text, challenge yourself to think like the instructor and underline or highlight information you believe is most likely to be used in exam questions. Then read the information aloud until you fully understand and remember it.

The **thymus gland** consists of two symmetrical lobes located in the mediastinum (midchest area). It is proportionately larger in infants and children and shrinks as people age. The main function of the thymus gland is to produce T lymphocytes that are necessary for the immune system. It plays an active role in the immune system in childhood but gets smaller and becomes less active as a person ages.

The **reproductive glands,** sometimes called the gonads, are the ovaries and testes. The ovaries are small, oval-shaped structures located on each side of the uterus in the lower abdominal cavity, attached to the broad ligament. The ovaries contain graafian follicles, in which are immature ova, or eggs. The **ovaries** produce an ovum during each menstrual cycle and secrete estrogen and progesterone. **Estrogen** helps develop secondary sexual characteristics in the female, including breasts and pubic hair. It also plays a vital role in the menstrual cycle and is important in the prevention of osteoporosis in postmenopausal women. **Progesterone** prepares the uterus for pregnancy and helps to support the developing fetus.

The **testes** are egg-shaped glands located in the scrotum of the male reproductive tract. The testes secrete **testosterone,** which is responsible for the development of male secondary sexual characteristics during puberty, such as deepening of the voice, growth of facial and pubic hair, and increased muscle development. It is also necessary in the production of sperm.

Almost all endocrine glands operate in a **negative feedback system** (Box 12-1). For example, the parathyroid glands secrete parathyroid hormone, which regulates blood calcium levels. A decrease in blood calcium level stimulates the parathyroid glands to secrete more parathyroid hormone; parathyroid hormone stimulates the bones to release more calcium into the blood and facilitates calcium uptake from the kidneys into the bloodstream. Thus, blood calcium levels are restored to normal. On the other hand, if blood calcium levels increase (above normal), the parathyroid glands decrease production of parathyroid hormone. Either way, the response of the parathyroid glands is a negative (opposite) response to the stimulus of a decrease or increase in blood calcium levels.

Flashpoint

As we age, our reproductive glands produce fewer hormones. This increases the risk for developing osteoporosis and causes uncomfortable symptoms in both women and men. Hormone replacement therapy (HRT) can replenish the body with adequate amounts of estrogen, progesterone, and testosterone.

Learning Style Tip

Noticing data patterns helps you recall them later. For example, note that the chemistry abbreviations for electrolytes are the same as the first letters in the combining forms. The prefix is the only thing that changes when describing high or low levels of electrolytes in the blood.

		high level in the blood	low level in the blood
potassium:	K	hyper**k**alemia	hypo**k**alemia
sodium:	Na	hyper**na**tremia	hypo**na**tremia
calcium:	Ca	hyper**cal**cemia	hypo**cal**cemia

Box 12-1 Negative Feedback System

Within the endocrine system, glands and hormones work together to maintain home-ostasis in the body by utilizing a negative feedback system. The system is called negative because it works by opposites to maintain a healthy balance of certain substances in the body. Each gland produces a hormone that serves to oppose another substance. The gland may increase or decrease production of the hormone to stimulate a corresponding decrease or increase of that substance. Thus, this system works much like a thermostat functions, activating the production of heat in response to falling temperatures (a decrease in the normal level) or decreasing heat production in response to normal or above-normal heat levels.

Structure and Function Practice Exercises

Fill in the Blanks

Choose the term that matches the description.

Exercise 1

Homeostasis	Circadian rhythm	Hypoglycemia
Hormones	Thyroid gland	Thymus gland
Endocrine glands	Parathyroid glands	Reproductive glands
Pituitary gland	Adrenal glands	Ovaries
Anterior lobe	Pancreas	Testes
Posterior lobe	Diabetes mellitus	Negative feedback system
Pineal gland	Hyperglycemia	

1. _____ Responsible for sexual maturation; plays a role in the metabolism of food and energy storage

2. _____ Produces T lymphocytes that are necessary for the immune system

3. _____ Located on top of each kidney; secrete the hormones epinephrine, aldosterone, cortisol and androgens

4. _____ The state of dynamic equilibrium

5. _____ Sleep-wake cycle

6. _____ Secretes the hormones insulin and glucagon, which work cooperatively to maintain healthy blood glucose levels

7. _____ The portion of the pituitary gland that secretes the hormones oxytocin and ADH

8. _____ Work in pairs to maintain a healthy balance to keep the body's internal environment healthy

9. _____ Secrete the hormones estrogen and progesterone

10. _____ Produces the hormones triiodothyronine and thyroxine that are responsible for growth throughout childhood and regulation of body metabolism

11. _____ Low blood sugar

12. _____ Located in the brain, above and behind the thalamus; produces the hormone melatonin

13. _____ Secrete the hormone testosterone

14. _____ The ovaries and testes; sometimes called the gonads

15. _____ The portion of the pituitary gland that secretes the hormones GH, TSH, FSH, LH, prolactin, and ACTH

16. _____ High blood sugar

17. _____ Structure attached to the lower surface of the hypothalamus in the brain; it controls all of the other glands in the body

18. _____ They secrete the hormone PTH, which helps to regulate calcium and phosphorus levels in the blood.

19. _____ A pathology in which blood sugar levels may widely fluctuate

20. _____ Each gland produces a hormone that serves to oppose another substance. The gland may increase or decrease production of the hormone to stimulate a corresponding decrease or increase of that substance.

Fill in the Blanks

Choose the hormone that matches the description.

Exercise 2

Growth hormone (GH)	Melatonin	Androgens
Thyroid-stimulating hormone (TSH)	Triiodothyronine (T3) and thyroxine (T4)	Insulin Glucagon
Follicle-stimulating hormone (FSH) and luteinizing hormone (LH)	Calcitonin Parathormone (PTH)	Estrogen Progesterone
Prolactin	Epinephrine Aldosterone	Testosterone

Adrenocorticotropic hormone (ACTH)	Cortisol
Oxytocin	
Antidiuretic hormone (ADH)	

1. _____ Acts on the liver to convert glycogen into glucose

2. _____ Acts on the uterus to promote contractions during labor and delivery

3. _____ Responsible for growth throughout childhood and regulation of body metabolism

4. _____ Promotes the growth of body structures, such as bones

5. _____ Produces sperm, deepening of the voice, growth of facial hair, and increased muscle development in the male

6. _____ Influences the body's natural circadian rhythm

7. _____ Acts on the adrenal glands to secrete glucocorticoids, including cortisol

8. _____ Enables the body to respond to stressful situations by converting glycogen into glucose for quick energy

9. _____ Affects the growth and functioning of the thyroid gland

10. _____ Regulates calcium and phosphorus levels in the blood

11. _____ Breaks carbohydrates down into glucose and stimulates cells to take up glucose from the blood

12. _____ Acts on the kidneys to increase the absorption of water

13. _____ Plays a vital role in the menstrual cycle and is important in the prevention of osteoporosis

14. _____ Act on the gonads to produce an ovum in the female and sperm in the male

15. _____ Works to decrease inflammation

16. _____ Plays a role in regulating and maintaining the body's water, sodium, and electrolyte balance

17. _____ Responsible for secondary sexual characteristics in females and males

18. _____   Necessary to prepare and maintain the uterus for a fertilized ovum

19. _____   Acts on the mammary glands to produce milk

20. _____   Also called parathyroid hormone; helps to regulate calcium and phosphorus levels in the blood

Fill in the Blanks

Label Figure 12-3 with the appropriate anatomical terms and combining forms.

Exercise 3

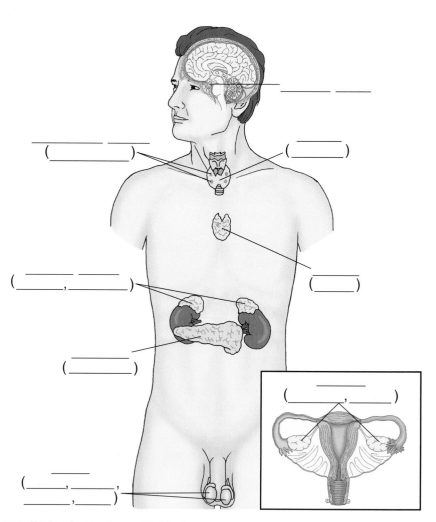

FIGURE 12-3 Endocrine system with blanks.

Combining Forms and Abbreviations

Combining Forms

Table 12-1 contains combining forms that pertain to the endocrine system, along with examples of terms that utilize the combining forms, and a pronunciation guide. Read aloud to yourself as you move from left to right across the table. Be sure to use the pronunciation guide so that you learn to say the terms correctly.

TABLE 12-1
COMBINING FORMS RELATED TO THE ENDOCRINE SYSTEM

Combining Form	Meaning	Example (Pronunciation)	Meaning of New Term
acr/o	extremities	acroanesthesia (ăk-rō-ăn-ĕs-THĒ-zē-ă)	absence of sensation in the extremities
aden/o	gland	adenopathy (ăd-ĕ-NŎP-ă-thē)	disease of a gland
adren/o	adrenal gland	adrenal (ăd-rē-năl)	pertaining to the adrenal gland
adrenal/o		adrenalectomy (ăd-rē-năl-ĔK-tō-mē)	excision or surgical removal of an adrenal gland
calc/o	calcium	hypercalcemia (hī-pĕr-kăl-SĒ-mē-ă)	condition of excessive calcium in the blood
gluc/o	glucose, sugar, sweet	glucogenesis (gloo-kō-JĔN-ĕ-sĭs)	creation of glucose
glucos/o		glucosuria (gloo-kō-SŪR-ē-ă)	sugar in the urine
glyc/o		glycemia (glī-SĒ-mē-ă)	sugar in the blood
glycos/o		glycosuria (glī-kō-SŪ-rē-ă)	sugar in the urine
home/o	same, unchanging	homeostasis (hō-mē-ō-STĀ-sĭs)	unchanging, stopping (maintenance of equilibrium)
hydr/o	water	hydrolysis (hī-DRŎL-ĭ-sĭs)	destruction of water
kal/i	potassium	hyperkalemia (hī-pĕr-kă-LĒ-mē-ă)	condition of excessive potassium in the blood
natr/o	sodium	natremia (nă-TRĒ-mē-ă)	condition of sodium in the blood
pancreat/o	pancreas	pancreatography (păn-krē-ă-TŎG-ră-fē)	process of recording the pancreas
parathyroid/o	parathyroid	parathyroidectomy (păr-ă-thī-royd-ĔK-tō-mē)	excision or surgical removal of a parathyroid gland

Continued

TABLE 12-1

COMBINING FORMS RELATED TO THE ENDOCRINE SYSTEM—cont'd

Combining Form	Meaning	Example (Pronunciation)	Meaning of New Term
thym/o	thymus	thymoma (thī-MŌ-mă)	tumor of the thymus
thyr/o	thyroid	thyrotoxicosis (thī-rō-tŏks-ĭ-KŌ-sĭs)	abnormal condition of poison in the thyroid
thyroid/o		thyroiditis (thī-royd-Ī-tĭs)	inflammation of the thyroid
toxic/o	toxin, poison	toxicologist (tŏks-ĭ-KŌL-ō-jĭst)	specialist in the study of toxins

IN A FLASH!

It's time to print out all of the Combining Form Flash Cards for Chapter 12 and run through them at least three times before you continue.

Abbreviations

Table 12-2 lists some of the most common abbreviations related to the endocrine system, as well as others often used in medical documentation.

TABLE 12-2

ABBREVIATIONS

ADH	antidiuretic hormone
BMI	body mass index
BMR	basal metabolic rate
Ca	calcium
CA	cancer
DI	diabetes insipidus
DKA	diabetic ketoacidosis
DM	diabetes mellitus
FBG, FBS	fasting blood glucose, fasting blood sugar
FSBS	finger stick blood sugar
GH	growth hormone
GTT	glucose tolerance test
HRT	hormone replacement therapy
IDDM	insulin-dependent diabetes mellitus (type 1 diabetes)
K	potassium

TABLE 12-2

ABBREVIATIONS—cont'd

Na	sodium
NIDDM	non–insulin-dependent diabetes mellitus (type 2 diabetes)
PTH	parathyroid hormone
T3, T4	triiodothyronine, thyroxine (thyroid hormones)
TSH	thyroid-stimulating hormone

 Learning Style Tip

With your study buddy, create a fun "abbreviation conversation" in which two people are talking in code. Use as many medical abbreviations as possible from this and other chapters. Take turns reciting each side of the conversation and review the meaning of any abbreviations you have forgotten.

IN A FLASH!

It's time to print out all of the Abbreviation Flash Cards for Chapter 12 and run through them at least three times before you continue.

Combining Forms and Abbreviations Practice Exercises

Fill in the Blanks

Fill in the blanks below using Table 12-1.

Exercise 4

1. Excision or surgical removal of a parathyroid gland _____

2. Excision or surgical removal of an adrenal gland _____

3. Disease of a gland _____

4. Specialist in the study of toxins _____

5. Condition of excessive calcium in the blood _____

6. Creation of glucose _____

7. Tumor of the thymus _____

8. Sugar in the urine _____

9. Pertaining to the adrenal gland _____

10. Inflammation of the thyroid _____

11. Process of recording the pancreas _____

12. Unchanging, stopping (maintenance of equilibrium) _____

13. Condition of excessive potassium in the blood _____

14. Condition of sodium in the blood _____

15. Abnormal condition of poison in the thyroid _____

Fill in the Blanks

Fill in the blanks below using Table 12-2.

Exercise 5

1. The abbreviation TSH stands for _____

   _____ _____.

2. The abbreviation CA stands for _____.

3. The abbreviation Ca stands for _____.

4. The thyroid hormones include _____ and

   _____.

5. The abbreviation for diabetes mellitus is _____.

6. There are two major forms of diabetes. One is NIDDM, which stands for

   _____ _____

   _____ _____.

7. Another form of diabetes is IDDM, which stands for

   _____ _____

   _____ _____.

8. The abbreviation GH stands for _____

   _____.

9. The abbreviation DKA stands for _____

   _____.

10. The abbreviation HRT stands for _____

_____ _____ .

Pathologies, Procedures, and Pharmacology

Pathology Terms

Table 12-3 includes terms that relate to diseases or abnormalities of the endocrine system. Use the pronunciation guide and say the terms aloud as you read them. This will help you get in the habit of saying them properly.

TABLE 12-3
PATHOLOGY TERMS

acromegaly (ăk-rō-MĔG-ă-lē)	type of hyperpituitarism in which an overactive pituitary gland after adulthood causes abnormal continued growth of bones and tissues of the face and extremities
Addison's disease (ĂD-ĭ-sŭnz dĭ-ZĒZ)	illness characterized by gradual adrenal-gland failure, resulting in insufficient production of steroid hormones and the need for hormone replacement therapy; also called *hypoadrenalism* and *adrenocortical insufficiency*
congenital hypothyroidism (kŏn-JĔN-ĭ-tăl hī-pō-THĪ-royd-ĭ-zum)	congenital condition of thyroid hormone deficiency, characterized by arrested physical and mental development; formerly called *cretinism*

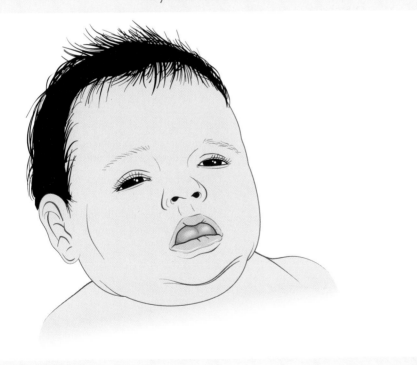

Congenital hypothyroidism.

Continued

TABLE 12-3

PATHOLOGY TERMS—cont'd

Cushing's disease (KOOSH-ĭngz dĭ-ZĒZ)	disorder caused by hypersecretion of cortisol by the adrenal gland, resulting in altered fat distribution and muscle weakness; also called *hyperadrenocorticism, hypercortisolism* and *hyperadrenalism*

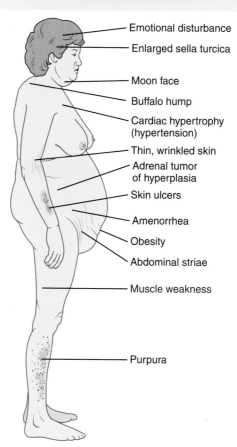

Emotional disturbance
Enlarged sella turcica
Moon face
Buffalo hump
Cardiac hypertrophy (hypertension)
Thin, wrinkled skin
Adrenal tumor of hyperplasia
Skin ulcers
Amenorrhea
Obesity
Abdominal striae
Muscle weakness
Purpura

Cushing's disease.

diabetes insipidus (dī-ă-BĒ-tēz ĭn-SĬP-ĭ-dŭs)	disorder unrelated to diabetes mellitus, characterized by excessive output of dilute urine
diabetic ketoacidosis (DKA) (dī-ă-BĚT-ĭk kē-tō-ă-sĭ-DŌ-sĭs)	condition of severe hyperglycemia
diabetes mellitus (DM) (dī-ă-BĒ-tēz mĕl-Ī-tŭs)	chronic metabolic disorder in which the pancreas secretes insufficient amounts of insulin or the body is insulin resistant

TABLE 12-3
PATHOLOGY TERMS—cont'd

dwarfism (DWĂRF-i-zum)	hyposecretion of growth hormone during childhood, resulting in an abnormally small adult

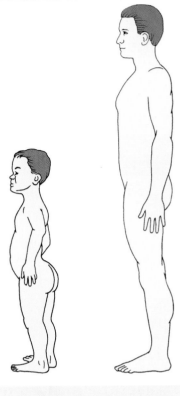

Dwarfism.

exophthalmos (ĕks-ŏf-THĂL-mōs)	abnormal protrusion of the eyeballs

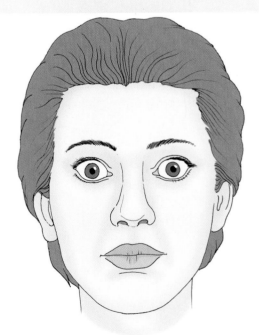

Exophthalmos.

TABLE 12-3
PATHOLOGY TERMS—cont'd

gestational diabetes (jĕs-TĀ-shŭn-ăl dī-ă-BĒ-tēz)	diabetes that begins during pregnancy due to insulin resistance and altered glucose metabolism
giantism (JĪ-ăn-tĭ-zum)	type of hyperpituitarism that causes hypersecretion of growth hormone during childhood, resulting in an abnormally large adult

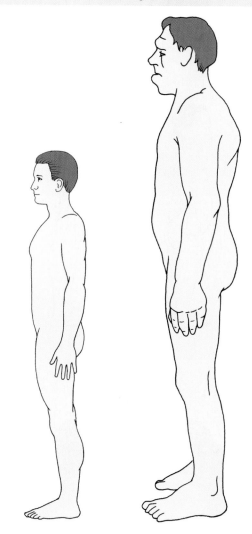

Giantism.

goiter (GOY-tĕr)	enlarged thyroid gland
Graves' disease (grāvz dĭ-ZĒZ)	hyperthyroidism caused by an autoimmune response, which may cause exophthalmos; also called *thyrotoxicosis*
Hashimoto's thyroiditis (hă-shē-MŌ-tōz thī-roy-DĪ-tĭs)	chronic, inflammatory condition that leads to the most common type of thyroiditis; also called *chronic lymphocytic thyroiditis* and *autoimmune thyroiditis*
hirsutism (HŬR-sūt-ĭ-zum)	male pattern of body-hair development in females

TABLE 12-3
PATHOLOGY TERMS—cont'd

hyperaldosteronism (hī-pĕr-ăl-dō-STĔR-ōn-ĭ-zum)	condition in which the adrenal glands release excessive aldosterone; also called *Conn's syndrome*
hyperparathyroidism (hī-pĕr-păr-ă-THĪ-royd-ĭ-zum)	condition in which the parathyroid glands produce an excessive amount of parathyroid hormone (PTH)
hypoparathyroidism (hī-pō-păr-ă-THĪ-royd-ĭ-zum)	condition in which the parathyroid glands are hypoactive and as a result the level of parathyroid hormones (PTH) is too low
myxedema (mĭks-ĕ-DĒ-mă)	severe form of hypothyroidism that develops in the older child or adult, causing nonpitting edema in connective tissue
nondiabetic hypoglycemia (nŏn-dī-ă-BĔT-ĭk hī-pō-glī-SĒ-mē-ă)	condition in which a nondiabetic person experiences mild symptoms associated with low blood glucose
panhypopituitarism (păn-hī-pō-pĭ-TŪ-ĭ-tăr-ĭ-zum)	condition resulting from diminished secretion of pituitary hormones; also called *underactive pituitary gland*
pheochromocytoma (fē-ō-krō-mō-sī-TŌ-mă)	tumor of the adrenal medulla (central part of the adrenal gland), usually benign but sometimes causing fluctuation of stress hormones like adrenaline
pituitary dwarfism (pĭ-TŪ-ĭ-tăr-ē dwărf-ĭ-zum)	type of hypopituitarism in which reduced growth and development occur due to deficiency of growth hormone in childhood
polydipsia (pŏl-ē-DĬP-sē-ă)	much (increased) thirst
polyphagia (pŏl-ē-FĀ-jē-ă)	much (increased) appetite
polyuria (pŏl-ē-Ū-rē-ă)	much (increased) urination
precocious puberty (prē-KŌ-shŭs PŪ-bĕr-tē)	premature onset of puberty with the appearance of secondary sex characteristics in young children
retinopathy (rĕt-ĭn-ŎP-ă-thē)	disease of the retina, often caused by diabetes
thyrotoxicosis (thī-rō-tŏks-ĭ-KŌ-sĭs)	severe episode of worsening symptoms of hyperthyroidism

Learning Style Tip

Choose several terms that interest you from Table 12-3 and enter them, one at a time, into an Internet image search engine such as Google Images. Examine the interesting variety of photos and illustrations that you find and see what you can learn from the images.

IN A FLASH!

It's time to print out all of the Pathology Terms Flash Cards for Chapter 12 and run through them at least three times before you continue.

Common Diagnostic Tests and Procedures

Average blood glucose (eAG): Reflection of the average blood glucose level over the past 2 to 3 months reported by the same units (mg/dL) seen on glucose meters; directly correlates to HbA1c results

Fasting blood glucose (FBG): Test of blood glucose levels after a fast of 8 to 12 hours, used to screen for diabetes; also called *FBS*, or *fasting blood sugar*

Finger stick blood sugar (FSBS): Test of blood glucose from a drop of capillary blood obtained by pricking the finger; also called *finger stick blood glucose (FSBG)*

Glycosylated hemoglobin (HbA1c): Reflection of the average blood glucose level over the past 2 to 3 months by measuring the amount of hemoglobin with sugar attached to it; reported as a percentage

Radioactive iodine uptake: Nuclear medicine study that measures how rapidly radioactive iodine is taken up from the blood after oral or intravenous administration

Thyroid function test: Reflection of thyroid function by measuring levels of thyroid-stimulating hormone (TSH), triiodothyronine (T3), and thyroxine (T4)

Thyroid scan: Radiographic evaluation of the thyroid after a radioactive substance is injected; identifies thyroid size, shape, position, and function

Thyroid-stimulating hormone (TSH): Measure of the ability of the thyroid gland to concentrate and retain circulating iodine for synthesis of thyroid hormone

A common area of confusion is between finger stick blood sugar (FSBS) and fasting blood sugar (FBS). Please note the following differences:

FBS: The person has fasted for a designated time, usually 8 to 12 hours. Blood is drawn from a vein with a needle and syringe or with a device called a Vacutainer (a needle attached to a vacuum-sealed tube). The blood specimen is tested in the laboratory.

FSBS: Blood sugar may be checked at any time but is usually checked just prior to meals. A drop of capillary blood is obtained by poking the tip of the finger with a lancet (tiny, sharp blade). The blood is tested immediately using an instrument called a glucometer (Fig. 12-4).

Flashpoint

"Fasting" before a blood test means having nothing to eat or drink, except for water, for a certain period of time. If you are instructed to fast for 8 or 12 hours, you may want to have your last meal by 8 p.m. and arrive at the laboratory for your blood draw by 8 a.m.

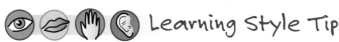 **Learning Style Tip**

If your instructor provides exam reviews, be sure to attend. They are your opportunity to review and reinforce information, identify correct answers on questions you missed, and ask questions.

Pharmacology

Table 12-4 provides a list of common endocrine system medications used to control blood sugar levels and treat abnormal hormone levels.

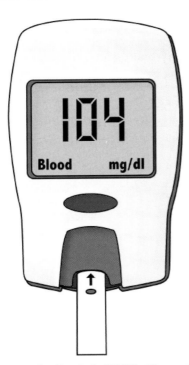

FIGURE 12-4 **Glucometer.** (From Eagle, S., et al. [2009]. *The professional medical assistant.* Philadelphia, PA: F. A. Davis Company, p. 535; with permission)

TABLE 12-4
PHARMACOLOGY

Therapeutic Classification	Generic Name	Brand Name	Common Use
Insulin	aspart	NovoLog	Insulin replacement; helps glucose get into cells
	lispro	Humalog	
	glargine	Lantus	
Combination isophane/ regular insulin	humulin	None	
	novolin	None	
Biguanide	metformin	Glucophage, Glumetza, Fortamet, Riomet	Controls (lowers) high blood sugar
Sulfonylurea	chlorpropamide	Diabinese	Increases insulin production by the pancreas
	glipizide	Glucotrol	
	glimepiride	Amaryl	
	glyburide	DiaBeta, Glynase, Micronase	
	tolbutamide	None	
	tolazamide	None	
Alpha-glucosidase inhibitor	acarbose	Precose	Slows digestion of complex carbohydrates
	miglitol	Glyset	
Meglitinide	repaglinide	Prandin	Increases insulin production by the pancreas
	nateglinide	Starlix	

Continued

TABLE 12-4

PHARMACOLOGY—cont'd

Therapeutic Classification	Generic Name	Brand Name	Common Use
Thiazolidinedione	pioglitazone	Actos	Lowers insulin resistance; reduces glucose
	rosiglitazone	Avandia	
Hormone	glucagon	None	Severe hypoglycemia treatment; increases blood glucose
Incretin mimetic	exenatide	Byetta	Increases insulin release
	liraglutide	Victoza	
Antithyroid agent	carbimazole	None	Decreases production of thyroid hormone
	methimazole	Tapazole	
	propylthiouracil	None	
Synthetic hormone	levothyroxine	Levothroid, Levoxyl, Synthroid, Unithroid	Replaces or provides more thyroid hormone
	liothyronine	Cytomel	
Growth hormone	somatropin	Genotropin, Humatrope, Norditropin, Nutropin, Serostim, Zorbtive	Treatment of growth failure; increases production of growth hormone
Growth hormone antagonist	bromocriptine	Parlodel	Decreases production of growth hormone
	lanreotide	Somatuline	
	octreotide	Sandostatin	
Prolactin inhibitors	bromocriptine		Decreases production of prolactin
	cabergoline	Dostinex	

Pathologies, Procedures, and Pharmacology Practice Exercises

Deciphering Terms

Write the correct meaning of these medical terms.

Exercise 6

1. pancreatic _____

2. acromicria _____

3. homeotherapy _____

4. adrenopathy _____

5. hyperkalemia _____

6. euglycemia _____

7. dysthymic _____

8. thyroidorrhexis _____

9. adenopathy _____

10. glucopenia _____

11. hypoglycemia _____

12. hypernatremia _____

13. glycosuria _____

14. toxicologist _____

15. hydrophobia _____

Fill in the Blanks

Fill in the blanks below.

Exercise 7

1. Chester has a condition caused by hyposecretion of growth hormone during his childhood. He has _____.

2. Abnormal protrusion of the eyeballs is known as _____.

3. Lonnie has a condition caused by hypersecretion of growth hormone during his childhood. He has _____.

4. Adreanna has exophthalmos caused by hyperthyroidism. She has

   _____ _____.

5. _____ _____ is a condition caused by hypersecretion of cortisol by the adrenal gland, which results in altered fat distribution and muscle weakness.

6. Benito has developed a severe form of hypothyroidism that causes nonpitting edema in connective tissue. He has _____.

7. Julia has _____ disease, in which gradual adrenal gland failure causes insufficient production of steroid hormones and the need for hormone replacement therapy.

8. _____ _____ is a congenital condition of thyroid hormone deficiency, characterized by arrested physical and mental development.

9. The hormone _____ plays a role in regulating and maintaining the body's water, sodium, and electrolyte balance.

10. _____ reflects the average blood glucose level over the past 3 to 4 months.

Multiple Choice

Select the one best answer to the following multiple-choice questions.

Exercise 8

1. Annette Vizzetti has insulin-dependent diabetes mellitus (IDDM). She is a regular patient at Valley Clinic and has come in today for a regular health check. The physician is interested in knowing what Ms. Vizzetti's average blood glucose levels have been for the last 2 to 3 months. Which of the following tests is the physician most likely to order?
   a. TSH
   b. GTT
   c. HbA1c
   d. fasting blood glucose

2. When Ms. Vizzetti was first diagnosed with IDDM, she complained to her physician of the three "polys," the classic signs of diabetes. Which of the following is **not** one of them?
   a. polyphagia
   b. polydipsia
   c. polyphasia
   d. polyuria

3. Normal blood glucose level is 60 to 99. When Ms. Vizzetti checks her glucose today, she notes that the result is 172. The correct medical term for this condition is:
   a. hypercalcemia
   b. hyperglycemia
   c. hyperkalemia
   d. hypernatremia

4. Ms. Singh has been ill for the past 2 days with stomach flu. Her symptoms include diarrhea and vomiting. She has not been able to keep food or fluids down and has become moderately dehydrated. Because of her diarrhea and poor intake, her blood potassium level is below normal. The correct term for this is:

   a. hyponatremia

   b. hypocalcemia

   c. hypokalemia

   d. hypoglycemia

5. Because Ms. Singh is dehydrated, her blood sodium level is higher than normal. The correct term for this is:

   a. hypernatremia

   b. hypercalcemia

   c. hyperkalemia

   d. hyperglycemia

Fill in the Blanks

Write the common use for the medication using Table 12-4.

Exercise 9

1. Glucotrol _____

2. Synthroid _____

3. carbimazole _____

4. Victoza _____

5. miglitol _____

6. somatropin _____

7. cabergoline _____

8. acarbose _____

9. Somatuline _____

10. Actos _____

CASE STUDY

Read the case study and answer the questions that follow. Most of the terms are included in this chapter. Refer to your medical dictionary for the other terms.

Diabetes

Marsha Bloom is a 43-year-old female with a history of good health other than mild obesity. She reported a recent 25-pound weight loss over 3 months without dieting. She described an increased appetite and states that she has been eating more than usual. She has also had polydipsia, polyphagia, and polyuria. Ms. Bloom complained of increasing fatigue in spite of getting 8 to 9 hours of sleep each night. Her greatest concern was a recent realization that her vision has worsened significantly. She described being unable to recognize her friend at the grocery store until she was just a few feet away from her. This is what prompted her to seek medical attention.

Ms. Bloom underwent a random blood glucose level test, a fasting blood glucose level test, and a glycosylated hemoglobin test. Diagnosis of diabetes is usually confirmed based on the classic symptoms and two separate fasting glucose levels of more than 126 mg/dL or a random glucose level over 200 mg/dL. In Ms. Bloom's case, the results of all three tests were elevated. Because of this, her physician started her on oral agents to control her blood glucose levels and referred her to a diabetic educator to learn more about her disease and develop a food and exercise plan.

Three months later, after meeting with the diabetic educator and being evaluated by her ophthalmologist, Ms. Bloom began a regular exercise program and made some positive changes in her diet. Over the past 3 months, she has lost another 20 pounds, has noted an improvement in her vision, and commented that her "poly" symptoms have resolved. Best of all, she states that her energy level has increased dramatically.

Non–insulin-dependent diabetes mellitus (NIDDM), also known as *type 2 diabetes,* is the most common form of diabetes, affecting an estimated 20 million Americans. Typical onset occurs after the age of 40, which explains why it has also been known as *adult-onset diabetes.* There appears to be a genetic tendency, because it runs in families. Sadly, the incidence of type 2 diabetes is rapidly growing in this country. This is thought to be a result of childhood and adult obesity as well as sedentary lifestyle.

Symptoms begin gradually and include the three "polys": *polydipsia, polyuria,* and *polyphagia.* Obesity is a common factor, yet, as blood sugar skyrockets out of control, individuals may begin to note an ability to eat more yet lose weight. They may also experience delayed wound healing. In NIDDM, the pancreas still produces some insulin; the problem may be a deficiency of insulin production or resistance to the insulin that is produced.

Case Study Questions

Exercise 10

1. Ms. Bloom experienced which of the following symptoms prior to diagnosis?
   a. decreased appetite
   b. decreased urination
   c. decreased visual acuity
   d. weight gain

2. Ms. Bloom's diagnosis of type 2 diabetes was confirmed by:
   a. a test that reveals the average blood glucose level over the past 3 to 4 months
   b. a test of a drop of capillary blood obtained by pricking her finger
   c. a test of her blood after a 1-hour fast
   d. all of these

Flashpoint

ChooseMyPlate.gov is a US Department of Agriculture (USDA) website that provides free education and interactive tools to encourage healthy eating, weight management, and physical activity.

3. Which of the following statements is true regarding NIDDM?
   a. It is the second most common form of diabetes.
   b. Onset is usually before the age of 40.
   c. Obesity is uncommon.
   d. There may be a genetic component.

4. Which of the following statements is true regarding NIDDM?
   a. The pancreas fails to produce insulin.
   b. The body may be resistant to the insulin that is produced.
   c. Exercise is not recommended for disease management.
   d. The primary form of treatment is injection of insulin.

5. Create a list of healthy foods and types of exercise that you enjoy.

6. A healthy diet and daily exercise can control the symptoms of type 2 diabetes. Use the list you created above to design a 3-day meal plan and exercise program.

End-of-Chapter Practice Exercises

Word Building

*Using **only** the word parts in the lists provided, create medical terms with the indicated meanings.*

Exercise 11

Prefixes	Combining Forms	Suffixes
eu-	acr/o	-centesis
hyper-	aden/o	-ectomy
hypo-	adrenal/o	-emia
	calc/o	-ic
	cyan/o	-ism
	dermat/o	-itis
	gluc/o	-kinesia
	hydr/o	-logy
	kal/i	-megaly
	natr/o	-meter
	pancreat/o	-oma
	parathyroid/o	-osis
	thym/o	-pathy
	thyr/o	-ptosis
	thyroid/o	-therapy
	toxic/o	

1. Study of poison _____

2. Tumor of a gland _____

3. Below-normal parathyroid (hormone) _____

4. Adrenal disease _____

5. Condition of excessive calcium in the blood _____

6. Measuring instrument for glucose _____

7. Water treatment _____

8. Abnormal condition of blueness of the extremities _____

9. Condition of excessive potassium in the blood _____

10. Inflammation of the pancreas _____

11. Pertaining to a good or normal thymus _____

12. Condition of excessive thyroid _____

13. Inflammation of the skin of the extremities _____

14. Condition of below-normal sodium in the blood _____

15. Excision or surgical removal of the thymus _____

16. Surgical puncture of the pancreas _____

17. Prolapse of the pancreas _____

18. Tumor of the thymus _____

19. Enlargement of the thyroid _____

20. Movement of the extremities _____

True or False

Decide whether the following statements are true or false.

Exercise 12

1. True   False   The abbreviation **TSH** stands for *thyroid-stimulating hormone.*

2. True   False   The abbreviation **ADH** stands for *adenopathy.*

3. True   False   The abbreviation **K** stands for *kidney.*

4. True   False   A **FBS** measures blood glucose levels after the patient has fasted for 8 to 12 hours.

5. True   False   The abbreviation **Na** stands for *natural.*

6. True   False   A **glycosylated hemoglobin** test reveals the average blood glucose level over the past 9 months.

7. True   False   The abbreviation **FSBS** stands for *fasting blood sugar.*

8. True   False   A **TSH** level may be drawn to check for hypothyroidism.

9. True False The abbreviation **PTH** stands for *parathyroid hormone.*

10. True False A **fasting blood sugar** is drawn after an 8- to 12-hour fast.

Deciphering Terms

Write the correct meaning of these medical terms.

Exercise 13

1. polyphagia _____

2. thyrotoxicosis _____

3. parathyroidectomy _____

4. polydipsia _____

5. glycolysis _____

6. pancreatorrhexis _____

7. hydrogenic _____

8. polyuria _____

9. pancreatopathy _____

10. microthymus _____

Multiple Choice

Select the one best answer to the following multiple-choice questions.

Exercise 14

1. Which of the following combining forms means *poison?*
   a. thyr/o
   b. thym/o
   c. toxic/o
   d. thyroid/o

2. Which of the following combining forms means *extremities?*
   a. kal/i
   b. calc/o
   c. acr/o
   d. natr/o

3. Which of the following combining forms means *sodium?*
   a. natr/o
   b. kal/i
   c. acr/o
   d. calc/o

4. Which of the following combining forms means *same, unchanging?*
   a. thym/o
   b. hydr/o
   c. aden/o
   d. home/o

5. Which of the following combining forms refers to the adrenal gland?
   a. aden/o
   b. thyroid/o
   c. adren/o
   d. acr/o

6. Which of the following abbreviations is related to body size?
   a. BMR
   b. BS
   c. BMI
   d. FBS

7. Which of the following abbreviations represents a hormone?
   a. GH
   b. HRT
   c. DI
   d. DKA

8. All of the following abbreviations represent electrolytes **except:**
   a. Na
   b. K
   c. T3
   d. Ca

9. Which of the following tests might be done to measure a patient's current blood sugar?

   a. DM

   b. FSBS

   c. TSH

   d. ADH

10. An individual suffering from a low hormone level may be administered:

    a. CA

    b. FBS

    c. HRT

    d. IDDM

11. A severe form of hypothyroidism that develops in the older child or adult and causes nonpitting edema in connective tissue is:

    a. myxedema

    b. Addison's disease

    c. Cushing's disease

    d. hirsutism

12. A condition of thyroid hormone deficiency characterized by arrested physical and mental development and formerly known as *cretinism* is:

    a. congenital hypothyroidism

    b. Hashimoto's thyroiditis

    c. dwarfism

    d. Graves' disease

13. A condition of severe hyperglycemia potentially leading to coma is:

    a. diabetes mellitus

    b. diabetes insipidus

    c. diabetic ketoacidosis

    d. nondiabetic hypoglycemia

14. A tumor of the adrenal medulla that is usually benign but may cause fluctuation of stress hormones like adrenaline is:

    a. exophthalmos

    b. pheochromocytoma

    c. goiter

    d. thyrotoxicosis

15. All of the following diagnostic tests are matched with the correct definition **except:**

   a. glycosylated hemoglobin: reflection of the average blood glucose level over the past 2 to 3 months

   b. thyroid scan: radiographic evaluation of the thyroid after a radioactive substance is injected; identifies thyroid size, shape, position, and function

   c. fasting blood glucose: test of blood glucose from a drop of capillary blood obtained by pricking the finger

   d. thyroid function test: reflection of thyroid function by measuring levels of thyroid-stimulating hormone (TSH), triiodothyronine (T3), and thyroxine (T4)

16. Which of the following terms means *excessive sensation in the extremities?*

   a. acroanesthesia

   b. adrenalodynia

   c. anacusis

   d. hyperacroesthesia

17. Which of the following terms means *creation of sugar?*

   a. glycolysis

   b. glucogenic

   c. glycogenesis

   d. glucokinesia

18. The term *adenopathy* means:

   a. disease of a gland

   b. pertaining to the adrenal gland

   c. abnormal condition of a gland

   d. pain in a gland

19. The term *hyperkalemia* means:

   a. condition of excessive calcium in the blood

   b. condition of excessive potassium in the blood

   c. condition of excessive sodium in the blood

   d. condition of excessive iron in the blood

20. Breakdown by the body of water molecules may be called:

   a. hydrogenesis

   b. hydrolysis

   c. hydrokinesis

   d. hydrophobia

SKELETAL AND MUSCULAR SYSTEMS

13

Chapter Outline

Structure and Function

The skeletal system and the muscular system work together in a complementary fashion to make movement possible. Neither system would be effective without the other. Bones of the skeletal system provide a strong framework for the muscles that are attached to them. When the muscles contract and relax in different combinations, they create a pulling effect on the bones that results in movement.

The Skeletal System

Structures of the skeletal system include bones, tendons, and ligaments (Fig. 13-1). **Bones** are composed of dense connective tissue, which includes bone cells in a matrix of the mineral calcium and collagen fibers. Bones are dynamic, living, ever-changing structures. Unlike the white, dry, dead bones you may have seen, living bones have a rich supply of blood vessels and nerves. If injured, they may hurt and bleed. The most common injuries to bones are fractures. This also means they have the ability to heal themselves. Important to the healing process is the development of **osteocytes,** new bone cells, which are constantly created through **osteogenesis.** New cells replace older ones that are injured or broken down as they age. Because bones are able to remodel themselves in this way, certain activities, such as weight lifting or weight-bearing exercise like jogging and walking, stimulate bones to become stronger and denser.

Flashpoint

Stresses on bone, such as weight bearing and muscle contractions, help bones to remain strong or become stronger.

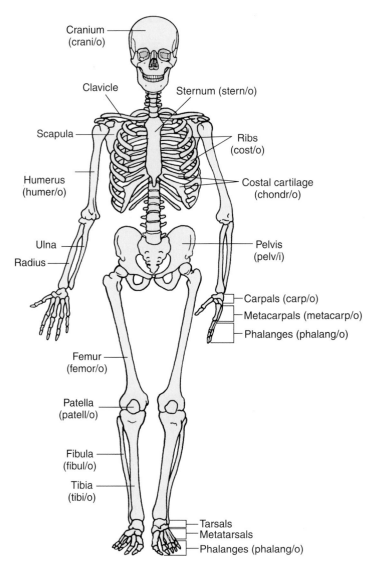

FIGURE 13-1 **The skeletal system.**

The **skeletal system** provides protection, movement, and a framework for the body. Bones that provide protection include those that make up the cranium; they are fused together to create a strong container for the brain. Other protective bones include those of the **vertebral column,** which protect the spinal cord and combine with the sternum and ribs to create the **thorax,** which protects the heart, great vessels, and lungs (Fig. 13-2).

The skeletal system also plays important roles in blood production and mineral regulation. Marrow, a soft substance within bone, performs **hematopoiesis,** or the production of red and white blood cells. This explains why a bone marrow transplant may be necessary for someone with a blood disorder such as leukemia.

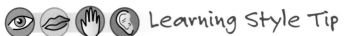 Learning Style Tip

Rewrite explanations, concepts, and definitions from this chapter in your own words. This forces you to think about what they really mean and to put them into simpler terms that you will remember. For verbal and auditory benefit, read your notes aloud and record your voice. This will enable you to study while you are driving or exercising.

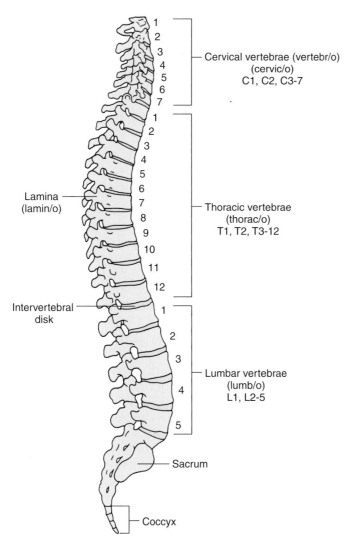

FIGURE 13-2 **The vertebral column.**

Bones store **essential minerals** such as calcium, phosphorus, and magnesium. These minerals are largely responsible for providing bones with strength and hardness. These same minerals are also necessary for nerve and muscle function, so they must be present in these tissues as well as in the blood. When dietary mineral intake is inadequate or the need for these minerals increases, as in puberty or pregnancy, the bones release their stores of minerals into the bloodstream for use. A decrease in bone strength and density may result if sufficient amounts of these minerals are not replenished. This loss of bone mass is called **osteoporosis.** A person with osteoporosis has a greater risk of fractures, especially at the hip and vertebral column. Other risk factors for *osteoporosis* include advanced age, menopause, sedentary lifestyle, high protein intake, prolonged use of certain medications, and some endocrine diseases.

Tendons are cords of fibrous connective tissue that attach muscles to bones. A tendon that attaches to a larger area of a bone is called an **aponeurosis.** This structure is flat or ribbonlike and larger than a typical tendon. Tendons do not contract or lengthen when muscles contract or relax, but they help to enable the bone's movement.

Ligaments are bands or sheets of strong, fibrous connective tissue that connect bones to other bones across joints. They provide joint stability and limit joint motion. They essentially hold joints together, allowing the attached muscles to move bones upon contraction while preventing the joint from falling apart.

A **joint** is a place where two bones meet. Bones enable movement at joints through attachments to muscles and tendons. There are three types of bone joints, sometimes called *articulations:*

Synarthrosis—an immovable joint, such as the sutures of the skull
Amphiarthrosis—a slightly movable joint, such as a vertebra
Diarthrosis—a freely movable joint, such as the hip joint

Some joints allow no movement, such as those between the bones of the skull. Diarthrosis, also known as synovial joints, allow for a great deal of movement, or **range of motion.** The shoulder joint allows the arm to raise overhead 180 degrees. The elbow can bend 145 degrees, and the knee can bend 130 degrees. The amount of range of motion *(ROM)* at a joint is measured with a **goniometer** (Fig. 13-3). Active range of motion *(AROM)* involves moving a body part as far as possible without assistance. If someone gets help moving the body part, it is called active assistive range of motion *(AAROM)*. If a person is completely relaxed while somebody else moves the body part, it is called passive range of motion *(PROM)*.

Synovial joints are surrounded by a joint capsule (Fig. 13-4). The structures of the joint capsule include the articular cartilage that protects the bone ends, the synovial fluid between the bone ends that lubricates and nourishes the articular cartilage, and the synovial membrane that secretes the synovial fluid. A disorder of these joints, called *osteoarthritis*, or degenerative joint disease *(DJD)*, commonly affects large weight-bearing joints such as the hip and knee. The articular cartilage deteriorates, allowing the bone ends to rub together, thus resulting in inflammation and pain. Risk factors for osteoarthritis include age, obesity, and overuse. If treatment measures are unsuccessful, and the pain becomes too great, a joint replacement may be necessary.

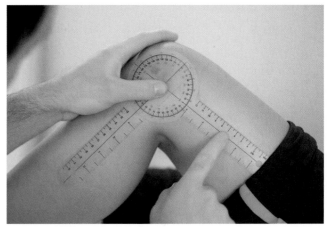

FIGURE 13-3 **Goniometer.** (Photograph © Thinkstock)

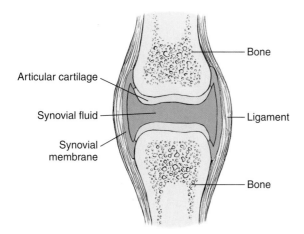

FIGURE 13-4 **Synovial joint.**

The Muscular System

Muscles are connective tissues made up of contractile fibers. They are covered by a fibrous membrane called a **fascia,** which is connective tissue arranged in sheets or bands. The fascia covers, separates, and supports muscle. Because muscle and fascia are connected, these two structures are commonly referred to as one: myofascia.

There are three types of muscle: striated (skeletal) muscle, sometimes called *voluntary muscle;* smooth muscle, sometimes called *involuntary muscle;* and cardiac muscle.

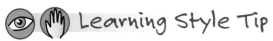 Learning Style Tip

Purchase an anatomy coloring book and use colored pencils or markers to complete it. Write the associated combining forms next to each muscle and bone as you color it.

Striated muscles are found in all skeletal muscles and also in the tongue, pharynx, and upper portion of the esophagus. The striations, or stripes, in this type of muscle are due to the bundled structure of the muscle fibers and their appearance under the microscope. This type of muscle is also sometimes called *voluntary muscle* because we are usually able to consciously move and control it. Skeletal muscles are involved in the movement of body parts, reflexive movements, and maintenance of posture. Examples of skeletal muscles are those that move the bones, eyeballs, and tongue. Skeletal muscles contract to create movement. The type and force of movement depends on the type of muscle and the force of muscle contraction. Through exercise, skeletal muscle can **hypertrophy,** or increase in size (Fig. 13-5). Skeletal muscles that are not used (for example, in a comatose patient) will **atrophy,** or decrease in size.

Muscle groups often work together to achieve both movement and stabilization. For example, the quadriceps muscles extend the knee while the hamstring muscles extend the hip, enabling us to stand up from a chair or walk up stairs. When this is occurring, other muscles in the trunk of the body contract to keep the body in a stable, upright position. Nerves bring signals to the muscle tissue from the brain and spinal cord to control muscle movement. Many muscles are required for movement such as walking. A person's

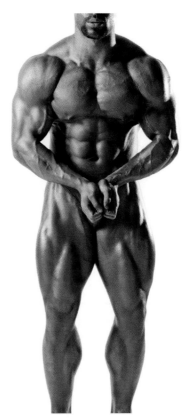

FIGURE 13-5 **Bodybuilder.** (Photograph © Thinkstock)

gait, or the manner and style in which the person walks, is coordinated by the skeletal muscles of the trunk, legs, and arms (Box 13-1). Even the muscles of the neck have a role in gait. Figure 13-6 illustrates the major muscles of the body.

In addition to fostering movement and providing support, skeletal muscles also produce heat as a by-product of their function. This is why a person feels hot and begins to perspire while exercising: The body has produced more heat than is needed, and natural cooling mechanisms kick in. This same principle works when a person is exposed to a cold environment and more body heat is needed. Without adequate clothing, body temperature drops, and shivering begins. Shivering is an involuntary increase in muscle activity that produces heat energy as a by-product, which warms the body.

Smooth muscle is found principally in the internal organs of the digestive tract, respiratory passages, the urinary bladder, and the walls of blood vessels. No cross striations appear on these muscle fibers. This type of muscle is arranged in sheets or layers. It is considered involuntary because it functions without the need for conscious thought. In the digestive tract, smooth muscle contracts to propel food through the alimentary canal to be broken down for digestion and absorption. In the walls of blood vessels, smooth muscle moves blood through the vessels to various parts of the body. Unlike skeletal muscle, smooth muscle's size and strength cannot be affected by exercise.

Cardiac (heart) muscle cells contain striations that appear similar to skeletal muscle cells. However, these muscle fibers are arranged in branching networks, rather than linear bundles. The branched structure allows them to connect with one another in a continuous network. Located at the connections are

Flashpoint

Heat is a natural by-product of muscle activity.

Box 13-1 Gait

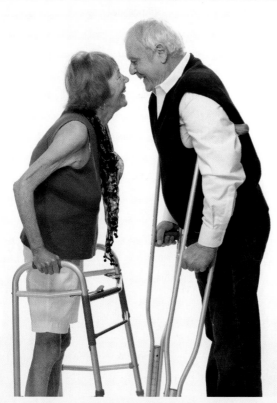

Gait with assistive devices. (Photograph © Thinkstock)

The manner in which a person walks, or the gait, is influenced by factors such as muscle weakness, pain, or injury to an area of the body. For example, while walking, weakness of the anterior ankle muscles may cause the foot to drag on the floor when moving the leg forward. To prevent this, a person will alter the gait pattern by either raising the hip higher or bending the knee further, allowing the foot to clear the floor. If there is pain in the hip, knee, or ankle, a person will alter the gait pattern by trying to put less weight on that leg, resulting in a limp. Having pain in the back may cause a person to walk with a stooped-forward posture. When a person has an injury to the leg such as a fracture, he or she may be wearing a cast or brace and may be limited in the amount of weight he or she is permitted to place on the leg. In many cases, there is a period where the injured person is not permitted to put any weight at all on the leg. This provides time for the tissues to heal undisturbed.

A doctor or physical therapist may recommend use of an assistive device to improve gait or increase safety while walking. If the doctor has instructed a person to be non–weight bearing (NWB), partial weight bearing (PWB), or toe touch weight bearing (TTWB) on a leg, an assistive device is required. Axillary crutches (AC) and front wheel walkers (FWW) are used when a person cannot put full weight on a leg. Canes can only be used when full weight bearing (FWB) is permitted. Assistive devices are used not only for people who are recovering from injuries or procedures but also for people with muscle weakness or pain. In addition, those with poor balance may use assistive devices to improve their safety by decreasing their risk of falls.

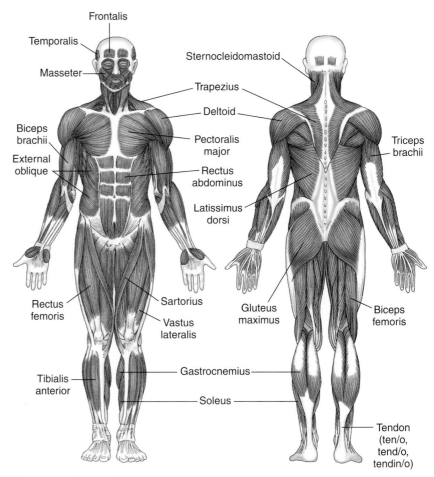

FIGURE 13-6 **The muscular system.**

intercalated discs, which increase the efficiency of electrical impulse transmission throughout the heart. Cardiac muscle works to pump blood through the heart and out to the body. Strong contractions of the heart muscle push blood through the circulatory system, supplying blood and oxygen to all the tissues of the body. Blood returns to the right side of the heart—which pumps it to the lungs, where it is reoxygenated—and then returns back to the left side of the heart. As with skeletal muscles, cardiac muscle's efficiency improves with use. Exercise that increases the heart rate increases the efficiency of the cardiac muscle.

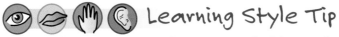 Learning Style Tip

Look at Figures 13-5 and 13-6. Name all of the muscles you can see on the bodybuilder. Next, using Figure 13-6 as a map, find all of the muscles on your own body, touching each one and saying its name aloud. Repeat this until you are able to do it without looking at Figure 13-6.

Structure and Function Practice Exercises

Fill in the Blanks

Choose the term that matches the description.

Exercise 1

Bones	Synarthrosis	Joints
Osteocytes	Amphiarthrosis	Muscles
Osteogenesis	Diarthrosis	Fascia
Skeletal system	Range of motion	Striated muscle
Vertebral column	Goniometer	Hypertrophy
Thorax	Osteoporosis	Atrophy
Hematopoiesis	Tendons	Gait
Essential minerals	Aponeurosis	Smooth muscle
	Ligaments	

1. _____ A disorder of decreased bone mass

2. _____ An immovable joint

3. _____ The sternum and the ribs

4. _____ Attach muscles to bones

5. _____ Connective tissues made up of contractile fibers

6. _____ New bone cells

7. _____ A freely movable joint

8. _____ Functions include protection, blood production, and mineral regulation

9. _____ Attach bones to other bones

10. _____ The space where two bones meet and where movement occurs

11. _____ Composed of dense connective tissue including cells in a matrix of calcium and collagen fibers

12. _____ Connective tissue arranged in sheets or bands which covers muscle tissue

13. _____ Bones that protect the spinal cord

14. _____ A device for measuring joint range of motion

15. _____ Decrease in size

16. _____ Calcium, phosphorus, and magnesium

17. _____ The production of red and white blood cells

18. _____ Muscle that is not controlled by conscious thought and is not affected by exercise

19. _____ Increase in size

20. _____ A slightly movable joint

21. _____ The amount of motion available at a joint

22. _____ A tendon that resembles a ribbon and attaches to a larger area of bone

23. _____ Creation of new bone cells

24. _____ The manner and style in which a person walks

25. _____ Considered voluntary muscle and is affected by exercise

Fill in the Blanks

Label Figure 13-7 with the appropriate anatomical terms and combining forms.

Exercise 2

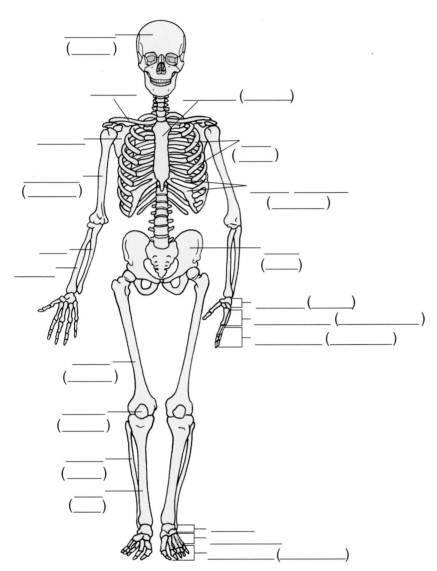

FIGURE 13-7 **Skeletal system with blanks.**

Fill in the Blanks

Label Figure 13-8 with the appropriate anatomical terms and combining forms.

Exercise 3

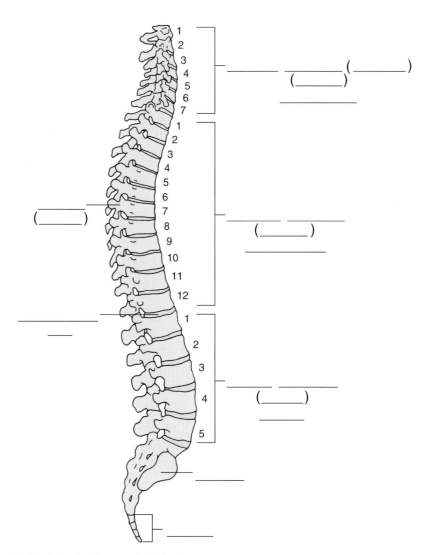

FIGURE 13-8 Vertebral column with blanks.

Fill in the Blanks

Label Figure 13-9 with the appropriate anatomical terms and combining forms.

Exercise 4

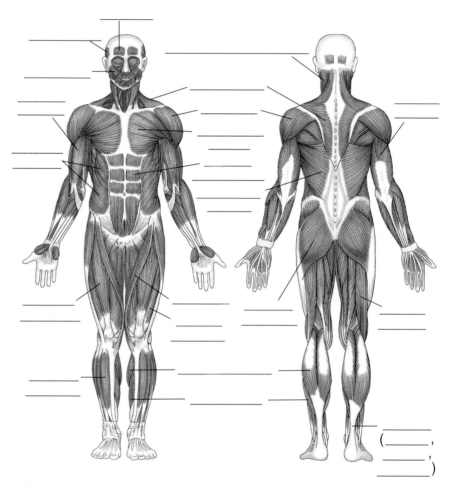

FIGURE 13-9 **Muscular system with blanks.**

Combining Forms and Abbreviations

Combining Forms

Table 13-1 contains combining forms that pertain to the musculoskeletal system, a combination of the skeletal and muscular systems, along with examples of terms that utilize the combining forms and a pronunciation guide. Read aloud to yourself as you move from left to right across the table. Be sure to use the pronunciation guide so that you can learn to say the terms correctly.

Flashpoint

Write the following numbers in a vertical pattern: 7, 12, 5, 5, 4. Repeat the numbers aloud until you have them memorized. Second, write the following terms next to each number from top to bottom: cervical, thoracic, lumbar, sacral, coccygeal. Third, repeat the numbers with each term top to bottom until you have them memorized. You have just memorized 33 bones of the body: the vertebrae—7 cervical, 12 thoracic, 5 lumbar, 5 sacral, and 4 coccygeal.

TABLE 13-1

COMBINING FORMS RELATED TO THE MUSCULOSKELETAL SYSTEM

Combining Form	Meaning	Example (Pronunciation)	Meaning of New Term
acr/o	extremities	acroanesthesia (ăk-rō-ăn-ĕs-THĒ-zē-ă)	absence of sensation in the extremities
ankyl/o	stiff joint	ankylosis (ăng-kĭ-LŌ-sĭs)	abnormal condition of a stiff joint
arthr/o	joint	arthrocentesis (ăr-thrō-sĕn-TĒ-sĭs)	surgical puncture of a joint
articul/o		articular (ăr-TĬK-ū-lăr)	pertaining to a joint
burs/o	bursa, sac	bursitis (bŭr-SĪ-tĭs)	inflammation of a bursa
carp/o	carpus	carpectomy (kăr-PĔK-tō-mē)	excision or surgical removal of a carpus
cervic/o	neck	cervicodynia (sĕr-vĭ-kō-DĬN-ē-ă)	pain of the neck
chondr/o	cartilage	chondrodysplasia (kŏn-drō-dĭs-PLĀ-zē-ă)	bad, painful, or difficult formation or growth of cartilage
cost/o	ribs	costochondritis (kŏs-tō-kŏn-DRĪ-tĭs)	inflammation of the ribs and cartilage
crani/o	cranium	craniocerebral (krā-nē-ō-sĕ-RĒ-brăl)	pertaining to the cranium and brain
fasci/o	fascia	fasciodesis (făsh-ē-ŎD-ĕ-sĭs)	binding or surgical fixation of a fascia
femor/o	femur	femorotibial (fĕm-ō-rō-TĬB-ē-ăl)	pertaining to the femur and tibia
fibul/o	fibula	fibular (FĬB-ū-lăr)	pertaining to the fibula
humer/o	humerus	humeral (HŪ-mĕr-ăl)	pertaining to the humerus
ili/o	ilium	iliolumbar (ĭl-ē-ō-LŬM-bar)	pertaining to the ilium and lower back
kinesi/o	movement	kinesiology (kĭ-nē-zē-ŎL-ō-jē)	study of movement
kyph/o	hump	kyphosis (kī-FŌ-sĭs)	abnormal condition of a hump
lamin/o	lamina	laminectomy (lăm-ĭ-NĔK-tō-mē)	excision or surgical removal of a lamina
lord/o	bent backward	lordoscoliosis (lōr-dō-skō-lē-Ō-sĭs)	abnormal condition of crookedness and backward bend
lumb/o	lower back	lumbodynia (lŭm-bō-DĬN-ē-ă)	pain of the lower back
menisc/o	meniscus	meniscectomy (mĕn-ĭ-SĔK-tō-mē)	excision or surgical removal of a meniscus

TABLE 13-1

COMBINING FORMS RELATED TO THE MUSCULOSKELETAL SYSTEM—cont'd

Combining Form	Meaning	Example (Pronunciation)	Meaning of New Term
metacarp/o	metacarpus	metacarpectomy (mĕt-ă-kăr-PĔK-tō-mē)	excision or surgical removal of a metacarpus
metatars/o	metatarsals, ankle	metatarsophalangeal (mĕt-ă-tăr-sō-fă-LĂN-jē-ăl)	pertaining to the ankle, metatarsals, and phalanges
muscul/o	muscle	musculoskeletal (mŭs-kū-lō-SKĔL-ĕ-tăl)	pertaining to the muscles and skeleton
my/o		myocardial (mī-ō-KĂR-dē-ăl)	pertaining to heart muscle
myel/o	spinal cord, bone marrow	myeloplegia (mī-ĕl-ō-PLĒ-jē-ă)	paralysis of the spinal cord
orth/o	straight	orthopnea (or-THŎP-nē-ă)	breathing in the straight position
oste/o	bone	osteolytic (ŏs-tē-ō-LĬT-ĭk)	pertaining to the destruction of bone
patell/a	patella	patellapexy (pă-TĔL-ă-pĕk-sē)	surgical fixation of the patella
patell/o		patelloptosis (pă-TĔL-ŏpt-ō-sis)	prolapse of the patella
pelv/i	pelvis	pelvimeter (pĕl-VĬM-ĕ-tĕr)	measuring instrument for the pelvis
phalang/o	phalanges	phalangitis (făl-ăn-JĪ-tĭs)	inflammation of the phalanges
pub/o	pubis	pubofemoral (pū-bō-FĔM-ōr-ăl)	pertaining to the pubis and femur
radi/o	radius	radioulnar (rā-dē-ō-ŬL-năr)	pertaining to the radius and ulna
sacr/o	sacrum	sacrodynia (sā-krō-DĬN-ē-ă)	pain of the sacrum
scoli/o	crooked, bent	scoliometer (skō-lē-ŎM-ĕt-ĕr)	measuring instrument for crookedness or bend
spondyl/o	vertebrae	spondylomalacia (spŏn-dĭ-lō-mă-LĀ-shē-ă)	softening of a vertebra
vertebr/o		vertebroplasty (vĕr-TĒ-brō-plăs-tē)	surgical repair of a vertebra
stern/o	sternum	sternocostal (stĕr-nō-KŎS-tăl)	pertaining to the sternum and ribs
sthen/o	strength	myasthenia (mī-ăs-THĒ-nē-ă)	condition of absence of muscle strength
synov/o	synovial membrane	synovectomy (sĭn-ō-VĔK-tō-mē)	surgical removal of a synovial membrane
synovi/o		synovioma (sĭn-ō-vē-Ō-mă)	tumor of a synovial membrane

Continued

TABLE 13-1

COMBINING FORMS RELATED TO THE MUSCULOSKELETAL SYSTEM—cont'd

Combining Form	Meaning	Example (Pronunciation)	Meaning of New Term
tars/o	ankle (tarsal bones)	tarsometatarsal (tăr-sō-mĕt-ă-TĂR-săl)	pertaining to the ankle
ten/o	tendon	tenodynia (tĕn-ō-DĬN-ē-ă)	pain of a tendon
tend/o		tendotome (TĔN-dō-tōm)	cutting instrument for a tendon
tendin/o		tendinous (TĔN-dĭ-nŭs)	pertaining to a tendon
thorac/o	thorax	thoracolumbar (thō-răk-ō-LŬM-bar)	pertaining to the thorax and lower back
tibi/o	tibia	tibiofibular (tĭb-ē-ō-FĬB-ū-lăr)	pertaining to the tibia and fibula
uln/o	ulna	ulnocarpal (ŭl-nō-KĂR-păl)	pertaining to the ulna and carpus

IN A FLASH!

It's time to print out all of the Combining Form Flash Cards for Chapter 13 and run through them at least three times before you continue.

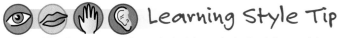 Learning Style Tip

Play instrumental music (without lyrics) while studying these terms. Repeatedly sing the terms and their meanings aloud along to the music until you can remember them. If the term describes an area of the body, touch that area on yourself, or point to it on another person, as you sing the term aloud.

Abbreviations

Table 13-2 lists some of the most common abbreviations related to the musculoskeletal system as well as others often used in medical documentation.

IN A FLASH!

It's time to print out all of the Abbreviations Flash Cards for Chapter 13 and run through them at least three times before you continue.

TABLE 13-2
ABBREVIATIONS

AAROM	active assistive range of motion	BE	below the elbow
ACL	anterior cruciate ligament	BK	below the knee
ADL	activity of daily living	BKA	below-the-knee amputation
AE	above the elbow	BMD	bone mineral density
AK	above the knee	C1–C7	first cervical vertebra, second cervical vertebra, etc.
AKA	above-the-knee amputation	DJD	degenerative joint disease (osteoarthritis)
AP	anteroposterior	DTR	deep tendon reflex
AROM	active range of motion	EMG	electromyography
AS	ankylosing spondylitis	Fx	fracture

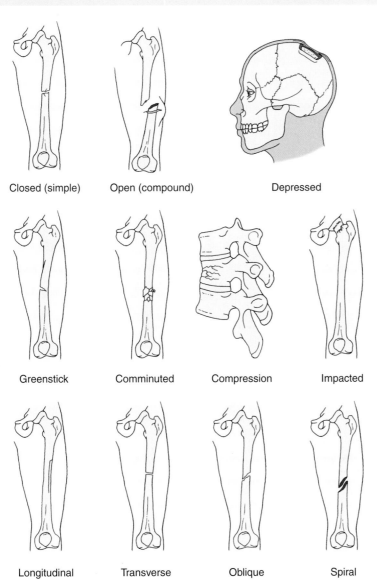

Closed (simple) Open (compound) Depressed

Greenstick Comminuted Compression Impacted

Longitudinal Transverse Oblique Spiral

Types of fractures.

Continued

TABLE 13-2
ABBREVIATIONS—cont'd

HNP	herniated nucleus pulposus	OT	occupational therapy, occupational therapist
IM	intramuscular	PROM	passive range of motion
JRA	juvenile rheumatoid arthritis	PT	physical therapy, physical therapist
L1–L5	first lumbar vertebra, second lumbar vertebra, etc.	RA	rheumatoid arthritis
LE	lower extremity	RLE	right lower extremity
LLE	left lower extremity	ROM	range of motion
LUE	left upper extremity	RUE	right upper extremity
MMT	manual muscle test	S1–S5	first sacral vertebra, second sacral vertebra, etc.
MVA	motor vehicle accident	T1–T12	first thoracic vertebra, second thoracic vertebra, etc.
NSAID	nonsteroidal anti-inflammatory drug	THA, THR	total hip arthroplasty, total hip replacement
OA	osteoarthritis	TKA, TKR	total knee arthroplasty, total knee replacement
ORIF	open reduction–internal fixation	UE	upper extremity
ortho	orthopedic		

Assistive Devices and Weight-Bearing Status

AC	axillary crutches	PUW	pick up walker
DME	durable medical equipment	PWB	partial weight bearing
FWB	full weight bearing	SBQC	small base quad cane
FWW	front wheel walker	SPC	single point cane
HW	hemi walker	TTWB	toe touch weight bearing
LBQC	large base quad cane	WBAT	weight bearing as tolerated
NWB	non–weight bearing	WC	wheelchair

Combining Forms and Abbreviations Practice Exercises

Fill in the Blanks

Fill in the blanks below using Table 13-1.

Exercise 5

1. pertaining to the tibia and fibula _____

2. inflammation of the phalanges _____

3. surgical repair of a vertebra _____

4. surgical fixation of the patella _____

5. pain in a tendon _____

6. pertaining to the femur and tibia _____

7. cutting instrument for a tendon _____

8. pertaining to a tendon _____

9. paralysis of the spinal cord _____

10. pertaining to the destruction of bone _____

11. excision or surgical removal of a metacarpus _____

12. pertaining to the humerus _____

13. pertaining to the sternum and ribs _____

14. measuring instrument for the pelvis _____

15. pertaining to the thorax and lower back _____

16. breathing in the straight position _____

17. pertaining to heart muscle _____

18. surgical puncture of a joint _____

19. excision or surgical removal of a carpus _____

20. bad, painful, or difficult formation or growth of cartilage _____

21. inflammation of the ribs and cartilage _____

22. pain of the neck _____

23. pertaining to the cranium and brain _____

24. pertaining to the fibula _____

25. excision or surgical removal of a lamina _____

26. pertaining to a joint _____

27. inflammation of a bursa _____

28. binding or surgical fixation of a fascia _____

29. pertaining to the ilium and lower back _____

30. abnormal condition of crookedness and backward bend _____

31. abnormal condition of a hump _____

32. pertaining to the muscles and skeleton _____

33. study of movement _____

34. measuring instrument for crookedness or bend _____

35. excision or surgical removal of a meniscus _____

36. pain of the sacrum _____

37. pertaining to the ulna and carpus _____

38. pain of the lower back _____

39. pertaining to the radius and ulna _____

40. excision or surgical removal of a synovial membrane _____

41. abnormal condition of a stiff joint _____

42. softening of a vertebra _____

43. pertaining to the pubis and femur _____

44. pertaining to the ankle _____

45. tumor of a synovial membrane _____

46. pertaining to the metatarsals and phalanges _____

Fill in the Blanks

Write the correct term next to each abbreviation using Table 13-2.

Exercise 6

1. LE _____

2. HNP _____

3. AC _____

4. OT _____

5. JRA _____

6. BE _____

7. Fx _____

8. AKA _____

9. NWB _____

10. RUE _____

11. FWW _____

12. PROM _____

13. WC _____   17. DME _____

14. DTR _____   18. SPC _____

15. ORIF _____   19. OA _____

16. PT _____   20. BMD _____

 Learning Style Tip

Write out poems or sayings that include the terms and definitions from this chapter that you need to remember. The sillier they are, the more likely you are to remember them. Read them aloud and repeat them over and over until you have them memorized.

Pathologies, Procedures, and Pharmacology

Pathology Terms

Table 13-3 includes terms that relate to diseases or abnormalities of the musculoskeletal system. Use the pronunciation guide and say the terms aloud as you read them. This will help you get in the habit of saying them properly.

TABLE 13-3	
PATHOLOGY TERMS	
adhesive capsulitis (ăd-HĒ-sĭv kăp-sū-LĪ-tĭs)	loss of range of motion in the shoulder; also called *frozen shoulder*
anterior cruciate ligament tear (ăn-TĒR-ē-ōr KROO-shē-āt LĬG-ă-mĕnt tār)	injury to one of the stabilizing ligaments of the knee, which originates on the anterior portion of the femur

Anterior cruciate ligament tear.

Continued

TABLE 13-3

PATHOLOGY TERMS—cont'd

bursitis (bŭr-SĪ-tĭs)	condition of inflammation of the tiny fluid-filled sacs that act as cushions and provide lubrication to decrease friction and irritation between structures such as bones, tendons, muscles, and skin
carpal tunnel syndrome (CTS) (KĂR-păl TŬN-ĕl SĬN-drōm)	compression of the median nerve, causing pain or numbness in the wrist, hand, and fingers

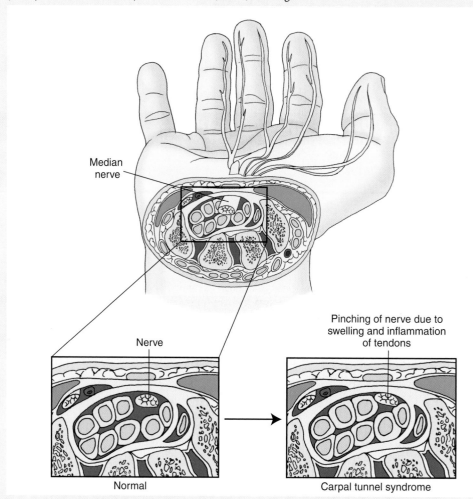

Carpal tunnel syndrome.

TABLE 13-3
PATHOLOGY TERMS—cont'd

claw toe (klaw tō)	condition in which the metatarsophalangeal (MTP) joint flexes dorsally while the other joint or joints in the toe flex toward the sole

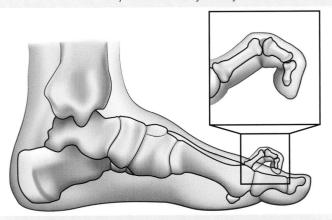

Claw toe.

contracture (kŏn-TRĂK-chūr)	fibrosis of connective tissue which decreases the mobility of a joint
crepitation (krĕp-ĭ-TĀ-shŭn)	grating sound from broken bones, or a clicking or crackling sound from joints
dislocation (dĭs-lō-KĀ-shŭn)	displacement or separation of a bone from its normal position where it articulates with another bone

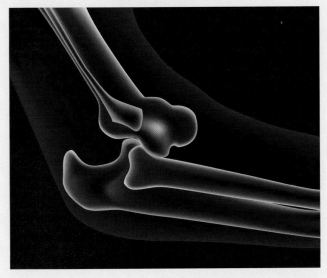

Dislocation.

electromyography (EMG) (ē-LEK-trō-mī-og-ră-fē)	test used to evaluate and record the electrical activity produced by skeletal muscles; used to diagnose neuromuscular disorders
fibromyalgia (fī-brō-mī-ĂL-jē-ă)	chronic condition marked by pain in the muscles, tendons, ligaments, and soft tissues of the body; also called *fibromyositis, fibrositis and myofibrositis*

Continued

TABLE 13-3
PATHOLOGY TERMS—cont'd

fracture (FRĂK-chūr)	condition in which a bone is broken or cracked

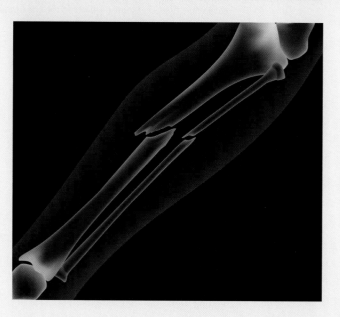

Fracture.

ganglion cyst (GĂNG-glē-ŏn sĭst)	condition in which one or more small benign tumors filled with a thick, colorless, gelatinous substance develop over a joint or tendon, usually on the wrist or back of the hand; sometimes called a *Bible cyst*

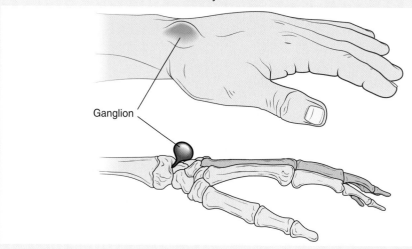

Ganglion

Ganglion cyst.

TABLE 13-3

PATHOLOGY TERMS—cont'd

gout (gowt)	hereditary form of arthritis, characterized by uric acid accumulation in the joints, especially in the great toe

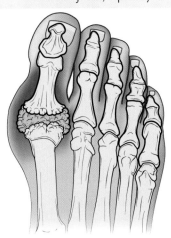

Gout affecting the great toe.

hallux rigidus (HĂL-ŭks RĬJ-ĭ-dŭs)	condition in which degenerative arthritis affects the metatarsophalangeal (MTP) joint at the base of the big toe, causing pain and stiffness
hallux valgus (HĂL-ŭks VĂL-gŭs)	condition in which the big toe is improperly aligned, pointing laterally toward the second toe and creating a large bump on the inner edge of the foot at the base of the big toe; commonly called *bunion*

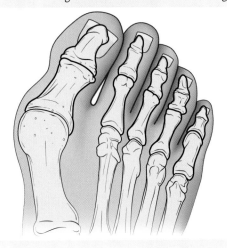

Hallux valgus.

Continued

TABLE 13-3

PATHOLOGY TERMS—cont'd

hammertoe (HĂM-ĕr-tō)	condition in which the toe is bent downward at the proximal interphalangeal (PIP) joint

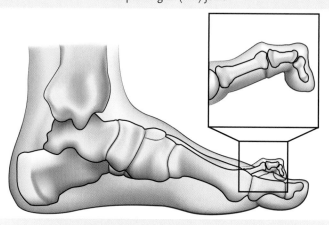

Hammertoe.

herniated disc (HĔR-nē-ā-tĕd dĭsk)	herniation of the soft center of an intervertebral disc

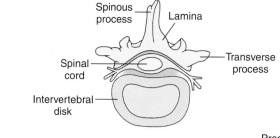

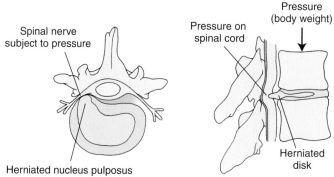

Herniated lumbar disk.

juvenile rheumatoid arthritis (JRA) (JŪ-vĕ-nĭl ROO-mă-toyd ăr-THRĪ-tĭs)	disorder similar to adult-onset RA, with earlier onset and more-severe symptoms

TABLE 13-3
PATHOLOGY TERMS—cont'd

kyphosis (kī-FŌ-sĭs)	abnormal increase in the curvature of the thoracic vertebrae, causing hunchback

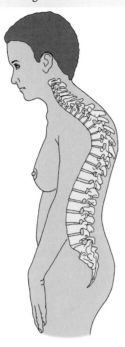

Kyphosis.

lordosis (lor-DŌ-sĭs)	abnormal increase in the curvature of the lumbar vertebrae, causing swayback

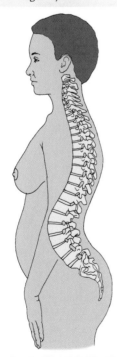

Lordosis.

Continued

TABLE 13-3

PATHOLOGY TERMS—cont'd

mallet toe (MĂL-ĕt- tō)	condition in which the toe is bent downward at the distal interphalangeal (DIP) joint

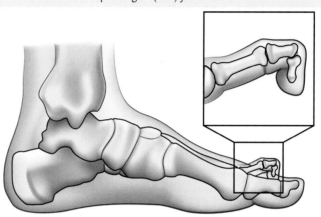

Mallet toe.

medial tibial syndrome (MĒ-dē-ăl TĬB-ē-ăl SĬN-drōm)	painful condition involving tiny tears in the muscles and tendons that attach to the anterior tibia (shin); commonly called *shin splints*
meniscal tear (měn- ĬS-kăl tār)	tear of one of the two C-shaped cartilage structures that serve to cushion and stabilize the knee joint, usually caused by a twisting force

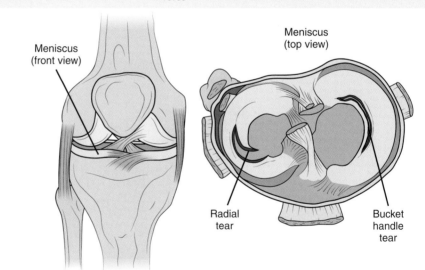

Meniscus (front view)

Meniscus (top view)

Radial tear

Bucket handle tear

Meniscal tear.

muscular dystrophy (MD) (MŬS-kū-lăr DĬS-trō-fē)	hereditary, progressive terminal disease that causes muscle atrophy and death, usually by age 20
myasthenia gravis (mī-ăs-THĒ-nē-ă GRĂV-ĭs)	autoimmune motor disorder that causes progressive muscle fatigue and weakness
osteitis deformans (äs-tē-ĬT-ŭs dē-FŌRM-ănz)	chronic condition in which the process of bone destruction and regrowth occurs abnormally, causing weak, fragile, enlarged, and misshapen bones; also called *Paget's disease*

TABLE 13-3
PATHOLOGY TERMS—cont'd

osteoarthritis (ŏs-tē-ō-ăr-THRĪ-tĭs)	condition of cartilage deterioration and joint inflammation marked by pain, stiffness, and decreased ROM, most commonly affecting synovial weight-bearing joints and vertebrae; also called *degenerative joint disease (DJD)*
osteomalacia (ŏs-tē-ō-măl-Ā-shē-ă)	condition of softening and weakening of the bones; when it occurs in children, it is called *rickets*
osteomyelitis (ŏs-tē-ō-mī-ĕl-Ī-tĭs)	acute or chronic infection within the bone, most commonly affecting the legs, arms, pelvis, and spine

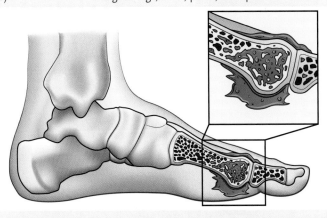

Osteomyelitis.

osteoporosis (ŏs-tē-ō-pōr-Ō-sĭs)	condition characterized by loss of bone mass throughout the skeleton

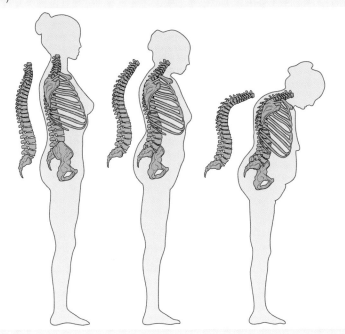

Osteoporosis.

Continued

TABLE 13-3
PATHOLOGY TERMS—cont'd

pathological fracture (păth-ō-LŎJ-ĭk-ăl FRĂK-chūr)	breaking of diseased, weakened bone from the stress of normal everyday activities
plantar fasciitis (PLĂN-tăr făs-ē-Ī-tĭs)	painful condition of the supporting structures of the arch of the foot, primarily the plantar fascia, a band of tissue that connects the heel with the toes

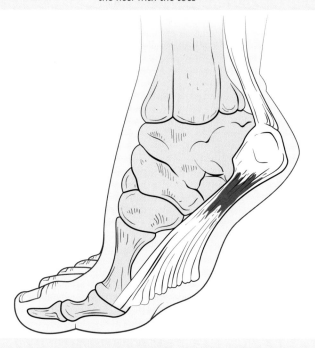

Plantar fasciitis.

rheumatoid arthritis (RA) (ROO-mă-toyd ăr-THRĪ-tĭs)	autoimmune arthritis that causes progressive joint pain and deformity and may affect organ systems

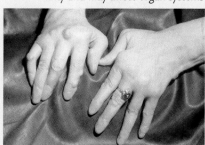

Rheumatoid arthritis. (From Dillon, P.M. [2008]. *Nursing health assessment.* Philadelphia, PA: F. A. Davis Company, p. 627; with permission)

TABLE 13-3
PATHOLOGY TERMS—cont'd

rotator cuff tear (RŌ-tā-tōr kŭf tār)	traumatic rip of one or more of the muscles or tendons within the rotator cuff of the shoulder

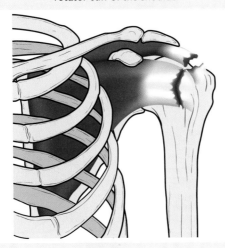

Rotator cuff tear.

scoliosis (sko-lē-Ō-sĭs)	abnormal S-shaped lateral curvature of the vertebrae

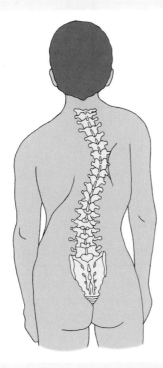

Scoliosis.

sprain (sprān)	complete or incomplete tear in the ligaments around a joint
strain (strān)	trauma to a muscle, and sometimes a tendon, due to violent contraction or excessive forcible stretching

Continued

TABLE 13-3

PATHOLOGY TERMS—cont'd

tendinitis (tĕn-dĭn-Ī-tĭs)	inflammation of a tendon due to overuse
thoracic outlet syndrome (TOS) (thō-RĂS-ĭk OWT-lĕt SĬN-drōm)	group of painful disorders involving compression of the nerves or vessels in the neck and arms

Scalene muscles

Clavicle

Nerve   Vein   Artery

Clavicle

Thoracic outlet syndrome.

IN A FLASH!

It's time to print out all of the Pathology Terms Flash Cards for Chapter 13 and run through them at least three times before you continue.

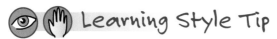 Learning Style Tip

Ask permission to spend time in the anatomy lab at your school. Locate the muscle and skeletal models and take turns applying temporary sticky labels to them with the appropriate names and associated combining forms. Take pictures of your work and use the pictures in later study sessions.

Common Diagnostic Tests and Procedures

Antinuclear antibody (ANA): Test to detect the presence of autoantibodies that may suggest an autoimmune disorder such as rheumatoid arthritis

Arthrography: Radiological examination of a joint after injection of a contrast fluid into the joint space

Bone marrow aspiration: Removal of a bone marrow specimen from the cortex of a flat bone for analysis

Bone scan: Use of a gamma camera to detect abnormalities in bone density after injection of radioactive material

C-reactive protein (CRP): Test to detect or monitor inflammatory conditions

Creatine kinase (CK): Test to measure isoenzyme that skeletal and cardiac muscles release into the blood when they are damaged

Cryotherapy: Application of cold, such as with ice compresses, to decrease inflammation and pain

Dual-energy x-ray absorptiometry (DEXA): Radiological evaluation of bone density to detect osteoporosis

Electromyogram (EMG): Record of skeletal-muscle electrical activity; used to diagnose neuromuscular disorders

Erythrocyte sedimentation rate (ESR, sed rate): Rate at which red blood cells settle in a tube of unclotted blood; an elevated ESR indicates inflammation

Rheumatoid factor: Blood test used to identify rheumatoid arthritis and other disorders

Total hip replacement (THR): Procedure to replace an arthritic hip with a prosthetic device to restore mobility and function; also referred to as total hip arthroplasty

Transcutaneous electrical nerve stimulation (TENS): Delivery of a mild electrical current to a painful area, to disrupt transmission of pain signals between the body and brain

Pharmacology

Table 13-4 provides a list of common musculoskeletal system medications.

TABLE 13-4

PHARMACOLOGY

Therapeutic Classification	Generic Name	Brand Name	Common Use
Osteoporosis Medications			
Bisphosphonate	alendronate	Fosamax	Increase bone density
	ibandronate	Boniva	
	risedronate	Actonel	
	zoledronic acid	Reclast	
Bone resorption inhibitor	denosumab	Prolia	Slow the formation and action of cells that break down bone
Calcitonin	thyrocalcitonin	Calcimar, Miacalcin	Regulate calcium levels
Parathyroid hormone and analog	teriparatide	Forteo	Stimulate bone growth and slow bone loss
Selective estrogen receptor modulator	raloxifene	Evista	Decrease bone breakdown which occurs after menopause
Other Medications			
Disease modifying anti-rheumatic drug (DMARD)	cyclophosphamide	Cytoxan	Slow the progression of rheumatoid arthritis
	methotrexate	Rheumatrex, Trexall	
Skeletal muscle relaxant	baclofen	Lioresal	Reduce tone in skeletal muscle; decrease muscle pain
	carisoprodol	Soma	
	chlorzoxazone	Parafon Forte	

Continued

TABLE 13-4

PHARMACOLOGY—cont'd

Therapeutic Classification	Generic Name	Brand Name	Common Use
	cyclobenzaprine	Flexeril	
	metaxalone	Skelaxin	
	methocarbamol	Robaxin	
	orphenadrine	Norflex	
	tizanidine	Zanaflex	
Uricosuric agent	probenecid	Probalan	Lower uric acid level in the body
Xanthine oxidase inhibitor	allopurinol	Zyloprim	Block the production of uric acid in the body
Xanthine oxidase inhibitor	febuxostat	Uloric	Block the production of uric acid in the body

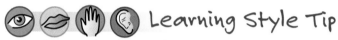 Learning Style Tip

Stress and anxiety can impair your ability to concentrate and remember what you study. Try beginning and ending your study sessions with a few minutes of soothing music or other relaxation techniques. Visualize yourself taking your exams with an alert mind, perfect recall, and clear focus. Visualize the grade you will earn and how good you will feel about your accomplishment.

Pathologies, Procedures, and Pharmacology Practice Exercises

Deciphering Terms

Write the correct meaning of these medical terms.

Exercise 7

1. paravertebral _____

2. supratibial _____

3. thoracic _____

4. tendolysis _____

5. sternotomy _____

6. phalangeal _____

7. patellofemoral _____

8. osteotomy _____

9. myopathy _____

10. myelosclerosis _____

11. lumbar _____

12. laminotome _____

13. radioulnar _____

14. cranioplasty _____

15. costochondritis _____

Fill in the Blanks

Fill in the blanks below.

Exercise 8

1. Suzanne has an abnormal S-shaped, lateral curvature of her spine. This
   condition is known as _____.

2. Another name for degenerative joint disease is _____.

3. Joseph has _____, an inflammatory condition that
   affects the tiny fluid-filled sacs located between structures such as bones,
   tendons, muscles, and skin.

4. When Howard climbs the stairs, his knees creak. This crackling sound is
   known as _____.

5. Lorinda spends much of her workday at a computer; as a result, she has
   developed _____ _____
   _____, which causes pain and numbness in her wrists,
   hands, and fingers due to compression of the median nerve.

6. Two different names for hip replacement are _____
   _____ _____ and
   _____ _____
   _____.

7. The physician ordered a(n) _____ x-ray, which will aim
   from front to back.

8. A(n) _____ records electrical activity of skeletal muscles. It is used to diagnose neuromuscular disorders.

9. An autoimmune form of arthritis that causes pain and deformity of joints and may involve organ systems is _____ arthritis.

10. When the leg is surgically removed from above the knee, it is known as a(n) _____ _____, abbreviated _____.

Multiple Choice

Select the one best answer to the following multiple-choice questions.

Exercise 9

1. Which of the following conditions is caused by compression of the median nerve, resulting in pain or numbness in the wrist, hand, and fingers?

   a. herniated disc

   b. myasthenia gravis

   c. gout

   d. carpal tunnel syndrome

2. Which of the following conditions is an autoimmune motor disorder that causes progressive muscle fatigue and weakness?

   a. myasthenia gravis

   b. gout

   c. carpal tunnel syndrome

   d. kyphosis

3. Martha Snyder has been diagnosed with rheumatoid arthritis. She most likely has which of the following complaints?

   a. arthralgia

   b. osteopenia

   c. arthrocentesis

   d. arthoclasia

4. The application of cold, such as with ice compresses, to decrease inflammation and pain is known as:

   a. arthrography

   b. cryotherapy

   c. dual-energy absorptiometry

   d. transcutaneous electrical nerve stimulation

5. Ilka Heidrick has myasthenia gravis. Which of the following is she most likely to experience?

    a.   increased energy level after exercise

    b.   progressive dementia

    c.   arthralgia

    d.   progressive fatigue

Fill in the Blanks

Using Table 13-4, write the therapeutic classification of the medication next to each generic or brand name.

Exercise 10

1. Boniva _____

2. Lioresal _____

3. raloxifene _____

4. methotrexate _____

5. metaxalone _____

6. Prolia _____

7. tizanidine _____

8. Uloric _____

9. teriparatide _____

10. Miacalcin _____

CASE STUDY

Read the case study and answer the questions that follow. Most of the terms are included in this chapter. Refer to your medical dictionary for the other terms.

Osteoarthritis

Michael Mayhew is a 59-year-old man with osteoarthritis of the knees. He has a history of bilateral knee injuries from college football as well as a 33-year career in construction. He has noticed a slow onset of symptoms, primarily over the past 10 years. His primary complaints were arthralgia and stiffness, especially first thing in the morning. Initial treatment was conservative and included decreased weight bearing, NSAIDs, physical therapy, and weight loss of 25 pounds. In spite of these measures, Mr. Mayhew continued to experience worsening symptoms over the next few years. Eventually, he underwent bilateral total knee replacement (TKR).

Follow-up note: Eight weeks after surgery, Mr. Mayhew stated he was pain free and had better use of his knees than he had in years.

Osteoarthritis, also known as *degenerative joint disease (DJD),* is the most common form of noninflammatory joint disease. The key feature of osteoarthritis is the wearing down and loss of cartilage in synovial joints. Osteoarthritis occurs most often after the age of 40 and involves joints that have had prior injuries or heavy chronic wear and tear. The most common joints involved are those of the hips, knees, hands, and spine. Pathological features include erosion of the articular cartilage, sclerosis of the bone beneath the cartilage, and formation of bone spurs. The primary symptom is joint pain when bearing weight. Management of osteoarthritis includes decreased weight-bearing activities, rest, NSAIDs, analgesics, glucosamine supplements, physical therapy, and weight loss (obesity is a common factor). If necessary, the patient may rely on assistive devices such as a cane, crutches, or walker. Surgery may eventually be necessary.

Case Study Questions

Exercise 11

1. Which of the following statements is true regarding Mr. Mayhew's experience?
   a. He had arthritis in his right knee only.
   b. The onset of his arthritis was sudden and severe.
   c. His symptoms were worse in the evening.
   d. He experienced stiffness in his knees in the morning.

2. What type of surgery did Mr. Mayhew have?
   a. repair of both knee joints
   b. replacement of both knee joints
   c. fixation of both knee joints
   d. fusion of both knee joints

3. Mr. Mayhew's primary symptom was arthralgia. This means:
   a. pain of a joint
   b. inflammation of a joint
   c. destruction of a joint
   d. softening of a joint

4. Which of the following statements is true regarding osteoarthritis?
   a. It is an uncommon form of arthritis.
   b. It is characterized by demineralization of the bones.
   c. It affects joints that have had prior injuries or heavy chronic wear and tear.
   d. It most commonly involves the shoulders, elbows, and wrists.

5. List the activities of daily living (ADLs) that were likely very painful for Mr. Mayhew just prior to his surgery.

6. Refer to your list of painful activities above. Suggest ways to perform these activities with less weight bearing on the knee joints.

7. Mr. Mayhew was instructed to decrease his weight-bearing activities and to lose weight. Since he should not be walking for exercise, what types of exercises could he do instead?

End-of-Chapter Practice Exercises

Word Building

*Using **only** the word parts in the lists provided, create medical terms with the indicated meanings.*

Exercise 12

Prefixes	Combining Forms	Suffixes
inter-	arthr/o	-al
para-	carp/o	-algia
sub-	cervic/o	-ar
	chondr/o	-dynia
	cost/o	-ectomy
	crani/o	-itis
	femor/o	-metry
	humer/o	-oma
	lamin/o	-pathy
	lumb/o	-penia
	metacarp/o	-plasty
	my/o	-plegia
	myel/o	-pnea
	orth/o	-tome
	oste/o	
	patell/o	
	pelv/i	
	stern/o	
	vertebr/o	

1. pertaining to the ribs and vertebrae _____

2. inflammation of a bone and joint _____

3. pertaining to a carpus _____

4. pertaining to beside or near the neck _____

5. pain of the cartilage _____

6. cutting instrument for a lamina _____

7. pertaining to between the ribs _____

8. surgical repair of the cranium _____

9. pertaining to the femur _____

10. disease of the humerus _____

11. pertaining to straight or upright _____

12. pain of the lower back _____

13. inflammation of a metacarpus _____

14. tumor of the bone marrow or spinal cord _____

15. paralysis of a muscle _____

16. pertaining to beneath the sternum _____

17. disease of a bone _____

18. excision or surgical removal of a patella _____

19. measurement of the pelvis _____

20. deficiency of bone _____

True or False

Decide whether the following statements are true or false.

Exercise 13

1. True   False   **BKA** is an abbreviation for *broken.*

2. True   False   **Gout** is a hereditary form of arthritis characterized by uric acid accumulation in the joints, especially in the great toe.

3. True   False   The abbreviation **IM** stands for *immobility.*

4. True   False   **Contracture** is fibrosis of connective tissue, which decreases mobility of a joint.

5. True   False   **Muscular dystrophy** is a hereditary, progressive terminal disease that causes muscle atrophy and death.

6. True   False   **Lordosis** is an abnormal increase in the curvature of the lumbar vertebrae, causing swayback.

7. True   False   The abbreviation **RA** stands for *rheumatoid arthritis.*

8. True   False   A **sprain** is an injury to a muscle or tendon.

9. True   False   **Kyphosis** is an abnormal increase in the curvature of the thoracic vertebrae, causing hunchback.

10. True   False   **Myasthenia gravis** is a grating sound from broken bones or a clicking or crackling sound from joints.

Deciphering Terms

Write the correct meaning of these medical terms.

Exercise 14

1. cervicitis —————————————————

2. metacarpophalangeal —————————————

3. arthrodynia ———————————————

4. osteoclasis ————————————————

5. extratibial ————————————————

6. thoracolumbar ——————————————

7. kinesimeter ————————————————

8. meniscal —————————————————

9. muscular —————————————————

10. puborectal ————————————————

Multiple Choice

Select the one best answer to the following multiple-choice questions.

Exercise 15

1. Which of the following terms means *treatment (using) movement?*
   a. kinesiotherapy
   b. kyphoplasty
   c. tarsokinesia
   d. tetrakinesis

2. Which of the following terms means *abnormal condition of a backward bend in the vertebrae?*
   a. stenosis
   b. spondylosis
   c. kyphosis
   d. lordosis

3. Which of the following terms means *drooping or prolapse of the tarsus?*

    a. dystocia

    b. tarsomegaly

    c. thoracopexy

    d. tarsoptosis

4. Which of the following terms means *pertaining to muscle and skin?*

    a. dermatomycosis

    b. myelocutaneous

    c. myoepithelium

    d. none of these

5. Which of the following terms means *pertaining to the sternum and around the heart?*

    a. sternopericardial

    b. retrosternal

    c. transcardiac

    d. substernal

6. The term *lordosis* indicates:

    a. pain of the lower back

    b. a pathological condition of the upper back

    c. an abnormal condition of the cervical and lumbar areas of the back

    d. inflammation of the cervical and lumbar areas of the back

7. The term *meniscocyte* indicates:

    a. a condition of fungus

    b. softening of the cartilage

    c. a hernia of a meniscus

    d. none of these

8. The term *puboprostatic* means:

    a. pertaining to the back of the pelvis

    b. pertaining to behind the patella

    c. pertaining to the pubis and prostate

    d. pertaining to disease of the prostate

9. Scoliokyphosis is:

    a.   a pathological condition of back curvature

    b.   an abnormal condition involving crookedness and a hump

    c.   a condition of crooked movement

    d.   none of these

10. The term *costochondritis* indicates:

    a.   a painful condition of the ribs

    b.   surgical puncture of the skin and ribs

    c.   cancer of the carpus

    d.   an abnormal condition of the ribs and cartilage

11. Which of the following tests will most likely identify the presence of inflammation?

    a.   erythrocyte sedimentation rate

    b.   creatine kinase

    c.   electromyogram

    d.   rheumatoid factor

12. Which of the following tests is most likely to identify osteoporosis?

    a.   bone marrow aspiration

    b.   dual-energy absorptiometry

    c.   bone scan

    d.   arthrography

13. Which of the following conditions causes loss of range of motion in the shoulder?

    a.   crepitation

    b.   hallux rigidus

    c.   adhesive capsulitis

    d.   osteitis deformans

14. All of the following disorders involve the feet **except:**

    a.   gout

    b.   plantar fasciitis

    c.   hallux valgus

    d.   ganglion cyst

15. All of the following disorders involve the arm or shoulder **except:**

    a. carpal tunnel syndrome

    b. adhesive capsulitis

    c. kyphosis

    d. rotator cuff tear

16. Which of the following abbreviations indicates a location on the lower extremities?

    a. AP

    b. AK

    c. BE

    d. AS

17. Which of the following abbreviations indicates an anatomical location?

    a. DTR

    b. IM

    c. UE

    d. OT

18. All of the following abbreviations indicate a surgical procedure **except:**

    a. TKR

    b. ADL

    c. AKA

    d. ORIF

19. All of the following abbreviations indicate a disease or disorder **except:**

    a. ROM

    b. DJD

    c. HNP

    d. Fx

20. All of the following abbreviations pertain to a type of arthritis **except:**

    a. OA

    b. RA

    c. JRA

    d. BKA

SPECIAL SENSES: EYES AND EARS 14

Chapter Outline

Structure and Function of the Eye

The eye is the sensory organ of sight. It is located within the orbital cavity of the face and is surrounded by protective structures including the eyebrows, eyelashes, and eyelids, which help keep foreign objects out of the eye.

The **eyeball** is a globe-shaped organ that consists of three layers (Fig. 14-1). These are the sclera, the outer portion; the choroid, the middle portion; and the retina, the inner portion. Each of these layers functions to protect the eye, provide vision, or communicate vision to the brain.

The outermost layer of the eye includes the sclera and cornea. The **sclera** has a distinctive white color. It provides strength, structure, and shape to the eye. At the front of the eye, the sclera bulges forward to become the **cornea,** which is transparent and allows light into the eye. A thin mucous membrane called the **conjunctiva** covers the outer surface of the eye and lines the eyelids. The conjunctiva contains many tiny blood vessels and secretory glands. These glands produce a clear, watery mucus that allows the eyelid to slide smoothly over the eye when you blink. When the eye is irritated, the tiny blood vessels dilate (enlarge) and become more prominent. This makes the whites of the eyes appear bloodshot or reddened.

The middle layer of the eyeball is the **choroid** layer. It is a dark-blue vascular layer between the sclera and retina that supplies blood to the entire eye. The **optic nerve,** which is attached to the retina, exits the posterior eye through an opening in the choroid and extends to the brain, where visual messages are delivered.

Flashpoint
Over-the-counter eyedrops that "get the red out" work by constricting (narrowing) the enlarged blood vessels in the irritated eye.

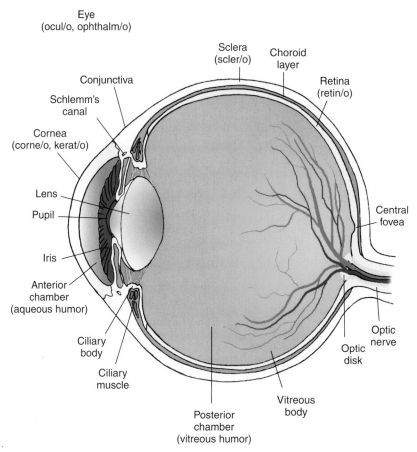

FIGURE 14-1 **The eyeball.**

Other structures in the choroid include the iris, pupil, ciliary body, lens, and suspensory ligaments. The **iris** is a circular structure that surrounds the pupil and gives the eyes their typical color. The **pupil** functions as an adjustable window that lets light into the inner structures of the eye. The iris contracts in low lighting, thereby dilating the pupil and making it appear bigger. This allows more light into the eye. In brightly lit environments, the iris expands, causing the pupil to constrict and appear smaller. This decreases the amount of light entering the eye. The **ciliary body** includes several **ciliary muscles,** including a circular muscle that lies posterior to the iris. It is attached to the **lens** by the **suspensory ligaments.** The lens is a clear, firm, transparent disk. With the help of ciliary muscles, the lens continually changes shape, enabling us to focus clearly on objects we are viewing. For near vision, the ciliary muscles contract, causing increased rounding of the lens; for far vision, they expand, causing flattening of the lens. This process is called **accommodation.** As we age, most of us develop *presbyopia,* which is an age-related decline in visual acuity. As this occurs, our lenses lose elasticity and are less able to accommodate for distance changes, especially close-up viewing. Because of this, many of us need corrective lenses by the time we reach our 40s or 50s. These lenses are mostly able to help make up for what our eyes' natural lenses can no longer do.

The innermost layer of the eye is the **retina.** It is responsible for the reception of visual impulses through the lens and the transmission of these impulses to the brain (Fig. 14-2). The retina is divided into two layers. The thin outer layer

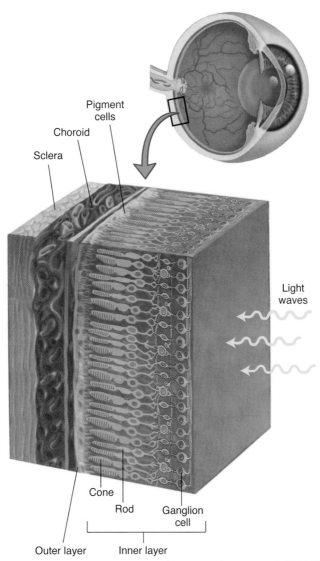

Pigment cells

Choroid

Sclera

Light waves

Cone

Rod

Ganglion cell

Outer layer

Inner layer

FIGURE 14-2 **Microscopic structures of the retina.** (From Eagle, S., et al. [2009]. *The professional medical assistant.* Philadelphia, PA: F. A. Davis Company, p. 748; with permission)

is red in color due to blood flow from its main central artery. It also contains pigment that protects the choroid and sclera from light at the back of the eye.

The thicker inner layer of the retina is the visual portion. It contains two types of visual receptors, called *rods and cones.* These are elongated nerve cells that are lined up along the posterior portion of the retina (Fig. 14-3). These visual receptors contain photopigments that undergo chemical changes when light strikes them. **Rods** detect the presence of light and function in dim lighting to produce images in black and white. **Cones** function in more brightly lit situations and detect color. A deficiency of cones results in *color deficiency,* often called *color blindness*—the inability to distinguish colors. As light waves from the anterior portion of the eye hit the retina, they stimulate rods and cones, which direct visual information to optic nerve fibers located on the inner surface of the thick inner layer of the retina.

Flashpoint

There are approximately 120 million rods and 6 million cones in the retina!

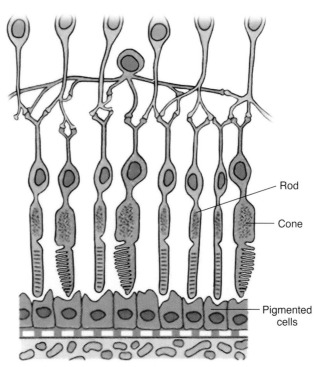

- Rod
- Cone
- Pigmented cells

FIGURE 14-3 Rods and cones. (From Eagle, S., et al. [2009]. *The professional medical assistant.* Philadelphia, PA: F. A. Davis Company, p. 748; with permission)

Optic nerve fibers transmit visual information via ganglion neurons, which converge at the optic disc. The optic disc, commonly called the *blind spot,* contains no rods or cones. The **optic nerve** gathers visual stimuli from the ganglion neurons and transmits this information to the brain for interpretation.

The eye contains two fluids, historically called humors. **Aqueous humor** is found in the posterior and anterior chambers. In the anterior chamber, aqueous humor provides nourishment for the lens and cornea. It drains through a small opening called the **Schlemm's canal**. In addition to aqueous humor, the posterior chamber also contains **vitreous humor.** Vitreous humor is a jellylike substance that fills the posterior chamber and gives shape to the eye. The aqueous humor, vitreous humor, and lens are all refractory structures that bend light rays to focus them sharply onto the retina.

Lacrimal glands are located on the superolateral (upper outer) side of the eye and open through the lacrimal duct at the medial (inner) side, next to the nose. They bathe, moisten, and lubricate the eye by producing tears that flow over the eye's surface. **Tears** also serve a protective role, containing a bacteria-killing enzyme, and wash away foreign debris (Box 14-1).

Flashpoint

The lacrimal gland is connected to the nose through the nasolacrimal duct and drains into the nasal cavity. This explains why our noses drip when our eyes produce tears.

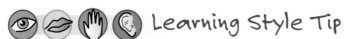 Learning Style Tip

Draw a vertical line down a sheet of paper. Write a series of "exam" questions on one half with the answers on the other. Cover the answer side so that you can't see it. Review the questions, looking at your answers only if you can't remember them. Repeat the process until you know all of the answers by heart. Remember to verbalize aloud if you are an auditory or verbal learner. Next, use the questions you created to quiz a group of classmates.

Box 14-1 Eye Safety

Our eyebrows, eyelashes, and eyelids help keep foreign objects out of our eyes but they cannot provide full protection from potential hazards. According to the American Optometric Association, thousands of eye injuries could be prevented each year by wearing proper eye protection. Potential eye hazards include *projectiles* (flying debris), *chemical* splashes or fumes, and *radiation,* such as light or lasers. Medical professionals may encounter any of these hazards but some are especially susceptible to *bloodborne pathogen* exposure. There are some infectious diseases that can be transmitted through blood or body fluid splashes, airborne droplets, or through touching the eyes with contaminated fingers.

The type of protective eyewear that should be worn depends on the type of hazard that may be encountered. Choices include safety glasses, goggles, face shields, and full-face respirators. It's important that the protective equipment fits well and is in good condition. The National Institute for Occupational Safety and Health reports that 90% of job-related eye injuries could have been prevented, or would have been less severe, if proper eye protection had been worn.

Structure and Function of the Ear

The **ear** is responsible for hearing, balance, and equilibrium. The structures of the ear are located in three main areas: the external, middle, and internal ear (Fig. 14-4).

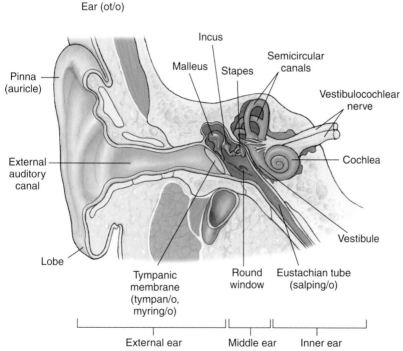

FIGURE 14-4 **The ear.**

The external ear is composed of the auricle, or **pinna,** which is the outer structure. It is made up of cartilage covered with skin and sits visibly outside of the head. It collects sound waves and channels them into the **external auditory canal,** which is a slender tube that leads to the middle ear. The canal is lined with modified sweat glands called *ceruminous glands* that secrete **cerumen,** a waxy substance that traps tiny foreign particles and prevents them from entering the ear's deeper structures.

At the inner end of the auditory canal is the **tympanic membrane (TM),** which is a thin, flat, irregularly shaped membrane commonly known as the *eardrum*. It creates a wall between the external and middle ear. Located within the middle ear is a downward-sloping canal called the **eustachian tube** that connects the middle ear to the throat. It allows air movement between the inner ear and outer atmosphere. When the eustachian tube is closed and the middle-ear pressure is greater or less than atmospheric pressure, we may describe our ears as feeling plugged. The pressure is relieved when the eustachian tube opens to allow air through. This is a common experience with altitude changes and explains the ear-popping sensation we experience when we travel over the mountains or ride in an airplane.

The TM is connected to the *malleus* (hammer), the first of three tiny **ossicles** (bones) also including the *incus* (anvil) and *stapes* (stirrup). The TM vibrates in response to sound waves, which causes movement of the ossicles. This in turn sends vibrations to the inner ear.

The anatomy of the inner ear is quite complex, with a mazelike design of twists and turns. Because of this, the inner ear is sometimes also called a **labyrinth.** The first structure of the inner ear is the **cochlea,** a tiny, circular, snail-shaped structure filled with fluid called **perilymph.** The inner surface of the cochlea is lined with a highly sensitive hearing structure called the **organ of Corti.** It contains nerve endings called *hair cells*, which are long, hairlike fibers that transmit impulses to the vestibulocochlear (auditory) nerve.

The cochlea receives vibration from the stapes through the oval window. These vibrations cause a disturbance of the perilymph, which in turn disturbs hair cells on the organ of Corti. The hair cells transmit impulses to the auditory nerve, where they are interpreted as sound. The round window is an opening in the lower part of the temporal bone, covered with a thin membrane. The **semicircular canals,** located behind the ossicles and two windows, contain perilymph and endolymph, a pale, transparent fluid. Together with the cochlea, these structures make up the **vestibular system.** They translate sound vibrations into nerve impulses that are sent to the brain via the **vestibulocochlear (auditory) nerve**.

Another function of the inner ear is to provide *equilibrium*, which is the sense of balance. **Static equilibrium** is feeling a sense of balance when we are at rest; **dynamic equilibrium** refers to our sense of balance when we are in motion. The vestibular system controls both forms of equilibrium. **Endolymph**, the pale transparent fluid within the labyrinth, responds to changes in body position based on gravity. The vestibulocochlear nerve transmits this information to the brain, and the brain interprets the body's position in space. Inflammation of the inner ear is called *labyrinthitis*.

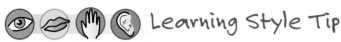 Learning Style Tip

Identify the time of the day you are best able to grasp and understand complex material. For most people, this is first thing in the morning, when they are rested. Spend at least 30 minutes each day at this time studying material you find most challenging. Also be sure to get plenty of sleep. Research shows that memory consolidation—the process of transferring information from short-term memory to long-term memory—occurs while we sleep.

Structure and Function Practice Exercises

Fill in the Blanks

Choose the term that matches the description.

Exercise 1

The Eye

Eyeball	Pupil	Rods
Sclera	Ciliary body	Cones
Cornea	Ciliary muscles	Aqueous humor
Conjunctiva	Lens	Schlemm's canal
Choroid	Suspensory ligaments	Vitreous humor
Optic nerve	Accommodation	Lacrimal glands
Iris	Retina	Tears

1. _____ Surrounds the pupil and gives eyes their color

2. _____ Innermost layer of the eye containing two types of visual receptors

3. _____ Fluid in the anterior chamber that provides nourishment for the lens and cornea and bends light rays to focus them sharply onto the retina

4. _____ White, outermost layer that provides strength, structure, and shape to the eye

5. _____ Cause the lens to change shape when they contract or expand

6. _____ Small opening for drainage of aqueous humor

7. _____ Fluid to bathe, moisten, and lubricate the eye; serve a protective role by killing bacteria and washing away foreign debris

8. _____ Attached to the retina; transmits visual information to the brain

9. _____ Dark-blue middle layer that supplies blood to the entire eye

10. _____ Attach the ciliary body and muscles to the lens

11. _____ Globe-shaped organ that consists of three layers

12. _____ Attached to the lens; includes several ciliary muscles

13. _____ Transparent bulge of the sclera that allows light into the eye

14. _____ Visual receptors in the retina that function in dim lighting to produce images in black and white

15. _____ The process of rounding and flattening of the lens that enables focus in both near and far vision

16. _____ Produce tears that flow over the eye's surface

17. _____ Dilates to allow more light to enter the eye; constricts to decrease the amount of light entering the eye

18. _____ Jellylike substance in the posterior chamber that gives shape to the eye and bends light rays to focus them sharply onto the retina

19. _____ Thin mucous membrane covering the outer surface of the eye that contains blood vessels and secretory glands

20. _____ Clear, firm, transparent disc in the middle layer that can change shape to allow vision at different distances

21. _____ Visual receptors in the retina that detect color and function in more brightly lit situations

Fill in the Blanks

Choose the term that matches the description.

Exercise 2

The Ear

Ear
Pinna
External auditory canal
Cerumen
Tympanic membrane

Eustachian tube
Ossicles
Labyrinth
Cochlea
Perilymph
Organ of Corti

Semicircular canals
Vestibular system
Vestibulocochlear (auditory) nerve
Static equilibrium
Dynamic equilibrium
Endolymph

1. _____ Cochlea vibrations cause a disturbance of this pale, transparent fluid, which in turn disturb hair cells on the organ of Corti, transmitting impulses to the auditory nerve.

2. _____ Waxy substance in the external auditory canal that traps tiny foreign particles and prevents them from entering the deeper structures

3. _____ Vibrations of the tympanic membrane cause these three tiny bones to move, which sends vibrations to the inner ear.

4. _____ Feeling a sense of balance when at rest or not moving

5. _____ Slender tube that runs from the external ear to the middle ear

6. _____ Translates sound vibrations into nerve impulses; controls both static and dynamic equilibrium

7. _____ Connects the middle ear to the throat; allows air movement between the inner ear and outer atmosphere

8. _____ Pale, transparent fluid within the labyrinth that responds to changes in body position based on gravity

9. _____ Made of cartilage covered with skin; collects sound waves and channels them into the external auditory canal

10. _____ Complex, mazelike anatomy of the inner ear

11. _____ Wall between the external and middle ear that is commonly known as the eardrum; vibrates in response to sound waves

12. _____ Located behind the ossicles, the oval window, and the round window; contains perilymph and endolymph; part of the vestibular system

13. _____ Sends nerve impulses to the brain

14. _____ Responsible for hearing, balance, and equilibrium

15. _____ Sense of balance when we are in motion

16. _____ Snail-shaped structure of the inner ear lined with the organ of Corti and filled with perilymph; part of the vestibular system

17. _____ Highly sensitive hearing structure lining the inner surface of the cochlea

Fill in the Blanks

Label Figure 14-5 with the appropriate anatomical terms and combining forms.

Exercise 3

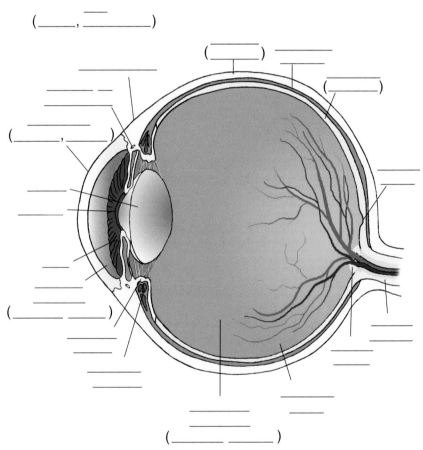

FIGURE 14-5 **Eyeball with blanks.**

Fill in the Blanks

Label Figure 14-6 with the appropriate anatomical terms and combining forms.

Exercise 4

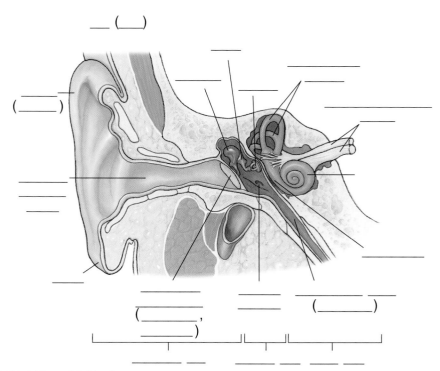

FIGURE 14-6 **Ear with blanks.**

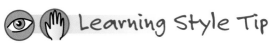

Learning Style Tip

Spend time in the anatomy lab (with permission) studying 3-D models of the eye and ear. Label the parts using removable sticky notes. Include the anatomical term and the associated combining forms.

Combining Forms and Abbreviations

Combining Forms

Table 14-1 contains combining forms that pertain to vision and hearing, along with examples of terms that utilize the combining forms and a pronunciation guide. Read aloud to yourself as you move from left to right across the table. Be sure to use the pronunciation guide so you can learn to say the terms correctly.

  Learning Style Tip

Associate visual images with terms you need to remember. Then link that visual image with the meaning of the term. For example, to remember the term *-centesis,* try picturing a penny (cent) with a large needle punctured through it. Share your images with your study buddies and ask them to share theirs with you.

IN A FLASH!
It's time to print out all of the Combining Form Flash Cards for Chapter 14 and run through them at least three times before you continue.

TABLE 14-1

COMBINING FORMS RELATED TO THE EYE AND EAR

Combining Form	Meaning	Example (Pronunciation)	Meaning of New Term
acous/o	hearing	acoustic (ă-KOOS-tĭk)	pertaining to hearing
audi/o		audiometry (aw-dē-ŎM-ě-trē)	measurement of hearing
blephar/o	eyelid	blepharoptosis (blĕf-ă-rō-TŌ-sĭs)	drooping or prolapse of the eyelid
conjunctiv/o	conjunctiva	conjunctivitis (kŏn-jŭnk-tĭ-VĪ-tĭs)	inflammation of the conjunctiva
corne/o	cornea	corneous (KŌR-nē-ŭs)	pertaining to the cornea
dacry/o	tear	dacryopyorrhea (dăk-rē-ō-pī-ō-RĒ-ă)	flow or discharge of pus in the tears
dipl/o	double	diploid (DĬP-loyd)	resembling double
ir/o	iris	irotomy (ī-RŎT-ō-mē)	cutting into or incision of the iris
irid/o		iridectome (ĭr-ĭ-DĚK-tōm)	cutting instrument for the iris
kerat/o	cornea, keratocele tissue	keratocele (kĕr-ĂT-ō-sēl)	hernia of the cornea
lacrim/o	lacrimal gland	lacrimal (LĂK-rĭm-ăl)	pertaining to the lacrimal glands

TABLE 14-1

COMBINING FORMS RELATED TO THE EYE AND EAR—cont'd

Combining Form	Meaning	Example (Pronunciation)	Meaning of New Term
myring/o	tympanic membrane	myringoplasty (mĭr-ĬN-gō-plăst-ē)	surgical repair of the tympanic membrane
tympan/o		tympanosclerosis (tĭm-pă-nō-sklĕ-RŌ-sĭs)	hardening of the tympanic membrane
ocul/o	eye	oculomycosis (ŏk-ū-lō-mī-KŌ-sĭs)	abnormal condition of eye fungus
ophthalm/o		ophthalmorrhexis (ŏf-thăl-mō-RĔK-sĭs)	rupture of the eye
optic/o		optician (ŏp-TĬSH-ăn)	specialist in eyes
ot/o	ear	otorrhea (ō-tō-RĒ-ă)	flow or discharge from the ear
phac/o	lens	phacotoxic (făk-ō-TŎK-sĭk)	poisonous to the lens
phak/o		phakolysis (făk-ŎL-ĭ-sĭs)	destruction of the lens
presby/o	old age	presbycusis (prĕz-bĭ-KŪ-sĭs)	old-age hearing
retin/o	retina	retinopexy (rĕt-Ĭ-nō-pĕk-sē)	surgical fixation of the retina
salping/o	tube (eustachian or fallopian)	salpingopharyngeal (săl-pĭng-gō-fă-RĬN-jē-ăl)	pertaining to the eustachian tube and pharynx
scler/o	sclera, hardening	scleral (sklĕr-ăl)	pertaining to the sclera

Abbreviations

Table 14-2 lists some of the most common abbreviations related to vision and hearing.

IN A FLASH!

It's time to print out all of the Abbreviation Flash Cards for Chapter 14 and run through them at least three times before you continue.

TABLE 14-2			
ABBREVIATIONS			
Eye			
AS, Ast	astigmatism	MD	macular degeneration
CAT	cataract	PERRLA	pupils are equal, round, reactive to light and accommodation
EM, em	emmetropia	RD	retinal detachment
EOM	extraocular movement	RK	radial keratotomy
G, glc	glaucoma	V, VA	visual acuity
LASIK	laser-assisted in-situ keratomileusis		
Ear			
AOM	acute otitis media	ENT	ears, nose, and throat
EENT	eyes, ears, nose, and throat	TM	tympanic membrane

Combining Forms and Abbreviations Practice Exercises

Fill in the Blanks

Fill in the blanks below using Table 14-1.

Exercise 5

1. flow or discharge from the ear _____

2. rupture of the eye _____

3. abnormal condition of eye fungus _____

4. hardening of the tympanic membrane _____

5. pertaining to hearing _____

6. measurement of hearing _____

7. hernia of the cornea _____

8. surgical fixation of the retina _____

9. pertaining to the sclera _____

10. drooping or prolapse of the eyelid _____

11. pertaining to the eustachian tube and pharynx _____

12. pertaining to the cornea _____

13. resembling double _____

14. surgical repair of the tympanic membrane _____

15. cutting into or incision of the iris _____

16. cutting instrument for the iris _____

17. poisonous to the lens _____

18. inflammation of the conjunctiva _____

19. pertaining to the lacrimal glands _____

20. flow or discharge of pus in the tears _____

21. specialist in eyes _____

23. old-age hearing _____

Fill in the Blanks

Fill in the blanks below using Table 14-2.

Exercise 6

1. Dr. Strouse specializes in treating EENT disorders. Therefore, she treats

   disorders of the _____, _____,

   _____, and _____.

2. When Dr. Strouse charts *PERRLA*, it means _____

   _____ _____,

   _____, _____

   _____ _____,

   and _____.

3. The abbreviations *Ast* and *AS* stand for _____.

4. Lisa has cataracts in both eyes. This condition is abbreviated

   _____.

5. The TM is found in the eye.

   a. True   b. False

6. The abbreviation LASIK stands for _____

   _____   _____

   _____   _____.

7. The abbreviation RK stands for retinal keratotomy.

   a. True   b. False

8. Glaucoma is abbreviated _____ or

   _____.

9. The abbreviation MD stands for macular detachment.

   a. True   b. False

10. Joann is taking a test to measure her visual acuity. This type of test is

   abbreviated _____ or _____.

Learning Style Tip

Inquire whether medical-terminology videos, audiotapes, or CDs are available for checkout at your college library. Search for free "apps" on your tablet or smartphone. They will most likely present information in a different manner than your classroom instructor did. By repeatedly exposing yourself to medical terms, in a variety of different ways, you increase your ability to learn and remember.

Pathologies, Procedures, and Pharmacology

Pathology Terms

Table 14-3 includes terms that relate to diseases or abnormalities of vision or hearing. Use the pronunciation guide and say the terms aloud as you read them. This will help you get in the habit of saying them properly.

IN A FLASH!

It's time to print out all of the Pathology Terms Flash Cards for Chapter 14 and run through them at least three times before you continue.

Common Diagnostic Tests and Procedures

Audiometry: Detailed measurement of hearing with an audiometer

   Cochlear implant: Surgical insertion into the cochlea of a device that receives sound and transmits signals to electrodes implanted within the cochlea, allowing hearing-impaired persons to perceive sound

TABLE 14-3

PATHOLOGY TERMS

Eye

amblyopia (ăm-blē-Ō-pē-ă)	disorder in which the brain disregards images from the weaker eye and relies on those from the stronger eye; sometimes called *lazy eye*
astigmatism (ă-STĬG-mă-tĭ-zum)	abnormal curvature of the cornea that distorts the visual image

A   Normal eye

B   Myopia

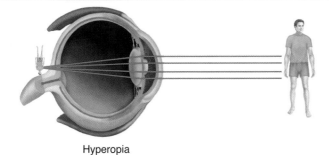

C   Hyperopia

D   Astigmatism

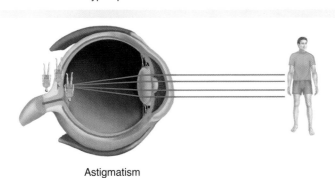

Astigmatism: Eyeball shape affects where the image is projected: (A) normal—on the retina; (B) myopia—in front of the retina; (C) hyperopia—behind the retina; (D) astigmatism—multiple images on the retina

Continued

TABLE 14-3
PATHOLOGY TERMS—cont'd
Eye

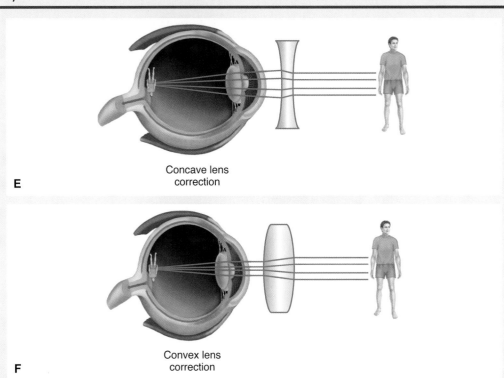

E   Concave lens
correction

F   Convex lens
correction

(E) concave lens correction for myopia; (F) convex lens correction for hyperopia. (From Eagle, S., et al. [2009]. *The professional medical assistant.* Philadelphia, PA: F. A. Davis Company, p. 757; with permission)

blepharitis (blĕf-ăr-Ī-tĭs)	noncontagious inflammation of the eyelash follicles and tiny oil glands along the margins of the eyelids

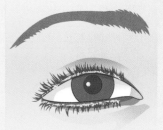

Blepharitis.

cataract (KĂT-ă-răkt)	cloudiness of the lens due to protein deposits as a result of aging, disease, or trauma or as a side effect of tobacco use or certain medications

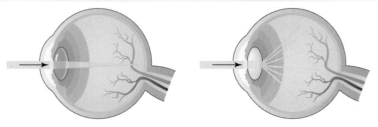

Normal lens   Clouded lens

Cataracts.

TABLE 14-3

PATHOLOGY TERMS—cont'd

Eye

central scotoma (SĔN-trăl skō-TŌ-mă)	blind spot in the center of the visual field surrounded by an area of normal vision
chalazion (kă-LĀ-zē-ōn)	small benign cyst in the eyelid formed by the distention of a meibomian gland (sebaceous gland of the eye) with secretions

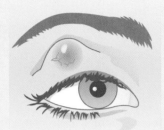

Chalazion.

conjunctivitis (kŏn-jŭnk-tĭ-VĪ-tĭs)	inflammation of the conjunctiva; also called *pinkeye*

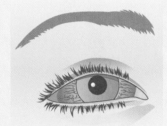

Conjunctivitis.

diabetic retinopathy (dī-ă-BĔT-ĭk rĕt-ĭn-ŎP-ă-thē)	progressive damage to microscopic vessels and other structures of the retina in patients with long-standing diabetes mellitus, which may result in blindness
ectropion (ĕk-TRŌ-pē-ŏn)	condition in which the lower eyelid is turned outward and droops more with aging

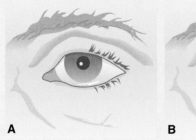 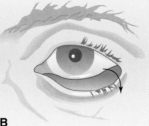

A   B

Ectropion: (A) normal eyelid, (B) ectropion.

Continued

TABLE 14-3
PATHOLOGY TERMS—cont'd

Eye

entropion (ĕn-TRŌ-pē-ŏn)	condition in which the eyelid edges are turned inward and rub against the surface of the eye, usually affecting the lower eyelid

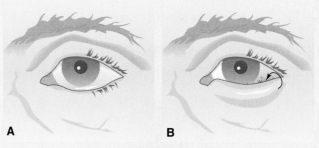

A   **B**

Entropion: (A) normal eyelid, (B) entropion.

glaucoma (acute) [glaw-KŌ-mă (a-KYÜT)]	type of glaucoma in which a sudden blockage of aqueous-humor outflow causes a rapid increase in intraocular pressure; can cause vision loss; also called *closed-angle glaucoma*

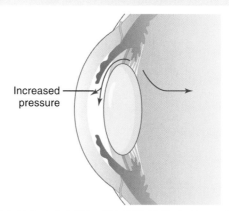

Increased pressure

Glaucoma (acute).

glaucoma (chronic) [glaw-KŌ-mă (KRÄ-nik)]	type of glaucoma in which the aqueous humor drains too slowly, leading to increasing intraocular pressure; can cause vision loss; also called *primary open-angle glaucoma*

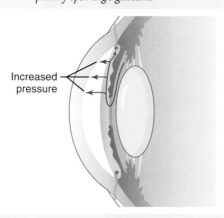

Increased pressure

Glaucoma (chronic).

TABLE 14-3

PATHOLOGY TERMS—cont'd

Eye

hordeolum (hor-DĒ-ō-lŭm)	infection of a sebaceous gland of the eyelid; also called a *stye*

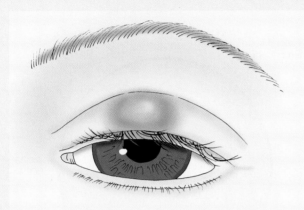

Hordeolum (stye).

hyperopia (hī-pĕr-Ō-pē-ă)	vision defect in which parallel rays focus behind the retina as a result of flattening of the globe of the eye or of an error in refraction; commonly called *farsightedness*

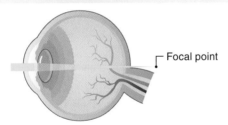

┌ Focal point

Hyperopia.

Continued

TABLE 14-3

PATHOLOGY TERMS—cont'd

Eye

hypertensive retinopathy (hī-pĕr-TĔN-sĭv rĕt-ĭn-ŎP-ă-thē)	destructive retinal changes caused by hypertension

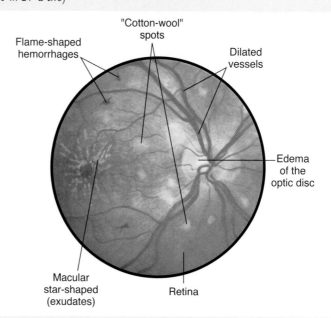

Hypertensive retinopathy. (From Eagle, S., et al. [2009]. *The professional medical assistant.* Philadelphia, PA: F. A. Davis Company, p. 756; with permission)

keratitis (kĕr-ă-TĪ-tĭs)	inflammation of the cornea, usually associated with decreased visual acuity, which may, if untreated, result in blindness
legal blindness (LĒ-gul BLĪND-nis)	loss in visual acuity that prevents a person from performing work requiring eyesight; defined as corrected visual acuity of 20/200 or less or a visual field of 20 degrees or less in the better eye
macular degeneration (MĂK-ū-lăr dĭ-jen-er-Ā-shŭn)	macular deterioration resulting in central vision loss, categorized as either atrophic (dry) or exudative (wet)

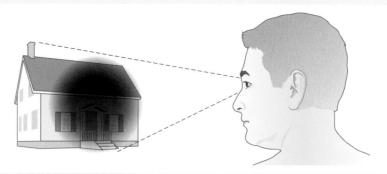

Macular degeneration.

TABLE 14-3

PATHOLOGY TERMS—cont'd

Eye

myopia (mī-Ō-pē-ă)	error of refraction in which light rays focus in front of the retina, enabling the person to see distinctly for only a short distance; commonly called *nearsightedness*

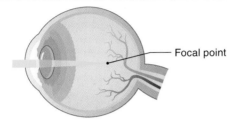
— Focal point

Myopia.

nystagmus (nĭs-TĂG-mŭs)	involuntary back-and-forth or cyclical movements of the eyes
ophthalmology (ŎP-thuh-mäl-ŭ-jē)	study of the structure, functions, and diseases of the eye
presbyopia (prĕz-bē-Ō-pē-ă)	permanent loss of accommodation of the lens of the eye that occurs as people enter their 40s, causing a marked inability to maintain focus on near objects
retinal detachment (RĔT-ĭ-năl dĭ-TACH-mŭnt)	separation of the inner sensory layer of the retina from the outer pigment layer, caused by a break in the inner layer that permits vitreous fluid to leak under the retina and lift off its innermost layer; may cause blindness

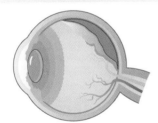

Retinal detachment.

Continued

TABLE 14-3
PATHOLOGY TERMS—cont'd

Eye

strabismus (stră-BĬZ-mŭs)	deviation or misalignment of eyes that may adversely affect depth perception; types include *exotropia* (eyes turned outward), *esotropia* (eyes turned inward), *hypertropia* (eyes turned upward), and *hypotropia* (eyes turned downward)

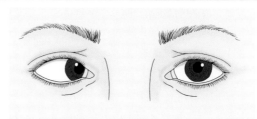

A   Esotropia

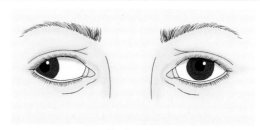

B   Exotropia

Strabismus: (A) esotropia, (B) exotropia.

uveitis (ū-vē-Ī-tĭs)	nonspecific term for any intraocular inflammatory disorder, which may affect the iris, ciliary body, choroid, or other parts of the eye

Ear

anacusis (ăn-ă-KŪ-sĭs)	total deafness
cholesteatoma (kō-lē-stē-ă-TŌ-mă)	condition in which a cyst develops in the middle ear

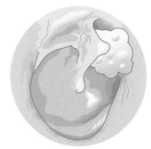

Cholesteatoma.

TABLE 14-3
PATHOLOGY TERMS—cont'd

Ear

labyrinthitis (lăb-ĭ-rĭn-THĪ-tĭs)	inflammation of the labyrinth within the inner ear; also called *otitis interna*
Ménière's disease (mān-ē-ĀRz dĭ-ZĒZ)	chronic, noncontagious disorder of the labyrinth that leads to progressive hearing loss, vertigo, and tinnitus; also called *labyrinthine hydrops*
otitis externa (ō-TĪ-tĭs ĕks-TĔR-nă)	acute inflammation or infection of the external auditory canal; also called *swimmer's ear*

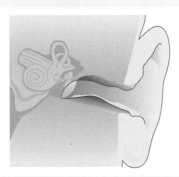

Otitis externa.

otitis media (ō-TĪ-tĭs MĒ-dē-ă)	inflammation or infection of the middle ear

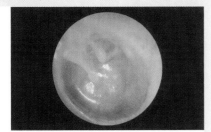 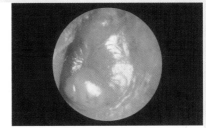

A Healthy tympanic membrane   B Infected tympanic membrane

Otitis media: (A) healthy tympanic membrane, (B) infected tympanic membrane.

otosclerosis (ō-tō-sklē-RŌ-sĭs)	chronic progressive deafness caused by spongy bone formation around the oval window with resulting ankylosis of the stapes
presbycusis (prĕz-bĭ-KŪ-sĭs)	progressive loss of hearing with aging
tinnitus (tĭn-Ī-tŭs)	perception of ringing, buzzing, tinkling, or hissing sound in the ear
vertigo (VĔR-tĭ-gō)	feeling of spinning or moving in space

Color vision tests: Use of multicolored charts to evaluate the patient's ability to recognize color (Fig. 14-7)

Corneal transplant (keratoplasty): Surgical replacement of a diseased cornea with a healthy one from a donor

Enucleation: Surgical removal of the entire eyeball

Laser-assisted in-situ keratomileusis (LASIK): Procedure in which a laser is used to alter the shape of the deep corneal layer after a top flap in the surface is opened

Laser photocoagulation: Destruction of areas of the retina with a laser beam

Phacoemulsification: Removal of the lens with an ultrasonic device to treat cataracts

Radial keratotomy: Incision into the outer portion of the cornea to flatten it and help correct nearsightedness

Refractive error test: Evaluation of the eye's ability to focus an image

Rinne test: Hearing test that compares bone conduction with air conduction, using a tuning fork (Fig. 14-8)

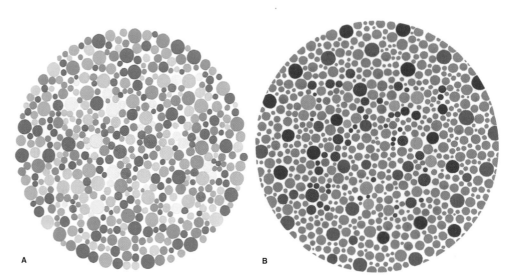

A   B

FIGURE 14-7 Color vision test.

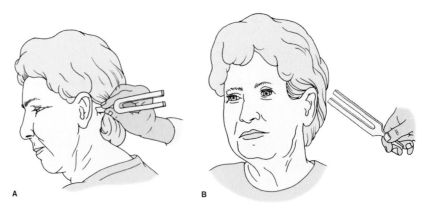

A   B

FIGURE 14-8 Rinne test.

Scleral buckling: Placement of a band of silicone around the eyeball to stabilize a detaching retina

Slit-lamp microscopy: Examination of the posterior surface of the cornea with a slit lamp

Tonometry: Measurement of intraocular tension to detect glaucoma

Tympanometry: Procedure for evaluation of the mobility and patency of the eardrum, detection of middle-ear disorders, and evaluation of the patency of the eustachian tube

Tympanoplasty: Reconstruction of a perforated tympanic membrane (Fig. 14-9)

Visual acuity test: Examination that identifies the smallest letters that can be correctly identified on a standardized Snellen's vision chart from 20 feet (Fig. 14-10)

Weber test: Hearing test that evaluates bone conduction using a tuning fork (Fig. 14-11)

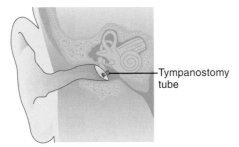

FIGURE 14-9 Tympanoplasty.

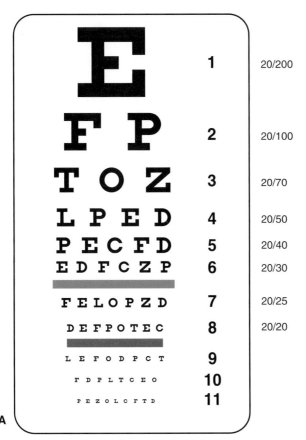

FIGURE 14-10 Visual acuity test: (A) Snellen chart with letters

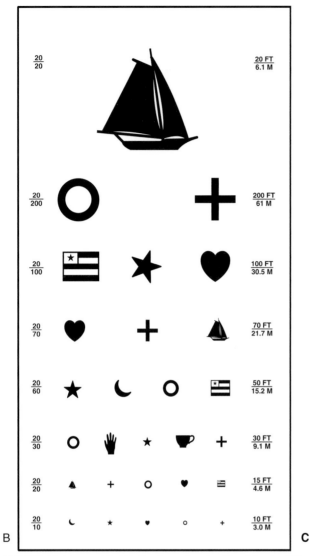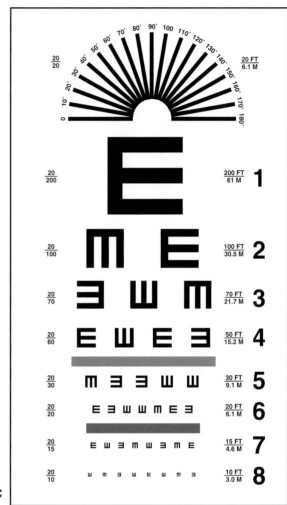

FIGURE 14-10—cont'd (B) Snellen chart with objects, (C) rotating "E" chart.

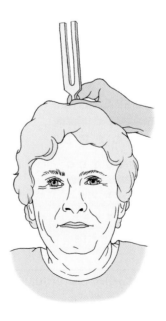

FIGURE 14-11 Weber test.

Learning Style Tip

Take timed (8- to 10-minute) study breaks every hour, during which you exercise. Studies show that exercise can help you think more clearly and decrease fatigue, tension, and anxiety. Study breaks can also help relieve symptoms of eyestrain such as burning, itching, watery or dry eyes, difficulty focusing, and headache.

Pharmacology

Table 14-4 provides a list of common eye and ear medications.

TABLE 14-4

PHARMACOLOGY

Therapeutic Classification	Generic Name	Brand Name	Common Use
Alpha agonists (ophthalmic)	alphagan	Brimonidine tartrate	Treatment of glaucoma: decrease fluid production and/or increase fluid drainage
	apraclonidine	Lopidine	
	dipivefrin ophthalmic	Propine	
	epinephrine ophthalmic	Epifrin	
Antibiotics (ophthalmic)	azithromycin	AzaSite	Treatment of ocular infections such as blepharitis, conjunctivitis, and keratitis: kill or inhibit spread of bacteria
	bacitracin	Bacticin	
	besifloxacin	Besivance	
	ciprofloxacin	Ciloxan	
	erythromycin ophthalmic	Ilotycin, Romycin	
	gatifloxacin ophthalmic	Zymaxid	
	levofloxacin ophthalmic	Iquix, Quixin	
	moxifloxacin hydrochloride ophthalmic	Moxeza, Vigamox	
	sulfacetamide sodium ophthalmic	AK Sulf, Bleph10, Ocusulf, Sturzsulf, Sulster	
	tobramycin ophthalmic	AKTob, Tobradex	
Antivertigo agents	dimenhydrinate	Dramamine	Treatment of motion sickness: minimize the effect of motion, reduce nausea and vomiting
	promethazine	Promethegan	
	scopolamine	Transderm	

Continued

TABLE 14-4
PHARMACOLOGY—cont'd

Therapeutic Classification	Generic Name	Brand Name	Common Use
Beta blockers (ophthalmic)	levobunolol HCL ophthalmic	Betagan	Treatment of glaucoma: decrease fluid production
	metipranolol	OptiPranolol	
	timolol hemihydrate	Betimol	
	timololmaleate ophthalmic	Timoptic-XE	
Carbonic anhydrase inhibitors: topical, oral, or intravenous	acetazolamide	Diamox	Treatment of glaucoma: decrease fluid production
	brinzolamide	Azopt	
	dorzolamide	Trusopt	
	methazolamide	Neptazane	
Cholinergics	pilocarpine	IsoptoCarpine, Pilocar, Pilopine	Treatment of glaucoma: increase fluid drainage
Cycloplegics and mydriatics	atropine	Isopto atropine	Dilate the pupil and/or temporary paralysis of accommodation during eye exam or procedure
	cyclopentolate	Cyclogyl	
	homatropine	Isopto homatropine	
	phenylephrine	Mydfrin	
	tropicamide	Mydriacyl	
Local anesthetics (ophthalmic)	lidocaine	Akten	Block pain signals in the eye before eye exam or surgical procedure
	proparacaine	Alcaine, Ocu-Caine, Ophthetic, Parcaine	
	tetracaine	Altacaine, Opticaine, TetraVisc	
NSAIDs (ophthalmic)	bromfenac	Prolensa, Xibrom	Decrease inflammation and reduce pain
	diclofenac	Voltaren	
	flurbiprofen	Ocufen	
	ketorolac tromethamine	Acular	
	nepafenac	Nevanac	
Prostaglandins (ophthalmic)	bimatoprost	Lumigan	Treatment of glaucoma: increase fluid drainage
	latanoprost	Xalatan	
	tafluprost	Zioptan	
	travoprost	Travatan Z	

Pathologies, Procedures, and Pharmacology Practice Exercises

Deciphering Terms

Write the correct meaning of these medical terms.

Exercise 7

1. keratoid _____

2. neoplasia _____

3. myringomycosis _____

4. tympanometry _____

5. retro-ocular _____

6. ophthalmoplegia _____

7. otoplasty _____

8. oculonasal _____

9. tympanic _____

10. keratotomy _____

11. blepharoptosis _____

12. ophthalmorrhea _____

13. intraocular _____

14. lacrimotome _____

15. phacosclerosis _____

Fill in the Blanks

Fill in the blanks below using Table 14-3.

Exercise 8

1. Kari wears corrective lenses because she has an abnormal curvature
   of the cornea that distorts her visual image. This is known as an

   _____.

2. Herbert has total deafness. The term for this is _____.

3. Hilda has hearing loss due to her advanced age. The term for this is

   _____.

4. Jack has _____ _____, which is a
   chronic, noncontagious disorder of the labyrinth that leads to progressive
   hearing loss, vertigo, and tinnitus.

5. _____ _____ is a condition of sudden
   blockage of aqueous-humor outflow that causes a rapid increase
   in intraocular pressure.

6. David is a farmer who has developed cloudiness of the lens due to
   protein deposits as a result of aging and tobacco use. This is called

   _____.

7. Monty has been a diabetic for 20 years and is developing the signs of
   _____ _____, which is vision loss
   due to his diabetes.

8. Blake has a condition that is causing central vision loss because
   of deterioration. This is known as _____

   _____.

9. Louise has an infection of a sebaceous gland of the eyelid. This is known
   as _____.

10. Dennis is experiencing vision loss in his left eye caused by a separation
    of the inner retinal layer from the outer layer. This is known as

    _____ _____.

11. _____ is a form of strabismus in which one or both eyes
    are turned outward.

12. _____ is a nonspecific term for any intraocular
    inflammatory disorder that may affect the iris, ciliary body, choroid,
    or other parts of the eye.

13. _____ is a condition of inflammation of the conjunctiva.

14. The type of vision loss associated with advancing age is

    _____.

15. _____ is a small benign cyst in the eyelid formed by the distention of a meibomian gland with secretions.

16. _____ is a cyst that develops in the middle ear.

Multiple Choice

Select the one best answer to the following multiple-choice questions.

Exercise 9

1. Which of the following conditions does **not** result in vision loss?

   a. presbycusis

   b. diabetic retinopathy

   c. retinal detachment

   d. glaucoma

2. Which of the following conditions results in an abnormal curvature of the cornea, distorting the visual image?

   a. presbycusis

   b. astigmatism

   c. cataract

   d. hordeolum

3. Albert Mills is an elderly man who experiences diminished hearing because of advanced age. This condition is known as:

   a. photophobia

   b. glaucoma

   c. presbycusis

   d. hordeolum

4. A type of blindness caused by diabetes is known as diabetic _____.

   a. retinopathy

   b. cataract

   c. macular degeneration

   d. Ménière's disease

5. Onset of blindness caused by increased intraocular pressure is known as:

   a. cataract

   b. macular degeneration

   c. hordeolum

   d. glaucoma

Fill in the Blanks

Using Table 14-4, write the therapeutic classification of the medication next to each generic or brand name.

Exercise 10

1. travoprost _____

2. atropine _____

3. Diamox _____

4. bacitracin _____

5. Prolensa _____

6. proparacaine _____

7. Pilopine _____

8. Vigamox _____

9. apraclonidine _____

10. dimenhydrinate _____

CASE STUDY

Read the case study and answer the questions that follow. Most of the terms are included in this chapter. Refer to your medical dictionary for the other terms.

Acute Otitis Media

Brad Stephens is a 5-year-old child with a medical history of chronic acute otitis media (AOM). With his first ear infection at 9 months of age, his symptoms were quite pronounced. He spiked a 104.5°F fever, ate and slept poorly, and was extremely fussy. However, with repeated episodes of AOM as he has aged, his symptoms have lessened significantly, making it difficult for his parents to know when he has an ear infection. Often his only symptom is fussiness. Brad has responded reasonably well in the past to antibiotics and decongestants, yet the infections frequently recur a short time later. At the age of 5, he still has one to two episodes of AOM each month. This raises concerns about hearing loss, so he was referred to an ENT specialist for consultation. The result was the decision to perform bilateral tympanotomy with tube placement.

Acute otitis media (AOM), the most common infection in infants and children, occurs when bacteria make their way from the oropharynx into the middle ear via the eustachian tube. Infections such as AOM often occur near the end of an upper respiratory infection (URI). Tissues are inflamed and edematous, and secretions are copious. Other risk factors for AOM include allergies and sinusitis. As infection sets in, the middle ear becomes inflamed, which causes edema and pressure in the middle ear. Serous fluid usually accumulates behind the TM as well. In some children, the eustachian tube does not readily open to allow passage of air or fluid to relieve this pressure. As a result, the TM begins to bulge outward. This pressure, along with inflammation, causes pain and a sensation of the ear being plugged. Hearing is temporarily impaired at this point. In severe cases, the TM becomes blistered or even ruptures, which results in scarring and varying amounts of hearing loss.

With mild cases of AOM, treatment may focus on relieving pain with analgesics, such as acetaminophen, and treating congestion. More-severe cases are treated with antibiotics. In the case of chronic AOM, surgery is considered. Surgery is generally a last resort and serves the purpose of buying time while the child grows and matures. In many cases, a child will outgrow ear infections as the structures of the middle ear and throat further develop and the eustachian tubes begin to work more effectively.

When a tympanotomy is performed, tiny tubes are inserted into the TM, which creates a windowlike opening between the middle and outer ear. This does not prevent AOM from occurring, but it does allow fluid and air to escape, reducing pressure in the middle ear and preventing rupture of the TM. This reduces the risk of permanent damage or hearing loss. An added advantage is that it becomes easier to recognize an infection, because drainage from the ear is easily observed. This allows for earlier treatment. The tiny tubes remain in place for 6 months to 2 years, eventually working their way out into the ear canal, at which time the TM heals itself.

Flashpoint

Small children can experience ear pain on an airplane due to the effects of changing air pressure on their developing eustachian tubes.

Case Study Questions

Exercise 11

1. Which of the following statements is true regarding Brad's experience?
   a. His symptoms worsened over time.
   b. Brad was referred to a physician who specialized in disorders of the ears, nose, and throat.
   c. Brad did not respond well to antibiotic therapy.
   d. His parents could easily tell when Brad had an ear infection.

2. Brad underwent a bilateral tympanotomy with tube placement. This procedure involves:
   a. Excision and removal of the eardrums
   b. Replacing the eardrums with tubes
   c. Creation of a mouthlike opening into the eustachian tube
   d. Cutting into the eardrums to place tubes

3. Which of the following statements is true regarding AOM?
   a. It is an uncommon type of infection in infants and children.
   b. It is contagious.
   c. It is caused when a virus attacks the middle ear.
   d. It is caused by bacterial growth in the middle ear.

4. Which of the following factors contributes to the development of AOM?
   a. A dry environment
   b. Failure of the outer ear canal to develop and work properly
   c. Allergies and sinusitis
   d. Accumulation of fluid in front of the TM

5. Which of the following statements is true regarding treatment of AOM?
   a. Antibiotics are always prescribed.
   b. Decongestants may be used.
   c. Surgery is common.
   d. Analgesics are seldom used.

6. Which of the following statements is true regarding the surgical procedure that Brad underwent?
   a. The purpose was to buy some time while the structures in his ear and throat further developed.
   b. The purpose was to repair the defect in his middle ear and cure his problem.
   c. The purpose was to restore his lost hearing.
   d. The purpose was to prevent the occurrence of AOM.

7. Which of the following statements is true regarding the tubes that are placed in the TM?
   a. They will be surgically removed once the ear has healed.
   b. They allow for the escape of fluid or air.
   c. They force the eustachian tube to work properly.
   d. They usually remain in place for 5 years.

8. Describe how chronic pain, such as a recurring earache, would affect your activities of daily living (ADLs).

9. Describe three or more ways in which hearing loss could affect a young child's ADLs.

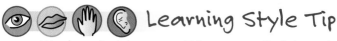 Learning Style Tip

Watch medical dramas on TV or rent medical-themed movies and write down medical terms as you hear them used. Keep this book and a medical dictionary handy to look up any terms you don't know. Read the definitions aloud.

End-of-Chapter Practice Exercises

Word Building

*Using **only** the word parts in the lists provided, create medical terms with the indicated meanings.*

Exercise 12

Prefixes	Combining Forms	Suffixes
an-	acous/o	-al
hyper-	audi/o	-ar
	blephar/o	-ectomy
	conjunctiv/o	-edema
	dipl/o	-ic
	irid/o	-itis
	kerat/o	-logy
	lacrim/o	-malacia
	myring/o	-metry
	nas/o	-oma
	ocul/o	-opia
	ophthalm/o	-osis
	ot/o	-pathy
	phac/o	-plasty

retin/o   -plegia
scler/o   -scope
tympan/o   -tic
                        -tomy

1. pertaining to absence of hearing _____

2. pertaining to the eye _____

3. swelling of the eyelid _____

4. excessive vision or far vision _____

5. study of the eye _____

6. inflammation of the cornea _____

7. double vision _____

8. cutting into or incision of the tympanic membrane _____

9. viewing instrument for the eye _____

10. disease of the retina _____

11. surgical repair of the sclera _____

12. surgical repair of the eye _____

13. pertaining to the ear _____

14. pertaining to the lacrimal gland and nose _____

15. softening of the lens _____

16. abnormal condition of the retina _____

17. tumor of the conjunctiva _____

18. excision or surgical removal of the iris _____

19. measurement of hearing _____

20. paralysis of the eye _____

True or False

Decide whether the following statements are true or false.

Exercise 13

1. True   False   The abbreviation **ENT** stands for *eyes, ears, nose, and throat.*

2. True   False   **Conjunctivitis** is a condition of inflammation of the conjunctiva.

3. True   False   The abbreviation **EM** stands for *extraocular movement.*

4. True   False   **Tinnitus** is a feeling of dizziness or vertigo.

5. True   False   **Strabismus** is a condition of blindness.

6. True   False   **Otosclerosis** causes progressive hearing loss.

7. True   False   **Vertigo** is ringing in the ears.

8. True   False   **Acute otitis media** is an infection of the outer ear.

9. True   False   The abbreviation **Ast** stands for *acoustic.*

10. True   False   **LASIK** is a procedure that improves vision.

Deciphering Terms

Write the correct meaning of these medical terms.

Exercise 14

1. dacryohemorrhea _____

2. iridomalacia _____

3. lacrimotomy _____

4. phacoid _____

5. presbycusis _____

6. retinopathy _____

7. dacryadenalgia _____

8. blepharospasm _____

9. iridoplegia _____

10. phakoma _____

Multiple Choice

Select the one best answer to the following multiple-choice questions.

Exercise 15

1. Which of the following terms means *absence of smell or odor?*

    a. anosmia

    b. anacusia

    c. anopia

    d. none of these

2. Which of the following terms means *excision or surgical removal of the tear gland?*

    a. cryoextraction

    b. dacryoadenectomy

    c. lacrimotomy

    d. cryosurgery

3. Which of the following terms means *disintegration of the lens?*

    a. phakolysis

    b. phacolysis

    c. both a and b

    d. phakomatosis

4. Which of the following terms means *specialist in the study of sound?*

    a. acoustic

    b. audiology

    c. audiometer

    d. none of these

5. Which of the following terms means *abnormal condition of hardening of the eardrum?*

    a. keratoscleritis

    b. tympanosclerosis

    c. phacosclerosis

    d. otosclerosis

6. Which of the following terms means *flow or discharge from the ear?*

    a. salpingorrhaphy

    b. dacryopyorrhea

    c. otorrhea

    d. iridorrhexis

7. The patient who needs a vision examination will visit an:

   a.   ophthalmologist

   b.   optician

   c.   ocularist

   d.   otologist

8. The term *hemiopia* means:

   a.   half vision

   b.   double vision

   c.   far or beyond vision

   d.   good or normal vision

9. The term *dysopia* means:

   a.   displacement in the position of the eyes

   b.   disturbance of sleep

   c.   distortion of smell perception

   d.   defective vision

10. The term *microblepharism* means:

   a.   condition of farsightedness

   b.   abnormal condition of large eyes

   c.   having same or equal eyelids

   d.   having abnormally small eyelids

11. The term *dacryoadenalgia* means:

   a.   pain in a lacrimal sac

   b.   pain in a lacrimal gland

   c.   a herniated protrusion of a lacrimal sac

   d.   hardening of a lacrimal gland

12. The term *diplopia* means:

   a.   near image

   b.   far view

   c.   double vision

   d.   two eyes

13. All of the following abbreviations pertain to conditions that cause vision loss or impairment **except:**

    a. Glc

    b. MD

    c. EOM

    d. RD

14. Which of the following abbreviations refers to a procedure that improves vision?

    a. AS

    b. LASIK

    c. CAT

    d. VA

15. All of the following abbreviations refer to the eyes **except:**

    a. ENT

    b. EM

    c. RK

    d. RD

16. Which of the following is a disorder in which the brain disregards images from a weaker eye and relies on those from the stronger eye?

    a. amblyopia

    b. astigmatism

    c. chalazion

    d. ectropion

17. Which of the following is an infection of a sebaceous gland of the eyelid?

    a. hordeolum

    b. keratitis

    c. cholesteatoma

    d. labyrinthitis

18. Which of the following is a feeling of spinning or moving in space?

    a. vertigo

    b. tinnitus

    c. otosclerosis

    d. Ménière's disease

19. An error in refraction is:

    a. myopia

    b. hypertropia

    c. presbyopia

    d. esotropia

20. Glaucoma has which of the following effects on the eye?

    a. cloudiness of the lens

    b. inflammation of the lid and eyelash follicles

    c. increased intraocular pressure

    d. loss of central vision

GLOSSARY OF STRUCTURE AND FUNCTION TERMS

This table contains a list of the medical terms used to complete the structure and function exercises in each chapter.

A

abdominal cavity: the cavity that contains the stomach, pancreas, liver, gallbladder, and large and small intestines

abrasion: area where skin has been scraped away

accommodation: the process of rounding and flattening of the lens that enables focus in both near and far vision

adrenocorticotropic hormone (ACTH): acts on the adrenal glands to secrete glucocorticoids, including cortisol

aldosterone: plays a role in regulating and maintaining the body's water, sodium, and electrolyte balance

alveoli: microscopic-sized air sacs

amphiarthrosis: a slightly movable joint

anatomical position: standing upright with the toes and the palms facing forward

androgens: responsible for secondary sexual characteristics in females and males

anterior lobe: the portion of the pituitary gland that secretes the hormones GH, TSH, FSH, LH, prolactin, and ACTH

antidiuretic hormone (ADH): acts on the kidneys to increase the absorption of water

aortic valve: exits the left ventricle into the aorta

apex: the largest part of the heart; the lower-left area

apical pulse: listening to this is considered the most-accurate method of measuring heart rate

aponeurosis: a tendon that resembles a ribbon and attaches to a larger area of bone

appendicular body: the arms and legs of the body

appendix: a structure that hangs from the cecum in which normal bacteria may be stored to repopulate the GI tract

aqueous humor: fluid in the anterior chamber that provides nourishment for the lens and cornea and bends light rays to focus them sharply onto the retina

areola: a region of pigmented tissue at the center surface of each breast

arterioles: tiny arteries

ascending colon: the structure that progresses upward from the cecum

atria: the two upper chambers of the heart

atrioventricular node: the "backup" pacemaker that transmits the SA node impulse to both ventricles

atrophy: decrease in size

auscultating: the term that means *listening to*

autonomic nervous system: the system that controls involuntary functions

axial body: the head, neck, and trunk portion of the body

axon: sends electrical impulses and transmits signals to other cells

B

basement membrane: place where new, living epidermal cells are produced

bicuspid valve: exits the left atrium into the left ventricle

bladder: a flexible, muscular container for urine

blood pH: the acidity or alkalinity in the blood

body planes: points of reference that are imaginary slices or cuts through the body that divide it vertically or horizontally

bolus: a rounded mass of chewed food that is ready to be swallowed

bones: composed of dense connective tissue including cells in a matrix of calcium and collagen fibers

brainstem: the essential pathway that conducts impulses between the brain and spinal cord

Braxton Hicks contractions: gentle contractions of the uterus at irregular intervals; also known as *false labor*

buccal cavity: the mouth

bulbourethral glands: lubricate the urethra and neutralize its acidic environment

C

calcitonin: regulates calcium and phosphorus levels in the blood

capillaries: blood enters these after leaving the arterioles; their walls are just one cell thick

cardiac cycle: the contraction and relaxation of the four heart chambers

cecum: the first part of the large intestine

cell body: houses all of the microscopic structures that keep the cell energized and functioning

cells: the structural units that form all body tissues

central nervous system (CNS): the brain and the spinal cord

cerebellum: responsible for posture, balance, and coordination

cerebrum: the largest portion of the brain

cerumen: waxy substance in the external auditory canal that traps tiny foreign particles and prevents them from entering the deeper structures

cervix: the narrowed section of the uterus that dilates during the birth process to allow delivery of the fetus

cholesterol: a fatty, plaque-like substance that can narrow or block coronary vessels

choroid: dark-blue middle layer that supplies blood to the entire eye

chyme: a more-liquid material made up of chewed food, saliva, and digestive juices

cilia: tiny hairs within the nasal cavity

ciliary body: attached to the lens; includes several ciliary muscles

ciliary muscles: cause the lens to change shape when they contract or expand

circadian rhythm: sleep-wake cycle

clitoris: elongated erectile tissue located beneath the anterior portion of the labia

cochlea: snail-shaped structure of the inner ear lined with the Organ of Corti and filled with perilymph; part of the vestibular system

conception: fertilization of the ovum

cones: visual receptors in the retina that detect color and function in more brightly lit situations

conjunctiva: thin mucous membrane covering the outer surface of the eye that contains blood vessels and secretory glands

connective tissue: acts to connect and support other body tissues

cornea: transparent bulge of the sclera that allows light into the eye

corpus albicans: the corpus luteum atrophies into this mass of fibrous tissue if conception does not occur

corpus callosum: divides the cerebrum into two hemispheres

corpus luteum: the remainder of the graafian follicle after ovulation

cortex: deep folds and shallow grooves on the surface of the cerebrum which increase its surface area

cortisol: works to decrease inflammation

cranial cavity: the cavity that contains the brain

cranium: the hard bones of the skull

cremasters: a muscle group that extends from the abdomen into the scrotum

crowning: when the top of the infant's head appears at the cervical opening

D

defecation: the process in which products of digestion move through the colon, the rectum, and the anus to be excreted as feces

dendrite: receives information and brings it to the cell body

dermatomes: areas of skin associated with specific spinal nerve roots

dermis: layer of skin that contains hair follicles, nerves, sweat glands, and sensory receptors

descending colon: the portion of the colon found along the left side of the abdomen

diabetes mellitus: a pathology in which blood sugar levels may widely fluctuate

diarthrosis: a freely movable joint

diastole: the lower blood pressure number that reflects the lowest pressure exerted against artery walls during ventricular relaxation

dilation: a term for expansion or opening of the cervix

dorsal cavity: the cavity that is located on the posterior or back part of the body

duodenum, jejunum, ileum: upper, middle, and end portion of the small intestine

dynamic equilibrium: sense of balance when we are in motion

E

ear: responsible for hearing, balance, and equilibrium

edema: swelling

effacement: a term for thinning of the cervix

electrolytes: the ions in bodily fluids

embryo: the zygote becomes this as all of the tissues and organs develop during the first 9 weeks

endocardium: the inner lining of the heart

endocrine glands: responsible for sexual maturation; play a role in the metabolism of food and energy storage

endolymph: pale, transparent fluid within the labyrinth that responds to changes in body position based on gravity

epicardium: the outer lining of the heart

epidermis: thin, outer layer of the skin

epididymis, vas deferens, and ejaculatory duct: spermatocytes will exit the testes through these ducts that join with the urethra

epiglottis: doorway to the trachea; a small flap of cartilage at the top of the esophagus that keeps food from entering the respiratory tract

epinephrine: enables the body to respond to stressful situations by converting glycogen into glucose for quick energy

epithelial tissue: forms the top layer of skin

erythema: redness

esophagus: a long, tubelike structure that passes through the diaphragm and connects to the stomach

essential minerals: calcium, phosphorus, and magnesium

estrogen: a hormone that prepares the uterus for a fertilized egg; plays a vital role in the menstrual cycle and is important in the prevention of osteoporosis

eustachian tube: connects the middle ear to the throat; allows air movement between the inner ear and outer atmosphere

exhalation: expiration

external auditory canal: slender tube that runs from the external ear to the middle ear

eyeball: globe-shaped organ that consists of three layers

F

fallopian tubes: two of these extend approximately 4 inches from the sides of the uterus toward the ovaries

fascia: connective tissue arranged in sheets or bands which covers muscle tissue

feces: the waste product that is excreted through the process of defecation

fertilization: when one sperm penetrates an egg and forms a zygote

fetus: at 9 weeks, the embryo is called this

filtrate: fluid that has been filtered by the walls of the glomerulus and Bowman's capsule

follicle-stimulating hormone (FSH): acts on the gonads to produce an ovum in the female and sperm in the male

follicular: the first phase of the menstrual cycle in which a woman is ovulating

foreskin: a fold of skin that covers the penis

frontal: the plane that divides the body into front and back portions; also known as the *coronal* plane

fundus, body, pylorus: the upper, middle, and lower portions of the stomach

G

gait: the manner and style in which a person walks

gallbladder: a small sac found on the inner surface of the liver which acts as a storage pouch for bile

gastric secretions: very acidic fluids that continue to break down food, preparing it for absorption within the intestines

gastrointestinal (GI) system: all structures of the alimentary canal, from the mouth to the anus, and the accessory organs

gestation: a term for pregnancy

glans penis: the distal, rounded end of the penis

glia: support cells that carry nutrients to neurons

glomerulus: capillary cluster within the Bowman's capsule

glucagon: acts on the liver to convert glycogen into glucose

glucose: sugar

goniometer: a device for measuring joint range of motion

graafian follicles: are found within the ovaries and contain the immature ova, or eggs

growth hormone: promotes the growth of body structures, such as bones

H

hair follicle: part of the hair that is buried in the skin

hair shaft: part of the hair that you can see which functions to filter dust and debris from the air

hard palate: divides the nasal cavity from the mouth

hematopoiesis: the production of red and white blood cells

hemodialysis: a process by which blood is filtered through a special membrane in a machine to remove excess fluid and wastes

homeostasis: the state of dynamic equilibrium in the internal environment of the body

hormones: chemicals secreted into the bloodstream that cause bodily reactions; work in pairs to maintain a healthy balance to keep the body's internal environment healthy

hyperglycemia: high blood sugar

hypertrophy: increase in size

hypoglycemia: low blood sugar

I

ileocecal valve: a valve through which products of digestion pass from the small intestine to the large intestine

ingestion: taking a bite of food

inhalation: inspiration

insulin: breaks carbohydrates down into glucose and stimulates cells to take up glucose from the blood

internal urinary sphincter: contracts to keep semen from entering the bladder and to keep urine from exiting the bladder

iris: surrounds the pupil and gives eyes their color

J

joints: the space where two bones meet and where movement occurs

K

kidneys: the key organs of the urinary system

L

labia: two layers of tissue that cover and protect the clitoris, the urethral meatus, and the vaginal opening

labyrinth: complex, mazelike anatomy of the inner ear

laceration: cut or tear in the flesh

lacrimal glands: produce tears that flow over the eye's surface

lactation: the production of breast milk to nourish the newborn baby

larynx: vibrates to create sound when we talk

lens: clear, firm, transparent disc in the middle layer that can change shape to allow vision at different distances

leukocytes: white blood cells

ligaments: attach bones to other bones

liver: the largest glandular organ of the body

lobes: division of the lungs; the right has three, and the left has two

lower airway: the bronchi and lungs

lower esophageal sphincter (LES): a muscular opening between the esophagus and the stomach that prevents backflow of gastric secretions

lunula: half-moon area at the base of the nail where new growth occurs

luteal phase: the second phase of the menstrual cycle in which the ovum is propelled toward the fallopian tube and conception may occur

lymph: clear, colorless, alkaline tissue fluid made up mostly of water, along with some protein, fats, white blood cells, and urea

lymph nodes: rich in specialized white blood cells; commonly called glands

lymphatic system: a part of the immune system that collects excess tissue fluid and returns it to circulation

lymphatic vessels: found throughout the body alongside arteries, veins, and capillaries

M

mature ovum: contains one-half of the necessary components of a new life and is produced by the ovaries every 28 days

mechanical digestion: the process in which food is broken down into smaller parts by the teeth and the tongue

mediastinum: the area slightly left of the center of the chest

medulla: the innermost part of the kidney

melanin: pigment that gives skin its color

melanocytes: pigment-producing skin cells

melatonin: influences the body's natural circadian rhythm

menarche: onset of menstruation

meninges: three membranes that protect the brain and spinal cord

menopause: the normal cessation of menses that occurs approximately 40 years after menarche

menstrual phase: the third phase of the menstrual cycle in which the uterus sheds the unneeded endometrial lining

menstruation: approximately every 28 days, the uterus sheds the layer of endometrial tissue that develops each month in preparation for pregnancy

metastasized: spread to another part of the body

micturition reflex: the urge to urinate

midline: an imaginary line that runs from the head to the feet and divides the body into right and left halves

motor impulses: information from the brain that travels to the rest of the body

motor nerves: nerves that control body movement

muscle tissue: composed of cells called contractile fibers

muscles: connective tissues made up of contractile fibers

myelin sheath: a special protective layer on the axon

myocardium: the middle, muscular layer of the heart

myotomes: groups of muscles associated with specific spinal nerve roots

N

nailbed: nails slide slowly over this layer of epithelial tissue as they grow

nares: nostrils

nasal septum: divides the nasal passages into left and right sides

nasopharynx: back of the nose

neck, axillae, groin, and abdomen: high numbers of lymph nodes are found in these areas

negative feedback system: each gland produces a hormone that serves to oppose another substance; the gland may increase or decrease production of the hormone to stimulate a corresponding decrease or increase of that substance

nephrons: microscopic structures located primarily within the outer cortex of the kidneys

nervous tissue: comprises the brain, spinal cord, and nerves for the entire body

neuron: a nerve cell

nipple: the center of the areola

O

occluded: the term that means *blocked*

optic nerve: attached to the retina; transmits visual information to the brain

oral cavity: the mouth

organ of Corti: highly sensitive hearing structure lining the inner surface of the cochlea

organs: two or more types of tissue that perform specialized functions

oropharynx: back of the mouth

ossicles: vibrations of the tympanic membrane cause these three tiny bones to move, which sends vibrations to the inner ear

osteocytes: new bone cells

osteogenesis: creation of new bone cells

osteoporosis: a disorder of decreased bone mass

ovaries: the oval-shaped structures on each side of the uterus that are the primary sex organs in females; secrete the hormones estrogen and progesterone

oxytocin: acts on the uterus to promote contractions during labor and delivery

P

pancreas: an organ that secretes substances which neutralize stomach acids and break down proteins, fats, and carbohydrates; secretes the hormones insulin and glucagon which work cooperatively to maintain healthy blood glucose levels

parasympathetic nervous system: the system that dominates during nonstressful times

parathormone (PTH): also called parathyroid hormone; helps to regulate calcium and phosphorus levels in the blood

parathyroid glands: they secrete the hormone PTH, which helps to regulate calcium and phosphorus levels in the blood

pelvic cavity: the cavity that contains the sigmoid colon, rectum, and bladder, and, in females, contains the uterus, fallopian tubes, and ovaries

pericardial fluid: a lubricant that reduces friction as the heart contracts and relaxes

pericardium: the fibrous membrane that encloses the heart

perilymph: cochlea vibrations cause a disturbance of this pale, transparent fluid, which in turn disturb hair cells on the organ of Corti, transmitting impulses to the auditory nerve

peripheral nervous system (PNS): the system that includes nerves in the arms and legs

peristalsis: muscular contractions that move the food bolus downward into the stomach and move chyme through the small intestine

peritoneal dialysis: a process by which blood is filtered through the patient's own membrane in the abdominal cavity to remove excess fluid and wastes

peritoneum: a membrane that lines the abdominal cavity

phagocytes: white blood cells that clean debris from lymph

phagocytosis: a process in which white blood cells engulf and destroy microorganisms, cell debris, and blood cells that are damaged, old, or abnormal

pharynx: funnel-shaped tissue at the back of the mouth which extends down to the esophagus

pH scale: a tool for measuring the acidity or alkalinity of a substance; used to measure the acid base which ranges from 0–14

pineal gland: located in the brain, above and behind the thalamus; produces the hormone melatonin

pinna: made of cartilage covered with skin; collects sound waves and channels them into the external auditory canal

pituitary gland: structure attached to the lower surface of the hypothalamus in the brain; controls all of the other glands in the body

placenta: organ of nutrition that begins forming early after conception and connects to the developing fetus through the umbilical cord

pleurae: membranes covering the lungs

pleural fluid: fluid between the visceral and parietal pleurae that acts as a sort of lubricant

posterior lobe: the portion of the pituitary gland that secretes the hormones oxytocin and ADH

progesterone: a hormone that is responsible for changes in the uterine lining in preparation for implantation of a developing embryo; necessary to prepare and maintain the uterus for a fertilized ovum

prolactin: acts on the mammary glands to produce milk

prostaglandin: stimulates smooth muscle contractions in the female reproductive tract to help move sperm

prostate gland: secretes fluid that helps to create a more-alkaline environment in the urethra

pulmonary arteries: they lead to the lungs and transport oxygen-poor blood

pulmonary valve: exits the right ventricle into the pulmonary arteries

pulmonary veins: they transport oxygen-rich blood to various parts of the body

pulse points: large arteries with a strong pulse that are easily palpated

pupil: dilates to allow more light to enter the eye; constricts to decrease the amount of light entering the eye

pyloric sphincter: releases chyme from the pylorus into the small intestine a little at a time

R

range of motion: the amount of motion available at a joint

recoil: the elastic quality that allows the lungs to expand and contract

referred pain: pain that is felt at an area of the body away from the actual injury site

reflex: action or response that happens so quickly one doesn't have time to think about it

renal failure: high blood pressure and type 2 diabetes are the most common causes

renal pelvis: the area where all of the calyces join

reproductive glands: the ovaries and testes; sometimes called the gonads

retina: innermost layer of the eye containing two types of visual receptors

retroperitoneal space: the space at the back of the abdomen just lateral to the spinal column; location in the back of the abdominal cavity

rods: visual receptors in the retina that function in dim lighting to produce images in black and white

rugae: folds that line the stomach allowing it to expand when we eat a large amount of food

S

sagittal: the plane that divides the body into right and left halves

saliva: a fluid secreted by the salivary glands which contains a chemical that starts to break down starches

Schlemm's canal: small opening for drainage of aqueous humor

sclera: white, outermost layer that provides strength, structure, and shape to the eye

scrotum: composed of two internal compartments and structures designed to maintain an optimal temperature for spermatogenesis

sebaceous glands: glands found at the base of hair follicles all over the body

sebum: substance secreted by oil glands

semicircular canals: located behind the ossicles, the oval window and the round window; contains perilymph and endolymph; part of the vestibular system

seminal vesicles: secrete fructose, prostaglandin, and other nutrients for sperm cells

sensory impulses: information from the rest of the body that travels to the brain

sensory nerves: gather information from the skin, muscles, and joints

septum: the thick layer of muscle tissue that divides the left and right sides of the heart

sigmoid colon: the portion of the colon that descends into the rectum

simple columnar: cells that are cylindrical in shape

simple cuboidal: cells that are cube shaped

simple squamous: cells that are flat in shape

sinoatrial node: the natural pacemaker for the heart

sinus cavities: air-filled spaces named maxillary, frontal, ethmoidal, and sphenoidal

skeletal system: functions include protection, blood production, and mineral regulation

skin: largest organ of the body with major functions of protection and temperature regulation

small intestine: a very long, narrow, tube-like structure in which the majority of digestion is completed and most nutrients are absorbed

smooth muscle: muscle that is not controlled by conscious thought and is not affected by exercise

spermatocytes: male reproductive cells

spermatogenesis: creation of sperm cells

spinal cord: the pathway for sensory impulses going to the brain and motor impulses coming from the brain

spleen: creates white blood cells and antibodies; acts as a type of storage container for blood and platelets

static equilibrium: feeling a sense of balance when at rest or not moving

striated muscle: considered voluntary muscle and is affected by exercise

subcutaneous layer: layer of skin that contains fat and provides insulation for deeper structures

sudoriferous glands: sweat glands

superior vena cava: lymph enters the circulatory system and combines with blood here

suspensory ligaments: attach the ciliary body and muscles to the lens

sympathetic nervous system: the system responsible for the physical changes of the fight-or-flight response

synarthrosis: an immovable joint

systole: the upper blood pressure number that reflects the highest pressure exerted against artery walls during ventricular contraction

T

T lymphocytes: white blood cells that are able to seek out and destroy abnormal cells

tears: fluid to bathe, moisten, and lubricate the eye; serve a protective role by killing bacteria and washing away foreign debris

tendons: attach muscles to bones

testes: located within the scrotum and contain the seminiferous tubules; secrete the hormone testosterone

testosterone: produces sperm, deepening of the voice, growth of facial hair, and increased muscle development in the male

thoracic cavity: the cavity that contains the lungs, heart, great vessels, trachea, and thymus

thorax: the sternum and the ribs

thymus gland: located above the heart and plays a role in immunity and protecting our bodies from cancer; produces T lymphocytes that are necessary for the immune system

thyroid gland: produces the hormones triiodothyronine and thyroxine, which are responsible for growth throughout childhood and regulation of body metabolism

thyroid-stimulating hormone (TSH): affects the growth and functioning of the thyroid gland

tissue: a group of similar cells that perform a specific function

tongue: allows us to taste food and helps to form chewed food into a bolus

tonsils and adenoids: lymph nodes in the throat

trachea: separates the upper and lower airways

transverse: the plane that divides the body into upper and lower portions; also known as the *horizontal* plane

transverse colon: the portion of the colon that passes horizontally across the uppermost part of the abdomen

tricuspid valve: exits the right atrium into the right ventricle

triiodothyronine (T3) and thyroxine (T4): responsible for growth throughout childhood and regulation of body metabolism

trimesters: three equal time periods in a pregnancy

tympanic membrane: wall between the external and middle ear that is commonly known as the eardrum; vibrates in response to sound waves

U

umbilical cord: contains two arteries, which supply oxygen and nutrients to the fetus, and one vein that removes carbon dioxide and wastes

upper airway: the mouth, nose, sinuses, and pharynx

urea: a waste product of protein metabolism

ureters: long, narrow tubes that drain urine from the renal pelvis to the urinary bladder

urethra: passageway for final urine elimination and emptying of the bladder; the exit passageway for both urine and semen

urinary system: the kidneys, ureters, bladder, and urethra

urine: the kidneys produce an average of 1 to 2 liters of this each day

uterus: houses and protects the developing fetus; its muscular tissue is able to expand as the fetus grows

uvula: soft tissue that hangs from the upper back of the mouth and prevents food from entering the nasal cavity as we eat

V

vagina: acts as the passageway for the penis during sexual intercourse and as the birth canal during the birth process

venae cavae: blood returns from the body to the right atrium through these inferior and superior structures

ventral cavity: the cavity that is located on the anterior or front side of the body

ventricles: the two lower chambers of the heart

venules: tiny veins

vertebral cavity: the cavity that contains the spinal column

vertebral column: bones that protect the spinal cord

vestibular system: translates sound vibrations into nerve impulses; controls both static and dynamic equilibrium

vestibulocochlear (auditory) nerve: sends nerve impulses to the brain

villi: fingerlike structures that increase the surface area of the small intestine

vitreous humor: jellylike substance in the posterior chamber that gives shape to the eye and bends light rays to focus them sharply onto the retina

vulva: the external structures of the female reproductive system

Z

zygote: contains 23 chromosomes from the ovum and 23 chromosomes from the sperm and will develop into an embryo and then a fetus

GLOSSARY OF WORD ELEMENTS

PART I: MEDICAL TO ENGLISH

PREFIXES			
a-	without, not, absence of	hyper-	excessive, above
ab-	away from	hypo-	below, beneath
ad-	toward	in-	without, not, absence of; in, within, inner
ambi-	both, both sides, around, about	infra-	below, beneath
an-	without, not, absence of	inter-	between
anti-	against	intra-	in, within, inner
auto-	self	iso-	same, equal
bi-	two	macro-	large
brady-	slow	mal-	bad, inadequate
circum-	around	micro-	small
con-	together, with	mono-	one, single
contra-	against, opposite	multi-	many, much
di-	twice, two, double	neo-	new
dia-	through, across	oligo-	deficiency
dys-	bad, painful, difficult	pan-	all
ec-	out, outside	para-	beside, near
ecto-	out, outside	peri-	beside, near
en-	in, within, inner	poly-	much, many
end-	in, within, inner	post-	after, following
endo-	in, within, inner	pre-	before
epi-	above, upon	pro-	before, forward
eso-	inward	quadri-	four
eu-	good, normal	re-	behind, back
ex-	away from, outside, external	retro-	behind, back
exo-	away from, outside, external	semi-	half
extra-	away from, outside, external	sub-	below, beneath
hemi-	half	super-	excessive, above

Continued

PREFIXES—cont'd

supra-	excessive, above	trans-	through, across
tachy-	rapid	tri-	three
tetra-	four	ultra-	beyond
tox-	toxin, poison	uni-	one, single

SUFFIXES

-ac	pertaining to	-emia	a condition of the blood
-acusia	hearing	-esthesia	sensation
-acusis	hearing	-gen	creating, producing
-al	pertaining to	-genesis	creating, producing
-algesia	pain	-genic	creating, producing
-algesic	pain	-genous	creating, producing
-algia	pain	-gram	record
-ar	pertaining to	-graph	recording instrument
-ary	pertaining to	-graphy	process of recording
-cele	hernia	-gravida	pregnant woman
-centesis	surgical puncture	-ia	condition
-cidal	destroying, killing	-ial	pertaining to
-cide	destroying, killing	-iasis	pathological condition or state
-clasis	to break	-iatrics	field of medicine
-clast	to break	-iatrist	specialist
-constriction	narrowing	-iatry	field of medicine
-cusis	hearing	-ic	pertaining to
-cyte	cell	-ical	pertaining to
-cytic	cell	-ician	specialist
-cytosis	a condition of cells	-ism	condition
-derma	skin	-ist	specialist
-desis	surgical fixation of bone or joint, binding, tying together	-itis	inflammation
-dilation	widening, stretching, expanding	-kinesia	movement
-dipsia	thirst	-kinesis	movement
-dynia	pain	-lepsy	seizure
-eal	pertaining to	-leptic	seizure
-ectasis	dilation, expansion	-lith	stone
-ectomy	excision, surgical removal	-logist	specialist in the study of
-edema	swelling	-logy	study of
-emesis	vomiting	-lysis	destruction

SUFFIXES—cont'd

-malacia	softening	-plastic	pertaining to formation or growth
-megaly	enlargement	-plasty	surgical repair
-meter	measuring instrument	-plegia	paralysis
-metry	measurement	-plegic	pertaining to paralysis
-necrosis	tissue death	-pnea	breathing
-oid	resembling	-pneic	pertaining to breathing
-ole	small	-prandial	meal
-ologist	specialist in the study of	-ptosis	drooping, prolapse
-ology	study of	-rrhage	bursting forth
-oma	tumor	-rrhagia	bursting forth
-opia	vision, view of	-rrhaphy	suture, suturing
-opsia	vision, view of	-rrhea	flow, discharge
-opsis	vision, view of	-rrhexis	rupture
-opsy	vision, view of	-salpinx	uterine (fallopian) tube
-ory	pertaining to	-sclerosis	abnormal condition of hardening
-osis	abnormal condition	-scope	viewing instrument
-osmia	smell, odor	-scopy	visual examination
-ous	pertaining to	-spasm	sudden involuntary contraction
-oxia	oxygen	-stasis	cessation, stopping
-paresis	slight or partial paralysis	-static	not in motion, at rest
-partum	childbirth, labor	-stenosis	narrowing, stricture
-pathy	disease	-stomy	mouthlike opening
-pause	cessation, stopping	-therapy	treatment
-penia	deficiency	-thorax	chest
-pepsia	digestion	-tic	pertaining to
-pexy	surgical fixation	-tocia	childbirth, labor
-phage	eating, swallowing	-tome	cutting instrument
-phagia	eating, swallowing	-tomy	cutting into, incision
-phasia	speech	-tous	pertaining to
-phobia	fear	-tripsy	crushing
-phonia	voice	-trophy	nourishment, growth
-phoria	feeling	-ule	small
-plasia	formation, growth	-uresis	urination
-plasm	formation, growth	-uria	urine

COMBINING FORMS

acous/o	hearing	carcin/o	cancer
acr/o	extremities	cardi/o	heart
aden/o	gland	carp/o	carpus
adenoid/o	adenoid	cec/o	cecum
adip/o	fat	cephal/o	head
adren/o	adrenal gland	cerebell/o	cerebellum
adrenal/o	adrenal gland	cerebr/o	brain
aer/o	air	cervic/o	cervix, neck
albino/o	white	cheil/o	lip
alveol/o	alveoli	chol/e	bile, gall
amni/o	amnion (amniotic sac), amniotic fluid	cholangi/o	bile duct
an/o	anus	cholecyst/o	gallbladder
andr/o	male	choledoch/o	common bile duct
angi/o	vessel	chondr/o	cartilage
ankyl/o	stiff joint	chromat/o	color
anter/o	anterior	cirrh/o	yellow
anthrac/o	coal, coal dust	col/o	colon
aort/o	aorta	colon/o	colon
append/o	appendix	colp/o	vagina
appendic/o	appendix	coni/o	dust
arteri/o	artery	conjunctiv/o	conjunctiva
arthr/o	joint	coron/o	heart
articul/o	joint	corne/o	cornea
ather/o	thick, fatty	cost/o	ribs
atri/o	atria	crani/o	cranium
audi/o	hearing	crypt/o	hidden
azot/o	nitrogenous compounds	cutane/o	skin
bacteri/o	bacteria	cyan/o	blue
balan/o	glans penis	cyst/o	bladder
bil/i	bile	cyt/o	cell
blephar/o	eyelid	dacry/o	tear
bronch/o	bronchus	dent/o	teeth
bronchi/o	bronchus	derm/o	skin
bronchiol/o	bronchiole	dermat/o	skin
bucc/o	cheek	diaphragmat/o	diaphragm
burs/o	bursa, sac	dipl/o	double
calc/o	calcium	dist/o	distal

COMBINING FORMS—cont'd

dors/o	dorsal	idi/o	unknown, peculiar
duoden/o	duodenum	ile/o	ileum
electr/o	electricity	ili/o	ilium
embry/o	embryo	immun/o	immune
encephal/o	brain	infer/o	inferior
enter/o	small intestine	ir/o	iris
epididym/o	epididymis	irid/o	iris
epiglott/o	epiglottis	jejun/o	jejunum
episi/o	vulva	kal/i	potassium
erythem/o	red	kerat/o	keratinized tissue, cornea
erythr/o	red	keton/o	ketone bodies (acids and acetones)
esophag/o	esophagus	kinesi/o	movement
eti/o	cause	kyph/o	hump
fasci/o	fascia	labi/o	lip
femor/o	femur	lact/o	milk
fet/o	fetus	lacrim/o	lacrimal gland
fibul/o	fibula	lamin/o	lamina
galact/o	milk	lapar/o	abdomen, abdominal wall
gangli/o	ganglion	laryng/o	larynx
gastr/o	stomach	later/o	lateral
gingiv/o	gums	leuk/o	white
gli/o	glue, gluelike	lex/o	word, phrase
glomerul/o	glomerulus	lingu/o	tongue
gloss/o	tongue	lip/o	fat
gluc/o	glucose, sugar, sweet	lith/o	stone
glucos/o	glucose, sugar, sweet	lob/o	lobe
glyc/o	glucose, sugar, sweet	lord/o	bent backward
glycos/o	glucose, sugar, sweet	lumb/o	lower back
gonad/o	gonads	lymph/o	lymph
gynec/o	woman, female	lymphaden/o	lymph gland
hem/o	blood	lymphangi/o	lymphatic vessel
hemat/o	blood	lymphocyt/o	lymph cell
hepat/o	liver	mamm/o	breast
hidr/o	sweat	mast/o	breast
home/o	same, unchanging	meat/o	meatus, opening
humer/o	humerus	medi/o	medial
hydr/o	water	melan/o	black
hyster/o	uterus	men/o	menses

Continued

COMBINING FORMS—cont'd

mening/o	meninges	ox/o	oxygen
meningi/o	meninges	pancreat/o	pancreas
menisci/o	meniscus	parathyroid/o	parathyroid
metacarp/o	metacarpus	patell/a	patella
metatars/o	metatarsals	patell/o	patella
metr/o	uterus	path/o	disease
morph/o	shape	pelv/i	pelvis
muc/o	mucus	pept/o	digestion
muscul/o	muscle	perine/o	perineum
my/o	muscle	peritone/o	peritoneum
myc/o	fungus	phac/o	lens
myel/o	spinal cord, bone marrow	phag/o	eating, swallowing
myring/o	tympanic membrane	phak/o	lens
narc/o	sleep, stupor	phalang/o	phalanges
nas/o	nose	phall/i	penis
nat/o	birth	pharyng/o	pharynx
natr/o	sodium	phas/o	speech
necr/o	dead	phleb/o	vein
nephr/o	kidney	phon/o	sound, voice
neur/o	nerve	pil/o	hair
noct/o	night	placent/o	placenta
ocul/o	eye	pleur/o	pleura
odont/o	teeth	pnea	breathing
olig/o	deficiency	pneum/o	lung, air
onych/o	nail	pneumon/o	lung, air
oophor/o	ovary	poster/o	posterior
ophthalm/o	eye	presby/o	old age
optic/o	eye	proct/o	rectum, anus
or/o	mouth	prostat/o	prostate
orch/o	testis	proxim/o	proximal
orchi/o	testis	psych/o	mind
orchid/o	testis	pub/o	pubis
orth/o	straight	pulmon/o	lung
oste/o	bone	py/o	pus
ot/o	ear	pyel/o	renal pelvis
ov/o	ovum	pylor/o	pylorus
ovari/o	ovary	radi/o	radius
ox/i	oxygen	radicul/o	nerve root

COMBINING FORMS—cont'd

rect/o	rectum	thalam/o	thalamus
ren/o	kidney	thorac/o	thorax
retin/o	retina	thromb/o	thrombus (clot)
rhin/o	nose	thym/o	thymus
rhytid/o	wrinkle	thyr/o	thyroid
sacr/o	sacrum	thyroid/o	thyroid
salping/o	tube (fallopian or eustachian)	tibi/o	tibia
scler/o	hardening, sclera	tonsill/o	tonsil
scoli/o	crooked, bent	ton/o	tension
seb/o	sebum	tox/o	toxin, poison
semin/o	sperm	toxic/o	toxin, poison
ser/o	serum	trache/o	trachea
sial/o	saliva, salivary gland	trich/o	hair
sigmoid/o	sigmoid colon	tympan/o	tympanic membrane
sinus/o	sinus	uln/o	ulna
son/o	sound	ur/o	urine
sperm/o	sperm	ureter/o	ureter
spermat/o	sperm	urethr/o	urethra
spin/o	spine	urin/o	urine
spir/o	breathing	uter/o	uterus
splen/o	spleen	vagin/o	vagina
spondyl/o	vertebrae	valv/o	valve
steat/o	fat	valvul/o	valve
stern/o	sternum	vas/o	vessel
sthen/o	strength	vascul/o	blood vessel
stomat/o	mouth, mouthlike opening	ven/o	vein
super/o	superior	ventr/o	ventral
synov/o	synovial membrane	ventricul/o	ventricle
synovi/o	synovial membrane	vertebr/o	vertebrae
tars/o	ankle (tarsal bones)	vesic/o	bladder
ten/o	tendon	vulv/o	vulva
tend/o	tendon	xanth/o	yellow
tendin/o	tendon	xer/o	dry
testicul/o	testis		

PART II: ENGLISH TO MEDICAL

Term	Prefix	Combining Form	Suffix
abdomen, abdominal wall		lapar/o	
abnormal condition			-osis
abnormal condition of hardening			-sclerosis
about	ambi-		
above	epi-, super-		
above	hyper-, supra-		
absence of	a-, an-, in-		
across	dia-, trans-		
adenoid		adenoid/o	
adrenal gland		adren/o, adrenal/o	
after	post-		
against	anti-, contra-		
air		aer/o, pneum/o, pneumon/o	
all	pan-		
alveoli		alveol/o	
amnion (amniotic sac)		amni/o	
amniotic fluid		amni/o	
ankle (tarsal bones)		tars/o	
anterior		anter/o	
anus		an/o, proct/o	
aorta		aort/o	
appendix		append/o, appendic/o	
around	ambi-, circum-		
artery		arteri/o	
at rest			-static
atria		atri/o	
away from	ab-, ex-, exo-, extra-		
back	re-, retro-		
bacteria		bacteri/o	
bad	dys-, mal-		
before	pre-, pro-		
behind	re-, retro-		
below	hypo-, sub-, infra-		
beneath	hypo-, sub-, infra-		

Term	Prefix	Combining Form	Suffix
bent		scoli/o	
bent backward		lord/o	
beside	para-, peri-		
between	inter-		
beyond	ultra-		
bile		bil/i, chol/e	
bile duct		cholangi/o	
binding			-desis
birth		nat/o	
black		melan/o	
bladder		cyst/o, vesic/o	
blood		hem/o, hemat/o	
blood vessel		vascul/o	
blue		cyan/o	
bone		oste/o	
bone marrow		myel/o	
both, both sides	ambi-		
brain		cerebr/o, encephal/o	
breast		mamm/o, mast/o	
breathing		spir/o	-pnea
bronchiole		bronchiol/o	
bronchus		bronch/o, bronchi/o	
bursa		burs/o	
bursting forth			-rrhage,-rrhagia
calcium		calc/o	
cancer		carcin/o	
carpus		carp/o	
cartilage		chondr/o	
cause		eti/o	
cecum		cec/o	
cell		cyt/o	-cyte,-cytic
cerebellum		cerebell/o	
cervix		cervic/o	
cessation			-pause,-stasis
cheek		bucc/o	
chest			-thorax
childbirth			-partum,-tocia
coal, coal dust		anthrac/o	

Continued

Term	Prefix	Combining Form	Suffix
colon		col/o, colon/o	
color		chromat/o	
common bile duct		choledoch/o	
condition			-ia,-ism
condition of cells			-cytosis
condition of the blood			-emia
conjunctiva		conjunctiv/o	
cornea		corne/o, kerat/o	
cranium		crani/o	
creating, producing			-gen,-genesis, -genic,-genous
crooked		scoli/o	
crushing			-tripsy
cutting instrument			-tome
cutting into			-tomy
dead		necr/o	
deficiency	oligo-	olig/o	-penia
destroying			-cidal,-cide
destruction			-lysis
diaphragm		diaphragmat/o	
difficult	dys-		
digestion		pept/o	-pepsia
dilation			-ectasis
discharge			-rrhea
disease		path/o	-pathy
distal		dist/o	
dorsal		dors/o	
double	di-	dipl/o	
drooping			-ptosis
dry		xer/o	
duodenum		duoden/o	
dust		coni/o	
ear		ot/o	
eating		phag/o	-phage,-phagia
electricity		electr/o	
embryo		embry/o	
enlargement			-megaly
epididymis		epididym/o	

Term	Prefix	Combining Form	Suffix
epiglottis		epiglott/o	
equal	iso-		
esophagus		esophag/o	
excessive	hyper-, super-, supra-		
excision			-ectomy
expanding			-dilation
expansion			-ectasis
external	ex-, exo-, extra-		
extremities		acr/o	
eye		ocul/o, ophthalm/o, optic/o	
eyelid		blephar/o	
fascia		fasci/o	
fat		adip/o, lip/o, steat/o	
fear			-phobia
feeling			-phoria
female		gynec/o	
femur		femor/o	
fetus		fet/o	
fibula		fibul/o	
field of medicine			-iatrics,-iatry
flow			-rrhea
following	post-		
formation			-plasia,-plasm
forward	pro-		
four	quadri-, tetra-		
fungus		myc/o	
gall		chol/e	
gallbladder		cholecyst/o	
ganglion		gangli/o	
gland		aden/o	
glans penis		balan/o	
glomerulus		glomerul/o	
glucose, sugar, sweet		gluc/o, glucos/o, glyc/o, glycos/o	
glue, gluelike		gli/o	
gonads		gonad/o	
good	eu-		

Continued

Term	Prefix	Combining Form	Suffix
growth			-plasia,-plasm,-trophy
gums		gingiv/o	
hair		pil/o, trich/o	
half	hemi-, semi-		
hardening		scler/o	
head		cephal/o	
hearing		acous/o, audi/o	-acusia,-acusis,-cusis
heart		cardi/o, coron/o	
hernia			-cele
hidden		crypt/o	
humerus		humer/o	
hump		kyph/o	
ileum		ile/o	
ilium		ili/o	
immune		immun/o	
in	en-, end-, endo-, in-, intra-		
inadequate	mal-		
incision			-tomy
inferior		infer/o	
inflammation			-itis
inner	en-, end-, endo-, in-, intra-		
inward	eso-		
iris		ir/o, irid/o	
jejunum		jejun/o	
joint		arthr/o, articul/o	
keratinized tissue		kerat/o	
ketone bodies (acids and acetones)		keton/o	
kidney		nephr/o, ren/o	
killing			-cidal,-cide
labor			-partum,-tocia
lacrimal gland		lacrim/o	
lamina		lamin/o	
large	macro-		
larynx		laryng/o	
lateral		later/o	
lens		phac/o, phak/o	

Term	Prefix	Combining Form	Suffix
lip		cheil/o, labi/o	
liver		hepat/o	
lobe		lob/o	
lower back		lumb/o	
lung		pneum/o, pneumon/o, pulmon/o	
lymph		lymph/o	
lymph cell		lymphocyt/o	
lymph gland		lymphaden/o	
lymphatic vessel		lymphangi/o	
male		andr/o	
many	multi-, poly-		
meal			-prandial
measurement			-metry
measuring instrument			-meter
meatus, opening		meat/o	
medial		medi/o	
meninges		mening/o, meningi/o	
meniscus		menisci/o	
menses		men/o	
metacarpus		metacarp/o	
metatarsals		metatars/o	
milk		galact/o, lact/o	
mind		psych/o	
mouth		or/o, stomat/o	
mouthlike opening		stomat/o	-stomy
movement		kinesi/o	-kinesia, -kinesis
much	multi-, poly-		
mucus		muc/o	
muscle		muscul/o, my/o	
nail		onych/o	
narrowing			-constriction, -stenosis
near	para-, peri-		
neck		cervic/o	
nerve		neur/o	
nerve root		radicul/o	
new	neo-		

Continued

Term	Prefix	Combining Form	Suffix
night		noct/o	
nitrogenous compounds		azot/o	
normal	eu-		
nose		nas/o, rhin/o	
not	a-, an-, in-		
not in motion			-static
nourishment			-trophy
odor			-osmia
old age		presby/o	
one	mono-, uni-		
opposite	contra-		
out	ec-, ecto-		
outside	ec-, ecto-, ex-, exo-, extra-		
ovary		oophor/o, ovari/o	
ovum		ov/o	
oxygen		ox/i, ox/o	-oxia
pain			-algesia, -algesic,-algia,-dynia
painful	dys-		
pancreas		pancreat/o	
paralysis			-plegia
parathyroid		parathyroid/o	
patella		patell/o, patell/a	
pathological condition or state			-iasis
peculiar		idi/o	
pelvis		pelv/i	
penis		phall/i	
perineum		perine/o	
peritoneum		peritone/o	
pertaining to			-ac,-al,-ar, -ary,-eal,-ial, -ic,-ical,-ory, -ous,-tic,-tous
pertaining to formation or growth			-plastic
pertaining to paralysis			-plegic
phalanges		phalang/o	
pharynx		pharyng/o	

Term	Prefix	Combining Form	Suffix
phrase		lex/o	
placenta		placent/o	
pleura		pleur/o	
poison, toxin	tox-	tox/o, toxic/o	
posterior		poster/o	
potassium		kal/i	
pregnant woman			-gravida
process of recording			-graphy
prolapse			-ptosis
prostate		prostat/o	
proximal		proxim/o	
pubis		pub/o	
pus		py/o	
pylorus		pylor/o	
radius		radi/o	
rapid	tachy-		
record			-gram
recording instrument			-graph
rectum		proct/o, rect/o	
red		erythem/o, erythr/o	
renal pelvis		pyel/o	
resembling			-oid
retina		retin/o	
ribs		cost/o	
rupture			-rrhexis
sac		burs/o	
sacrum		sacr/o	
saliva		sial/o	
salivary gland		sial/o	
same	iso-	home/o	
sclera		scler/o	
sebum		seb/o	
seizure			-lepsy,-leptic
self	auto-		
sensation			-esthesia
serum		ser/o	
shape		morph/o	
sigmoid colon		sigmoid/o	

Continued

Term	Prefix	Combining Form	Suffix
single	mono-, uni-		
sinus		sinus/o	
skin		cutane/o, derm/o, dermat/o	-derma
sleep		narc/o	
slight or partial paralysis			-paresis
slow	brady-		
small	micro-		-ole,-ule
small intestine		enter/o	
smell			-osmia
sodium		natr/o	
softening			-malacia
sound		phon/o, son/o	
specialist			-iatrist,-ician, -ist
specialist in the study of			-logist,-ologist
speech		phas/o	-phasia
sperm		semin/o, sperm/o, spermat/o	
spine		spin/o	
spinal cord		myel/o	
spleen		splen/o	
sternum		stern/o	
stiff joint		ankyl/o	
stomach		gastr/o	
stone		lith/o	-lith
stopping			-pause,-stasis
straight		orth/o	
strength		sthen/o	
stretching			-dilation
stricture			-stenosis
study of			-logy,-ology
stupor		narc/o	
sudden involuntary contraction			-spasm
sugar		gluc/o, glyc/o, glycos/o	
superior		super/o	
surgical fixation			-pexy
surgical fixation of bone or joint			-desis

Term	Prefix	Combining Form	Suffix
surgical puncture			-centesis
surgical removal			-ectomy
surgical repair			-plasty
suture, suturing			-rrhaphy
swallowing		phag/o	-phage,-phagia
sweat		hidr/o	
swelling			-edema
synovial membrane		synov/o, synovi/o	
tear		dacry/o	
teeth		dent/o, odont/o	
tendon		ten/o, tend/o, tendin/o	
tension		ton/o	
testis		orch/o, orchi/o, orchid/o, testicul/o	
thalamus		thalam/o	
thick, fatty		ather/o	
thirst			-dipsia
thorax		thorac/o	
three	tri-		
thrombus (clot)		thromb/o	
through	dia-, trans-		
thymus		thym/o	
thyroid		thyr/o, thyroid/o	
tibia		tibi/o	
tissue death			-necrosis
to break			-clasis,-clast
together	con-		
tongue		gloss/o, lingu/o	
tonsil		tonsill/o	
toward	ad-		
trachea		trache/o	
treatment			-therapy
tube (fallopian or eustachian)		salping/o	
tumor			-oma
twice	di-		
two	bi-, di-		
tying together			-desis
tympanic membrane		myring/o, tympan/o	

Continued

Term	Prefix	Combining Form	Suffix
ulna		uln/o	
unchanging		home/o	
unknown		idi/o	
upon	epi-		
ureter		ureter/o	
urethra		urethr/o	
urination			-uresis
urine		ur/o, urin/o	-uria
uterine (fallopian) tube			-salpinx
uterus		hyster/o, metr/o, uter/o	
vagina		colp/o, vagin/o	
valve		valv/o, valvul/o	
vein		phleb/o, ven/o	
ventral		ventr/o	
ventricle		ventricul/o	
vertebrae		spondyl/o, vertebr/o	
vessel		angi/o, vas/o	
view of			-opia,-opsia, -opsis,-opsy
viewing instrument			-scope
vision			-opia,-opsia, -opsis,-opsy
visual examination			-scopy
voice		phon/o	-phonia
vomiting			-emesis
vulva		episi/o, vulv/o	
water		hydr/o	
white		albin/o, leuk/o	
widening			-dilation
with	con-		
within	en-, end-, endo-,	in-, intra-	
without	a-, an-, in-		
woman		gynec/o	
word		lex/o	
wrinkle		rhytid/o	
yellow		cirrh/o, xanth/o	

GLOSSARY OF PATHOLOGY TERMS

A

abortion (ă-BOR-shŭn): spontaneous or therapeutic loss of a pregnancy at less than 20 weeks; also called *miscarriage*

abrasion (ă-BRĀ-zhŭn): scraping away of skin or mucous membranes

abruptio placentae (ă-BRŬP-shē-ō plă-SĔN-tă): sudden, premature detachment of the placenta from the uterine wall

achalasia (ăk-ă-LĀ-zē-ă): dilation and expansion of the lower esophagus, due to pressure from food accumulation

acne (ĂK-nē): disease of the sebaceous (oil) glands and hair follicles in the skin, marked by plugged pores, pimples, cysts, and nodules on the face, neck, chest, back, and other areas

acquired immune deficiency syndrome (AIDS) (ă-KWĪRD ĭm-ŪN dē-FĬSH-ĕn-sē SĬN-drōm): late-stage infection with the human immunodeficiency virus (HIV) which progressively weakens the immune system

acromegaly (ăk-rō-MĔG-ă-lē): type of hyperpituitarism in which an overactive pituitary gland after adulthood causes abnormal continued growth of bones and tissues of the face and extremities

actinic keratosis (ăk-TĬ-nĭk kĕr-ă-TŌ-sĭs): precancerous condition in which rough, scaly patches of skin develop, most commonly on sun-exposed areas such as the scalp, neck, face, ears, lips, hands, and forearms; also known as *solar keratosis*

acute bronchitis (ă-KŪT brŏng-KĪ-tĭs): infection and inflammation of bronchial airways

acute respiratory distress syndrome (ARDS) (ă-KŪT RĔS-pĭr-a-tor-ē dĭs-TRĔS SĬN-drōm): acute, life-threatening condition of lung injury that develops secondary to some other lung trauma or disorder

Addison's disease (ĂD-ĭ-sŭnz dĭ-ZĒZ): illness characterized by gradual adrenal-gland failure, resulting in insufficient production of steroid hormones and the need for hormone-replacement therapy; also called *hypoadrenalism*

adhesive capsulitis (ăd-HĒ-sĭv kăp-sū-LĪ-tĭs): loss of range of motion in the shoulder; also called *frozen shoulder*

allergic rhinitis (ă-LĔR-jĭk rī-NĪ-tĭs): inflammation of the nasal membranes, caused by allergies

alopecia (ă-lō-PĒ-shē-ă): autoimmune disease that results in loss of hair; alopecia areata causes patchy hair loss from the scalp; alopecia totalis causes total scalp hair loss; alopecia universalis causes total body hair loss

Alzheimer's disease (ĂLTS-hī-mĕrz dĭ-ZĒZ): form of chronic, progressive dementia caused by the atrophy of brain tissue

amblyopia (ăm-blē-Ō-pē-ă): disorder in which the brain disregards images from the weaker eye and relies on those from the stronger eye; sometimes called *lazy eye*

amenorrhea (ă-mĕn-ō-RĒ-ă): absence of menses in a woman between the ages of 16 and 40

amyotrophic lateral sclerosis (ALS) (ă-mī-ō-TRŌ-fĭk LĀ-tĕr-ăl sklĕ-RŌ-sĭs): chronic, progressive, degenerative neuromuscular disorder that destroys motor neurons of the body; also called *Lou Gehrig's disease*

anacusis (ăn-ă-KŪ-sĭs): total deafness

anaphylaxis (ăn-ă-fĭ-LĂK-sĭs): life-threatening systemic allergic reaction to a substance to which the body was previously sensitized

anemia (ă-NĒ-mē-ă): group of disorders generally defined as a reduction in the mass of circulating red blood cells

aneurysm (ĂN-ū-rĭ-zum): weakening and bulging of part of a vessel wall

angina (ăn-JĪ-nă): heart pain or other discomfort felt in the chest, shoulders, arms, jaw, or neck, caused by insufficient blood and oxygen to the heart; usually a symptom of heart disease

ankylosing spondylitis (AS) (ăng-kĭ-LŌ-sing spŏn-dĭl-Ī-tĭs): inflammatory response that causes degenerative changes in the spinal vertebrae, sacroiliac joints; and connective tissues, such as tendons, ligaments, hips, shoulders, knees, feet, and ribs, and in the tissues of the lungs, eyes, and heart valves

anorexia nervosa (ăn-ō-RĔK-sē-ă nĕr-VŌ-să): physical and psychiatric disorder that involves a combination of an intense fear of weight gain, distorted body image, and self-imposed starvation

anterior cruciate ligament tear (ăn-TĒR-ē-ōr KROO-shē-āt LĬG-ă-mĕnt tār): injury to one of the stabilizing ligaments of the knee, which originates on the anterior portion of the femur

appendicitis (ă-pĕn-dĭ-SĪ-tĭs): inflammation of the appendix

arrhythmia (ă-RĬTH-mē-ă): loss of heart rhythm (rhythmic irregularity)

arteriosclerosis (ăr-tē-rē-ō-sklĕ-RŌ-sĭs): thickening, loss of elasticity, and loss of contractility of arterial walls; commonly called *hardening of the arteries*

asbestosis (ăs-bĕ-STŌ-sĭs): respiratory disease caused by chronic or repetitive inhalation of asbestos fibers

ascites (ă-SĪ-tēz): accumulation of serous fluid in the peritoneal (abdominal) cavity

asthma (ĂZ-mă): disease marked by episodic narrowing and inflammation of the airways, resulting in wheezing, shortness of breath (SOB), and cough

astigmatism (ă-STĬG-mă-tĭ-zum): abnormal curvature of the cornea that distorts the visual image

atelectasis (ăt-ĕ-LĔK-tă-sĭs): partial collapse of the alveoli and tiny airways of the lung

atherosclerosis (ăth-ĕr-ō-sklĕ-RŌ-sĭs): the most-common form of arteriosclerosis, marked by deposits of cholesterol, lipids, and calcium on the walls of arteries, which may restrict blood flow

atrial fibrillation (AF, A-fib) (Ā-trē-ăl fĭ-brĭl-Ā-shŭn): common irregular heart rhythm marked by uncontrolled atrial quivering and a rapid ventricular response

autoimmune hemolytic anemia (aw-tō-ĭm-MŪN hē-mō-LĬT-ĭk ă-NĒ-mē-ă): group of disorders that occur when the immune system misidentifies red blood cells (RBCs) as foreign and creates autoantibodies that attack them

B

bacterial cystitis (bak-TIR-ē-ul sĭs-TĪ-tĭs): inflammation of the bladder caused by bacterial infection, commonly coexisting with bacterial urethritis, both of which together constitute a urinary tract infection (UTI), sometimes referred to as a *bladder infection*

balanoposthitis (băl-ă-nō-pŏs-THĪ-tĭs): inflammation of the glans penis and foreskin covering the glans penis; also called *balanitis*

Bartholin's gland cyst (BĂR-tō-lĭnz glănd sĭst): blockage of one or both Bartholin's glands, causing inflammation and tenderness

basal cell carcinoma (BĀ-săl sĕl kăr-sĭ-NŌ-mă): common type of skin cancer that typically appears as a small, shiny papule and eventually enlarges to form a whitish border around a central depression or ulcer that may bleed

Bell's palsy (bĕlz PAWL-zē): form of facial paralysis, usually unilateral and temporary

benign prostatic hypertrophy (bē-NĪN prŏs-TĂT-ĭc hī-PĔR-trŏ-fē): noncancerous enlargement of the prostate gland, common in elderly men

blepharitis (blĕf-ăr-Ī-tĭs): noncontagious inflammation of the eyelash follicles and tiny oil glands along the margins of the eyelids

bowel obstruction (BOW-ĕl ŏb-STRŬK-shŭn): partial or complete blockage of the small or large intestine; common causes include volvulus, intussusception, tumors, and adhesions (scar tissue)

brain abscess (brān ĂB-sĕs): collection of pus anywhere within the brain

brain attack (brān ă-TĂK): damage or death of brain tissue caused by interruption of blood supply due to a clot or vessel rupture; also known as *stroke* or *cerebrovascular accident (CVA)*

brain tumor (brān TŪ-mŏr): any type of abnormal mass growing within the cranium

bruit (bruw-ē): soft blowing sound caused by turbulent blood flow in a vessel

bulimia nervosa (bū-LĬM-ē-ă nĕr-VŌ-să): physical and psychiatric disorder that involves a combination of obsessively eating huge quantities of food with purging behaviors

bulla (BŬ-lă): large blister or skin vesicle filled with fluid

burn (bŭrn): type of thermal injury to the skin caused by a variety of heat sources; classified according to severity as first-degree (superficial), second-degree (partial-thickness), and third-degree (full-thickness)

bursitis (bŭr-SĪ-tĭs): condition of inflammation of the tiny fluid-filled sacs that act as cushions and provide lubrication to decrease friction and irritation between structures such as bones, tendons, muscles, and skin

C

callus (KĂ-lŭs): thickened, hardened, toughened area of skin caused by frequent or chronic pressure or friction

***Campylobacter* infection (kăm-pǐ-lō-BĂK-tĕr ĭn-FĔK-shŭn):** infection with *Campylobacter* organisms via contaminated food or water, resulting in intestinal illness

candidiasis (kăn-dǐ-DĪ-ă-sĭs): vaginal fungal infection caused by *Candida albicans,* with key symptoms including itching, burning, and a thick, curdy discharge; also known as a vaginal *yeast infection*

carbuncle (KĂR-bŭng-kul): very large furuncle or cluster of connected furuncles

cardiac tamponade (KĂR-dē-ăk tăm-pŏn-ĀD): serious condition in which the heart becomes compressed from an excessive collection of fluid or blood between the pericardial membrane and the heart

cardiomyopathy (kăr-dē-ō-mī-ŎP-ă-thē): group of conditions in which the heart muscle has deteriorated and functions less effectively

cardiopulmonary resuscitation (CPR) (KĂR-dē-ō-pŭl-mō-nĕ-rē rē-SUS-ĭ-tā-shun): a skill often taught in first-aid courses that helps restore a victim's breathing and circulation

carpal tunnel syndrome (KĂR-păl TŬN-ĕl SĬN-drōm): compression of the median nerve, causing pain or numbness in the wrist, hand, and fingers

cataract (KĂT-ă-răkt): cloudiness of the lens due to protein deposits as a result of aging, disease, or trauma or as a side effect of tobacco use or certain medications

celiac disease (SĒ-lē-ăk dǐ-ZĒZ): disorder in which the lining of the small intestine is damaged due to dietary factors, resulting in impaired nutrient absorption

cellulitis (sĕl-ū-LĪ-tĭs): potentially serious bacterial skin infection marked by pain, redness, edema, warmth, and fever

central scotoma (SĔN-trăl skō-TŌ-mă): blind spot in the center of the visual field surrounded by an area of normal vision

cerebral concussion (sĕ-RĒ-brăl kŏn-KŬ-shŭn): vague term referring to a brief loss of consciousness or brief episode of disorientation or confusion following a head injury

cerebral contusion (sĕ-RĒ-brăl kŏn-TOO-zhŭn): bruising of brain tissue

cerebral palsy (CP) (sĕ-RĒ-brăl PAWL-zē): group of motor-impairment syndromes caused by lesions or abnormalities of the brain arising in the early stages of development

cerebrovascular accident (CVA) (sĕr-ĕ-brō-VĂS-kū-lăr AK-sĭ-dĕnt): damage or death of brain tissue caused by interruption of blood supply due to a clot or vessel rupture; also called *stroke* or *brain attack*

chalazion (kă-LĀ-zē-ōn): small benign cyst in the eyelid formed by the distention of a meibomian gland with secretions

chlamydia (klă-MĬD-ē-ă): the most-common STI, a bacterial vaginal infection caused by *Chlamydia trachomatis*

cholecystitis (kō-lē-sĭs-TĪ-tĭs): inflammation of the gallbladder, usually secondary to the presence of gallstones

cholelithiasis (kō-lă-lǐ-THĪ-ăs-ĭs): condition in which gallstones are present in the gallbladder, liver, or biliary ducts

cholesteatoma (kō-lē-stē-ă-TŌ-mă): condition in which a cyst develops in the middle ear

chronic fatigue syndrome (CFS) (KRŎN-ĭk fă-TĒG SĬN-drōm): complex chronic disorder marked by severe fatigue unrelieved by rest, often worsened by mental or physical activity; sometimes called *chronic fatigue and immune dysfunction syndrome (CFIDS)*

chronic hypoxia (KRŎN-ĭk hī-PŎKS-ē-ă): a chronic lack of oxygen; as gas exchange becomes less effective, breathing becomes more and more difficult; eventually the person becomes dependent on oxygen

chronic mucocutaneous candidiasis (CMC) (KRŎN-ĭk mū-kō-kū-TĀ-nē-ŭs kăn-dĭ-DĪ-ă-sĭs): group of disorders in which persistent or recurrent *Candida* fungal infections develop on the skin, nails, or mucous membranes

chronic obstructive pulmonary disease (COPD) (KRŎN-ĭk ŏb-STRUK-tĭv PŬL-mō-nĕ-rē dǐ-ZĒZ): group of diseases in which alveolar air sacs are destroyed and chronic, severe SOB results

cirrhosis (sǐ-RŌ-sĭs): chronic liver disease characterized by scarring and loss of normal structure

claw toe (klaw tō): condition in which the metatarsophalangeal (MTP) joint flexes dorsally while the other joint or joints in the toe flex toward the sole

coal worker's pneumoconiosis (CWP) (KŌL WER-kerz nū-mō-kō-nē-Ō-sĭs): a type of pneumoconiosis caused by inhalation of coal dust; often called *black lung*

comedo (KŎ-mē-dō): blackhead

congenital hypothyroidism (kŏn-JĔN-ĭ-tăl hī-pō-THĪ-royd-ĭ-zum): congenital condition of thyroid hormone deficiency, characterized by arrested physical and mental development; formerly called *cretinism*

congestive heart failure (CHF) (kŭn-JES-tĭv hărt FĀL-yĕr): inability of the heart to pump enough blood to meet the needs of the body, resulting in lung congestion and dyspnea; also called *heart failure (HF)*

conjunctivitis (kŏn-jŭnk-tĭ-VĪ-tĭs): inflammation of the conjunctiva; also called *pinkeye*

contracture (kŏn-TRĂK-chŭr): fibrosis of connective tissue which decreases the mobility of a joint

contusion (kŏn-TOO-zhŭn): discoloration of the skin; bruise

cor pulmonale (kor pŭl-mă-NĂL-ē): condition of right ventricular enlargement or dilation from increased right ventricular pressure; also called *pulmonary heart disease* or *right-sided heart failure*

corn (kōrn): small callus that develops on smooth, hairless skin surfaces, such as the backs of fingers or toes, in response to pressure and friction; hard corns typically develop on the sides of feet and tops of toes; soft corns usually develop between toes

coronary artery disease (CAD) (KOR-ō-nă-rē ĂR-tĕr-ē dĭ-ZĒZ): narrowing of the lumen of heart arteries due to arteriosclerosis and atherosclerosis

coryza (kŏ-RĪ-ză): acute inflammation of the nasal mucosa; the common cold

crackles (KRĂ-kuls): abnormal crackly lung sound—like the sound of Rice Krispies—heard with a stethoscope, caused by air passing over retained secretions or by the sudden opening of collapsed airways

crepitation (krĕp-ĭ-TĀ-shŭn): grating sound from broken bones, or a clicking or crackling sound from joints

Crohn's disease (krōnz dĭ-ZēZ): disorder involving inflammation and edema deep into the layers of the lining of any part of the GI tract

croup (croop): acute viral disease, usually in children, marked by a barking, "seal-like" cough and respiratory distress

cryptorchidism (krĭpt-ŎR-kĭd-ĭ-zum): failure of one or both testes to descend into the scrotum

Cushing's disease (KOOSH-ĭngz dĭ-ZĒZ): disorder caused by hypersecretion of cortisol by the adrenal gland, resulting in altered fat distribution and muscle weakness; also called *hypercortisolism* and *hyperadrenalism*

cyst (sĭst): fluid- or solid-containing pouch in or under the skin

cystic fibrosis (SĬS-tĭk fĭ-BRŌ-sĭs): fatal genetic disease that causes frequent respiratory infections, increased airway secretions, and COPD in children

D

decubitus ulcer (dē-KŪ-bĭ-tŭs ŬL-sĕr): area of injury and tissue death caused by unrelieved pressure which impedes circulation in the skin and underlying tissues; also called *pressure ulcer* or *bedsore*

deep vein thrombosis (DVT) (dēp vān thrŏm-BŌ-sĭs): development of a blood clot in a deep vein, usually in the legs; also known as *thrombophlebitis*

delirium (dě-LĬR-ē-ŭm): acute, reversible state of agitated confusion, marked by disorientation, hallucinations, or delusions

dementia (dē-MĔN-shē-ă): progressive neurological disorder, with numerous causes, in which an individual suffers an irreversible decline in cognition due to disease or brain damage; sometimes called *senility*

depression (dē-PRĔSH-ŭn): mood disorder marked by loss of interest or pleasure in living

deviated septum (DĒ-vē-ā-tĕd SĔP-tŭm): condition in which the nasal septum is displaced to the side, causing the two nares (nasal passages) to be unequal

diabetes insipidus (dī-ă-BĒ-tēz ĭn-SĬP-ĭ-dŭs): disorder unrelated to diabetes mellitus, characterized by excessive output of dilute urine

diabetic ketoacidosis (dī-ă-BĔT-ĭk kĒ-tō-ă-sĭ-DŌ-sĭs): condition of severe hyperglycemia

diabetes mellitus (DM) (dī-ă-BĒ-tēz mĕl-Ī-tŭs): chronic metabolic disorder in which the pancreas secretes insufficient amounts of insulin or the body is insulin resistant

diabetic nephropathy (dī-ă-BĔT-ĭk nĕ-FRŎP-ă-thē): kidney disease associated with diabetes that results in inflammation, degeneration, and sclerosis of the kidneys

diabetic retinopathy (dī-ă-BĔT-ĭk rĕt-ĭn-ŎP-ă-thē): progressive damage to microscopic vessels and other structures of the retina in patients with long-standing diabetes mellitus, which may result in blindness

dislocation (dĭs-lō-KĀ-shŭn): displacement or separation of a bone from its normal position where it articulates with another bone

disseminated intravascular coagulation (DIC) (dĭ-SEM-ĭ-nāt-ĕd ĭn-tră-VĂS-kū-lăr kō-ăg-ū-LĀ-shŭn): serious condition that arises as a complication of another disorder, in which widespread, unrestricted microvascular blood clotting occurs; primary symptom is hemorrhage

diuresis (dī-ū-RĒ-sĭs): abnormal secretion of large amounts of urine

diverticulitis (dī-vĕr-tĭk-ū-LĪ-tĭs): inflammation of one or more diverticula (tiny pouches in the intestinal wall)

diverticulosis (dī-vĕr-tĭk-ū-LŌ-sĭs): condition in which diverticula form in the intestinal wall due to increased pressure

dwarfism (DWÅRF-i-zum): hyposecretion of growth hormone during childhood, resulting in an abnormally small adult

dysmenorrhea (dĭs-mĕn-ō-RĒ-ă): pain in the lower abdominopelvic area and other discomfort associated with menses

E

***E. coli* O157: H7 infection (ē KŌ-lī ĭn-FĔK-shŭn):** dangerous strain of *Escherichia coli* that produces toxins which can severely damage the intestinal lining, resulting in bloody diarrhea

ecchymosis (ĕ-kĭ-MŌ-sĭs): discoloration of the skin; bruise

eclampsia (ĕ-KLĂMP-sē-ă): complication of pregnancy characterized by severe hypertension, seizures, and possible coma

ectopic pregnancy (ĕk-TŎ-pĭk PRĔG-năn-sē): implantation of a fertilized ovum somewhere other than in the uterus, often in the fallopian tube; also called *tubal pregnancy*

ectropion (ĕk-TRŌ-pē-ŏn): condition in which the lower eyelid is turned outward and droops more with aging

eczema (ĔK-zĕ-mă): inflammatory skin condition marked by red, hot, dry, scaly, cracked, and itchy skin

embolus (ĔM-bō-lŭs): undissolved matter floating in blood or lymph fluid that may cause an occlusion and infarct

emesis (ĔM-ĕ-sĭs): vomiting

emphysema (ĕm-fĭ-SĒ-mă): disorder marked by abnormal increase in the size of air spaces distal to the terminal bronchiole and destruction of the alveolar walls, resulting in loss of normal elasticity and progressive dyspnea

empyema (ĕm-pī-Ē-mă): collection of infected fluid (pus) between the two pleural membranes that line the lungs

encephalitis (ĕn-sĕf-ă-LĪ-tĭs): inflammation of the brain; often combined with meningitis and then called *encephalomeningitis*

endocarditis (ĕn-dō-kăr-DĪ-tĭs): infection of the inner lining of the heart that may cause

vegetations to form within one or more heart chambers or valves

endometriosis (ĕn-dō-mē-trē-Ō-sĭs): growth of endometrial tissue in abnormal sites in the lower abdominopelvic area

end-stage renal disease (ESRD) (END-stāj RĒ-năl dĭ-ZĒZ): final phase of kidney disease

entropion (ĕn-TRŌ-pē-ŏn): condition in which the eyelid edges are turned inward and rub against the surface of the eye, usually affecting the lower eyelid

enuresis (ĕn-ū-RĒ-sĭs): involuntary urination during sleep; also called *bedwetting*

epidermoid cyst (ĕ-pĭ-DĔR-moyd sĭst): small sac or pouch below the skin surface containing a thick, cheesy substance; appears pale white or yellow but can be darker in dark-skinned people

epididymitis (ĕp-ĭ-dĭd-ĭ-MĪ-tĭs): acute or chronic inflammation or infection of the epididymis, a tubular structure on the posterior surface of the testicle

epidural hematoma (ĕp-ĭ-DŪR-ăl hē-mă-TŌ-mă): collection of blood between the dura mater and the skull

epilepsy (ĔP-ĭ-lĕp-sē): chronic disorder of the brain marked by recurrent seizures, which are repetitive abnormal electrical discharges within the brain

epistaxis (ĕp-ĭ-STĂK-sĭs): episode of bleeding from the nose; commonly known as a *nosebleed*

Epstein-Barr virus (EBV) (ĔP-stēn-BÅR VĪ-rŭs): acute infection that causes sore throat, fever, fatigue, and enlarged lymph nodes; also called *mononucleosis*

erectile dysfunction (ED) (ĕ-RĔK-tĭl dĭs-FŬNK-shŭn): general term that describes a number of disorders, all of which impact the ability of a man to attain an erection adequate to achieve a satisfactory sexual experience; also called *impotence*

esophageal varices (ē-sŏf-ă-JĒ-ăl VĂR-ĭ-sēz): varicose veins of distal end of the esophagus

esophagitis (ē-sŏf-ă-JĪ-tĭs): inflammation of the lower esophageal lining

exophthalmos (ĕks-ŏf-THĂL-mōs): abnormal protrusion of the eyeballs

F

fibrillation (fĭ-brĭl-Ā-shŭn): quivering of heart muscle fibers instead of an effective heartbeat

fibrocystic breast disease (fĭ-brō-SĬS-tĭk brĕst dĭ-ZĒZ): presence of multiple lumps in the breast, consisting of fibrous tumors or fluid-filled cysts

fibromyalgia (fī-brō-mī-ĂL-jē-ă): chronic condition marked by pain in the muscles, tendons, ligaments, and soft tissues of the body

fissure (FĬ-shūr): small, cracklike break in the skin

folliculitis (fō-lǐ-kū-LĬ-tǐs): inflammation of hair follicles, marked by rash with small red bumps, pustules, tenderness, and itching; common on the neck, axillae, and groin area

food poisoning (fūd POY-zun-ing): common term for a number of illnesses caused by eating food contaminated with bacterial or toxic organisms; sometimes called *dysentery*

fracture (FRĂK-chūr): condition in which a bone is broken or cracked

frequency (FRĒ-kwun-sē): need to urinate more often than normal

frostbite (FRŎST-bīt): injury that occurs when skin tissues are exposed to temperatures cold enough to cause them to freeze

functional incontinence: involuntary urine leakage after failing to reach a toilet in time

furuncle (FŪR-ŭng-kul): infection of a hair follicle and nearby tissue, also called a *boil*; more invasive than folliculitis because it involves the sebaceous gland

G

ganglion cyst (GĂNG-glē-ŏn sĭst): condition in which one or more small, benign tumors filled with a thick, colorless, gelatinous substance develop over a joint or tendon, usually on the wrist or back of the hand; sometimes called a *Bible cyst*

gastritis (gǎs-TRĪ-tǐs): inflammation of the stomach's mucosal lining

gastroenteritis (gǎs-trō-ĕn-tĕr-Ī-tǐs): inflammation of the stomach and intestines; often referred to as the *stomach flu* (although influenza is not the cause)

gastroesophageal reflux disease (GERD) (gǎs-trō-ě-sŏf-ă-JĒ-ăl RĒ-flŭks dǐ-ZĒZ): backflow of acidic gastric contents into the esophagus, causing esophagitis

gestational diabetes (jěs-TĀ-shŭn-ăl dī-ă-BĒ-tēz): development of type 2 diabetes mellitus that begins during pregnancy in a woman who did not have diabetes before becoming pregnant; due to insulin resistance and altered glucose metabolism

giantism (JĪ-ăn-tǐ-zum): type of hyperpituitarism that causes hypersecretion of growth hormone during childhood, resulting in an abnormally large adult

glaucoma (acute) [glaw-KŌ-mă (ă-KŪT)]: type of glaucoma in which a sudden blockage of aqueous-humor outflow causes a rapid increase in intraocular pressure; also called *closed-angle glaucoma*

glaucoma (chronic) [glaw-KŌ-mă (KRŎN-ĭk)]: type of glaucoma in which the aqueous humor drains too slowly, leading to increasing intraocular pressure; also called *primary open-angle glaucoma*

glomerulonephritis (acute) [glō-měr-ū-lō-ně-FRĪ-tǐs (ă-KŪT)]: type of nephritis (kidney infection) in which the glomeruli are the key structures affected; also called *acute nephritic syndrome*

glomerulonephritis (chronic) [glō-měr-ū-lō-ně-FRĪ-tǐs (KRŎN-ĭk)]: condition in which the glomeruli suffer gradual, progressive, destructive changes, with a resulting loss of kidney function; also called *chronic nephritis*

glucosuria (gloo-kō-SŪ-rē-ă): sugar in the urine

glycosuria (glī-kō-SŪ-rē-ă): sugar in the urine

goiter (GOY-těr): enlarged thyroid gland

gonorrhea (gŏn-ō-RĒ-ă): STI caused by *Neisseria gonorrhoeae* that results in inflammation of mucous membranes

gout (gowt): hereditary form of arthritis, characterized by uric acid accumulation in the joints, especially in the great toe

graft-versus-host disease (GVHD) (grăft VĚR-sŭz hōst dǐ-ZĒZ): complication of bone-marrow transplantation in which lymphoid cells from donated tissue attack the recipient and cause damage to the skin, liver, GI tract, and other tissues

Graves' disease (grăvz dǐ-ZĒZ): hyperthyroidism caused by an autoimmune response, which may cause exophthalmos

Guillain-Barré syndrome (GBS) (gē-YĂ-băr-RĀ SĬN-drōm): acute inflammatory disorder that causes rapidly progressing paralysis (which is usually temporary) and sometimes also sensory symptoms; also known as *acute inflammatory demyelinating polyneuropathy*

H

hallux rigidus (HĂL-ŭks rǐ-JĬD-ŭs): condition in which degenerative arthritis affects the metatarsophalangeal (MTP) joint at the base of the big toe, causing pain and stiffness

hallux valgus (HĂL-ŭks VĂL-gŭs): condition in which the big toe is improperly aligned, pointing laterally toward the second toe and creating a large bump on the inner edge of the foot at the base of the big toe; commonly called *bunion*

hammertoe (HĂM-ĕr-tō): condition in which the toe is bent downward at the proximal interphalangeal (PIP) joint

Hashimoto's thyroiditis (hă-shē-MŌ-tōz thī-roy-DĪ-tĭs): chronic, inflammatory condition that leads to the most-common type of thyroiditis; also called *chronic lymphocytic thyroiditis*

heart failure (HF) (hărt FĀL-yĕr): inability of the heart to pump enough blood to meet the needs of the body, resulting in lung congestion and dyspnea; also called *congestive heart failure*

hemoptysis (hē-MŎP-tĭ-sĭs): coughing up blood from the respiratory tract

hemorrhoids (HĔM-ō-roydz): internal or external varicose veins of the anal area

hemothorax (hē-mō-THŌ-răks): condition in which blood or bloody fluid has collected within the intrapleural space, causing lung compression and respiratory distress

hepatitis (hĕp-ă-TĪ-tĭs): chronic inflammation of the liver, caused by one of several viruses (types A, B, C, D, or E)

herpes genitalis (HĔRP-ēs jĕn-ĭ-TĂL-ĭs): STI caused by herpes simplex virus type 2 that results in painful vesicles; commonly called *genital herpes*

hernia (HĔR-nē-ă): protrusion of a structure through the wall that normally contains it

herniated disc (HĔR-nē-ā-tĕd dĭsk): herniation of the soft center of an intervertebral disc

hiatal hernia (hī-Ā-tăl HĔR-nē-ă): protrusion of a portion of the stomach through the diaphragm into the chest cavity; also called *hiatus hernia*

hirsutism (HŬR-sūt-ĭ-zum): male pattern of body-hair development in females

histoplasmosis (hĭs-tō-plăz-MŌ-sĭs): systemic respiratory disease caused by *Histoplasma capsulatum*, a fungus found in soil contaminated with bird droppings

Hodgkin's disease (HŎJ-kĭnz dĭ-ZĒZ): type of lymphatic cancer; also called *lymphoma*

hordeolum (hor-DĒ-ō-lŭm): infection of a sebaceous gland of the eyelid; also called a *stye*

human papillomavirus (HPV) (HŪ-măn păp-ĭ-LŌ-măVĪ-rŭs): STI caused by the human papillomavirus that results in painless, cauliflower-like warts; a cause of cervical cancer in women

Huntington's disease (HUN-ting-tunz dĭ-ZĒZ): hereditary, progressive, degenerative nervous disorder that leads to bizarre, involuntary movements and dementia

hydronephrosis (hī-drō-nĕf-RŌ-sĭs): condition in which the renal pelvis and calyces become distended and dilated and begin to atrophy due to urine outflow obstruction

hyperaldosteronism (hī-pĕr-ăl-dō-STĔR-ōn-ĭ-zum): condition in which adrenal glands release excessive aldosterone; also called *Conn's syndrome*

hypercapnia (hī-pĕr-KĂP-nē-ă): chronic retention of CO_2, causing symptoms of mental cloudiness and lethargy

hyperopia (hī-pĕr-Ō-pē-ă): vision defect in which parallel rays focus behind the retina as a result of flattening of the globe of the eye or of an error in refraction; commonly called *farsightedness*

hyperparathyroidism (hī-pĕr-păr-ă-THĪ-royd-ĭ-zum): condition in which the parathyroid glands produce an excessive amount of parathyroid hormone (PTH)

hypertension (hī-pĕr-TĔN-shŭn): blood pressure that is consistently higher than 140 systolic, 90 diastolic, or both

hypertensive retinopathy (hī-pĕr-TĔN-sĭv rĕt-ĭn-OP-ă-thē): destructive retinal changes caused by hypertension

hypoparathyroidism (hī-pō-păr-ă-THĪ-royd-ĭ-zum): condition in which the parathyroid glands are hypoactive and as a result the level of parathyroid hormones (PTH) is too low

I

idiopathic thrombocytopenic purpura (ITP) (ĭd-ē-ō-PĂTH-ĭk thrŏm-bō-sī-tō-PĒ-nĭk PŬR-pū-ră): disorder in which a deficiency of platelets results in abnormal blood clotting, marked by tiny purple bruises (purpura) that form under the skin

impetigo (ĭm-pĕ-TĪ-gō): bacterial skin infection marked by yellow to red weeping, crusted, or pustular lesions; common in children

impotence (ĬM-pŏ-tĕns): inability of a male to achieve or maintain erection

incision (ĭn-SĬ-zhŭn): surgical cut in the flesh

infertility (ĭn-fĕr-TIL-ĭ-tē): inability to achieve pregnancy after trying to conceive for a period of 1 year or more; may be primary, which is an inability to conceive a first child, or secondary, which is infertility in a woman who has previously conceived

influenza (ĭn-floo-ĔN-ză): common, contagious, acute viral respiratory illness; commonly called the *flu*

interstitial cystitis (IC) (ĭn-tĕr-STISH-ăl sĭs-TĪ-tĭs): chronic inflammatory condition of the bladder lining not caused by infection or other identified pathology

interstitial nephritis (ĭn-tĕr-STĬSH-ăl nĕf-RĪ-tĭs): pathological changes in renal tissue that destroy nephrons and impair kidney function

intussusception (ĭn-tŭ-sŭ-SĔP-shŭn): slipping or telescoping of a portion of the bowel into itself

irritable bowel syndrome (ĬR-ĭt-ă-bul BOW-ĕl SĬN-drōm): chronic condition characterized by alternating episodes of constipation and diarrhea

ischemia (ĭs-KĒ-mē-ă): temporary reduction in blood supply to a localized area of tissue

J

jaundice (JAWN-dĭs): condition marked by yellow staining of body tissues and fluids as a result of excessive levels of bilirubin in the blood

juvenile rheumatoid arthritis (JRA) (JŪ-vĕ-nīl ROO-mă-toyd ăr-THRĪ-tĭs): disorder similar to adult-onset RA, with earlier onset and more-severe symptoms

K

keratitis (kĕr-ă-TĪ-tĭs): inflammation of the cornea, usually associated with decreased visual acuity, which may, if untreated, result in blindness

kyphosis (kī-FŌ-sĭs): abnormal increase in the curvature of the thoracic vertebrae, causing hunchback

L

labyrinthitis (lăb-ĭ-rĭn-THĪ-tĭs): inflammation of the labyrinth within the inner ear; also called *otitis interna*

laceration (lăs-ē-RĀ-shŭn): cut or tear in the flesh

laryngitis (lăr-ĭn-JĪ-tĭs): condition of inflammation of the larynx, evidenced by a temporary hoarseness or loss of the voice

legal blindness (LĒ-gul BLĪND-nis): loss in visual acuity that prevents a person from performing work requiring eyesight; defined as corrected visual acuity of 20/200 or less or a visual field of 20 degrees or less in the better eye

legionellosis (lē-jŭ-nĕ-LŌ-sĭs): bacterial lung infection caused by the bacterium *Legionella pneumophila*

lordosis (lor-DŌ-sĭs): abnormal increase in the curvature of the lumbar vertebrae, causing swayback

Lyme disease (līm dĭ-ZĒZ): bacterial infection transmitted by ticks, marked by erythema migrans, a circular rash that slowly expands and enlarges; untreated disease causes multisystem symptoms

lymphosarcoma (lĭm-fō-săr-KŌ-mă): cancer of lymphatic tissue not related to Hodgkin's disease

M

macular degeneration (MĂK-ū-lăr dĭ-jen-er-Ā-shŭn): macular deterioration resulting in central vision loss, categorized as either atrophic (dry) or exudative (wet)

macule (MĂ-kūl): flat, discolored spot on the skin, such as a freckle

malabsorption syndrome (măl-ăb-SŌRP-shŭn SĬN-drōm): inadequate absorption of nutrients from the intestinal tract, especially the small intestine

malignant hypertension (mă-LĬG-nănt hī-pĕr-TĔN-shŭn): rare, life-threatening type of hypertension evidenced by optic-nerve (eye) edema and extremely high systolic and diastolic blood pressure

malignant melanoma (mă-LĬG-nănt mĕ-lă-NŌ-mă): aggressive form of skin cancer that often begins as various-colored, asymmetrical lesions larger than 6 mm in size

mallet toe (măl-ĕt tō): condition in which the toe is bent downward at the distal interphalangeal (DIP) joint

malnutrition (măl-nū-TRĬ-shŭn): nutritional deficiency due to inadequate intake or absorption of protein, vitamins, minerals, or other vital nutrients

medial tibial syndrome (MĒ-dē-ăl TĬB-ē-ăl SĬN-drōm): painful condition involving tiny tears in the muscles and tendons that attach to the anterior tibia (shin); commonly called *shin splints*

melasma (mĕ-LĂZ-mă): development of irregular areas of darker-pigmented skin on the forehead, nose, cheek, and upper lip; also called *chloasma* or the *mask of pregnancy*

Ménière's disease (măn-ē-ĀRZ dĭ-ZĒZ): chronic, noncontagious disorder of the labyrinth that leads to progressive hearing loss, vertigo, and tinnitus

meningitis (mĕn-ĭn-JĬT-ĭs): infection and inflammation of the meninges, the spinal cord, and cerebral spinal fluid (CSF), usually caused by an infectious illness; often combined with encephalitis and then called *encephalomeningitis*

meniscal tear (mĕn-ĬS-kăl tār): tear of one of the two C-shaped cartilage structures that serve to cushion and stabilize the knee joint, usually caused by a twisting force

migraine headache (MĪ-grān HED-āk): familial disorder marked by episodes of severe throbbing headache that is commonly unilateral and sometimes disabling

mitral regurgitation (MĪ-trăl rē-gŭr-jĭ-TĀ-shŭn): condition in which the mitral valve does not close tightly, allowing blood to flow backward into the left atrium; also called *mitral insufficiency* or *mitral incompetence*

mitral stenosis (MĪ-trăl stĕ-NŌ-sĭs): condition in which the mitral valve fails to open properly, thereby impeding normal blood flow and increasing pressure within the left atrium and lungs

multiple sclerosis (MS) (MŬL-tĭ-pul sklĕ-RŌ-sĭs): disease involving progressive myelin degeneration, which results in loss of muscle strength and coordination

murmur (MŬR-mŭr): blowing or swishing sound in the heart, due to turbulent blood flow or backflow through a leaky valve

muscular dystrophy (MD) (MŬS-kū-lăr DĬS-trŏ-fē): hereditary, progressive, terminal disease that causes muscle atrophy and death, usually by age 20

myasthenia gravis (mī-ăs-THĒ-nē-ă GRĂV-ĭs): autoimmune motor disorder that causes progressive muscle fatigue and weakness

myocardial infarction (MI) (mī-ō-KĂR-dē-ăl ĭn-FĂRK-shŭn): death of heart-muscle cells due to occlusion of a vessel; commonly called *heart attack*

myocarditis (mī-ō-kăr-DĪ-tĭs): condition in which the middle layer of the heart wall becomes inflamed

myopia (mī-Ō-pē-ă): error of refraction in which light rays focus in front of the retina, enabling the person to see distinctly for only a short distance; commonly called *nearsightedness*

myxedema (mĭks-ĕ-DĒ-mă): severe form of hypothyroidism that develops in the older child or adult, causing nonpitting edema in connective tissue

N

nasal polyps (NĀ-zul PŎL-ĭps): rounded tissue growths on the nasal or sinus mucosa

nephrotic syndrome (nĕ-FRŎT-ĭk SĬN-drōm): uncommon disorder marked by massive proteinuria, edema, hypoalbuminemia (low blood albumin), hyperlipidemia (high blood lipids), and hypercoagulability (high tendency to form blood clots)

neural tube defect (NUR-ul TŬB DĒ-fekt): incomplete closure of the spinal canal, which may allow protrusion of the spinal cord and meninges at birth, leading to paralysis; also known as *spina bifida*

neurogenic bladder (nū-rō-JĚN-ĭk BLĂD-ĕr): bladder dysfunction (retention, incontinence, or altered capacity) due to disease or injury of the central nervous system (CNS) or certain peripheral nerves

nondiabetic hypoglycemia (nŏn-dī-ă-BĚT-ĭk hī-pō-glī-SĒ-mē-ă): condition in which a nondiabetic person experiences mild symptoms associated with low blood glucose

non-Hodgkin's lymphoma (nŏn-HŎJ-kĭnz lĭm-FŌ-mă): group of more than 30 types of malignancies of B and T lymphocytes

nystagmus (nĭs-TĂG-mŭs): involuntary back-and-forth or cyclical movements of the eyes

O

obstructive sleep apnea (OSA) (ŏb-STRŬK-tĭv slēp ăp-NĒ-ă): dysfunctional breathing that occurs when the upper airway is intermittently blocked during sleep

oral herpes (OR-ăl HĔR-pēz): vesicular eruption in or on the mouth caused by herpes virus; also called *herpes labialis* or *cold sore*

oral thrush (OR-ăl thrŭsh): infection of the skin or mucous membrane with any species of candida, but mainly *Candida albicans*; also called *candidiasis*

orchitis (or-KĪ-tĭs): acute or chronic condition of inflammation of one or both testicles, caused by (usually viral) infection

orthopnea (ōr-THŎP-nē-ă): labored breathing that occurs when lying flat and improves when sitting up

osteitis deformans (äs-tē-ĪT-ŭs dē-FŌRM-ănz): chronic condition in which the process of bone destruction and regrowth occurs abnormally, causing weak, fragile, enlarged, and misshapen bones; also called *Paget's disease*

osteoarthritis (ŏs-tē-ō-ăr-THRĪ-tĭs): condition of cartilage deterioration and joint inflammation marked by pain, stiffness, and decreased ROM, most commonly affecting synovial weight-bearing joints and vertebrae

osteomalacia (ŏs-tē-ō-măl-Ā-shē-ă): condition of softening and weakening of the bones; when it occurs in children, it is called *rickets*

osteomyelitis (ŏs-tē-ō-mī-ĕl-Ī-tĭs): acute or chronic infection within the bone, most commonly affecting the legs, arms, pelvis, and spine

osteoporosis (ŏs-tē-ō-pōr-Ō-sĭs): condition characterized by loss of bone mass throughout the skeleton

otitis externa (ō-TĪ-tĭs ĕks-TĚR-nă): acute inflammation or infection of the external auditory canal; also called *swimmer's ear*

otitis media (ō-TĪ-tĭs MĒ-dē-ă): inflammation or infection of the middle ear

otosclerosis (ō-tō-sklē-RŌ-sĭs): chronic progressive deafness caused by spongy bone formation around the oval window with resulting ankylosis of the stapes

ovarian cyst (ō-VĀ-rē-ăn sĭst): sac of fluid or semisolid mass that grows within the ovary

P

palsy (PAWL-zē): partial or complete loss of motor function resulting in paralysis

pancreatitis (păn-krē-ă-TĪ-tĭs): acute or chronic inflammation of the pancreas

panhypopituitarism (păn-hī-pō-pĭ-TŪ-ĭ-tăr-ĭ-zum): condition resulting from diminished secretion of pituitary hormones; also called *underactive pituitary gland*

papule (PĂP-ūl): small, raised spot or bump on the skin, such as a mole

Parkinson's disease (PĂR-kĭn-sŏnz dĭ-ZĒZ): progressive, degenerative disorder that results in tremors, gait changes, and occasionally dementia

paronychia (păr-ō-NĬK-ē-ă): acute or chronic infection of the margins of the fingernail or toenail, marked by warmth, erythema, edema, pus, throbbing, pain, or tenderness; causes the nail to become discolored and thickened

pathological fracture (păth-ō-LŎJ-ĭk-ăl FRĂK-chŭr): breaking of diseased, weakened bone from the stress of normal, everyday activities

pediculosis (pĕ-dĭk-ū-LŌ-sĭs): infestation of head, body, or pubic lice, marked by itching, the appearance of lice on the body, and eggs (nits) attached to hair shafts

pelvic inflammatory disease (PID) (PĔL-vĭk ĭn-FLĂ-mă-tōr-ē dĭ-ZĒZ): any acute or chronic infection of the female reproductive system, including the uterus, fallopian tubes, and ovaries

peptic ulcer (PĔP-tĭk ŬL-sĕr): inflamed lesion in the gastric or duodenal lining

pericarditis (pĕr-ĭ-kăr-DĪ-tĭs): acute or chronic condition in which the fibrous membrane surrounding the heart becomes inflamed

peripheral artery disease (PAD) (pĕr-ĬF-ĕr-ăl ĂR-tĕr-ē dĭ-ZĒZ): condition of partial or complete obstruction of the arms or legs; similar to peripheral vascular disease (PVD), which includes both arteries and veins

peripheral neuropathy (pĕr-ĬF-ĕr-ăl nū-RŎP-ă-thē): dysfunction of nerves that transmit information to and from the brain and spinal cord, characterized by pain, altered sensation, and muscle weakness

peritonitis (pĕr-ĭ-tō-NĪ-tĭs): inflammation of the organs and structures within the peritoneal cavity

pernicious anemia (pĕr-NĬSH-ŭs ă-NĒ-mē-ă): chronic form of megaloblastic anemia (producing many large, immature, dysfunctional RBCs), caused by a deficit in the absorption of vitamin B$_{12}$, that reduces the body's ability to produce sufficient numbers of healthy RBCs

petechiae (pĕ-TĒ-kē-ē): tiny red or purple hemorrhagic spots (singular *petechia*)

phagocytosis (făg-ō-sī-TŌ-sĭs): process in which specialized white blood cells (phagocytes) engulf and destroy microorganisms, foreign antigens, and cell debris

pharyngitis (făr-ĭn-JĪ-tĭs): inflammation of the pharynx; commonly called a *sore throat*

pheochromocytoma (fē-ō-krō-mō-sī-TŌ-mă): tumor of the adrenal medulla (central part of the adrenal gland), usually benign but sometimes causing fluctuation of stress hormones like adrenaline

phimosis (fī-MŌ-sĭs): stenosis or narrowing of the foreskin opening of the penis

photophobia (fō-tō-FŌ-bē-ă): excessive sensitivity to light

pituitary dwarfism (pĭ-TŪ-ĭ-tăr-ē DWĂRF-ĭ-zum): type of hypopituitarism in which reduced growth and development occur due to deficiency of growth hormone in childhood

placenta previa (plă-SĔN-tă PRĒ-vē-ă): implantation of the placenta in the lower uterine segment rather than the central or upper portion of the uterine wall, which may cause maternal hemorrhage during labor

plantar fasciitis (PLĂN-tăr făs-ē-Ī-tĭs): painful condition of the supporting structures of the arch of the foot, primarily the plantar fascia, a band of tissue that connects the heel with the toes

pleural effusion (PLOO-răl ĕ-FŪ-zhŭn): excess collection of fluid in the intrapleural space

pleurisy (PLOO-rĭs-ē): condition in which the pleurae become inflamed, causing sharp inspiratory chest pain; also called *pleuritis*

pneumoconiosis (nū-mŏ-kō-nē-Ō-sĭs): any disease of the respiratory tract caused by chronic or repetitive inhalation of dust particles

***Pneumocystis carinii* pneumonia (nŭ-mō-SĬS-tĭs kă-RĪ-nē-ī nŭ-MŌ-nē-ă):** a type of pneumonia associated with AIDS

pneumonia (nŭ-MŌ-nē-ă): bacterial or viral infection of the lungs

pneumothorax (nū-mō-THŌ-răks): condition in which air collects in the intrapleural space; categorized as open, closed, spontaneous, or tension, and commonly called *collapsed lung*

poliomyelitis (pōl-ē-ō-mī-ĕl-Ī-tĭs): inflammation of the spinal cord, caused by a virus, which may result in spinal and muscular deformity and paralysis

polycystic kidney disease (PKD) (pŏl-ē-SĬS-tĭk KĬD-nē dĭ-ZĒZ): group of hereditary, progressive disorders in which cysts (small sacs of fluid) form in the kidneys, eventually destroying them

polycythemia vera (pŏl-ē-sī-THĒ-mē-ă VĒ-ră): chronic disorder marked by increased number and mass of all bone marrow cells, especially RBCs, with increased blood viscosity and a tendency to develop blood clots

polydipsia (pŏl-ē-DĬP-sē-ă): much (increased) thirst

polymyositis (PM) (pŏl-ē-mī-ō-SĪ-tĭs): disorder that causes the slow onset of muscle weakness and pain in the muscles of the trunk and progresses to affect muscles of the neck, shoulders, back, hip, and possibly hands and fingers

polyphagia (pŏl-ē-FĀ-jē-ă): much (increased) appetite

polyuria (pŏl-ē-Ū-rē-ă): much (increased) urination

precocious puberty (prē-KŌ-shŭs PŪ-bĕr-tē): premature onset of puberty with the appearance of secondary sex characteristics in young children

premenstrual syndrome (prē-MĔN-stroo-ăl SĬN-drŏm): range of symptoms occurring 7 to 14 days before menstruation, including fluid retention, bloating, temporary weight gain, breast tenderness, headaches, depression, irritability, diarrhea, constipation, and appetite changes

presbycusis (prĕz-bĭ-KŪ-sĭs): progressive loss of hearing with aging

presbyopia (prĕz-bē-Ō-pē-ă): permanent loss of accommodation of the lens of the eye that occurs as people enter their 40s, causing a marked inability to maintain focus on near objects

prostatitis (prŏs-tă-TĪ-tĭs): acute or chronic inflammation of the prostate gland

pseudomembranous enterocolitis (soo-dō-MĔM-brăn-ŭs ĕn-tĕr-ō-kō-LĪ-tĭs): inflammatory condition of both small and large bowels that results in severe watery diarrhea; also commonly called *C. difficile colitis*

psoriasis (sō-RĪ-ă-sĭs): chronic, inflammatory skin disorder marked by the development of silvery-white scaly plaques or patches with sharply defined borders and reddened skin beneath

pulmonary embolism (PE) (PŬL-mō-nĕ-rē ĔM-bō-lĭ-zum): sudden obstruction of a pulmonary blood vessel by debris, blood clots, or other matter

pulmonary tuberculosis (TB) (PŬL-mō-nĕ-rē tū-bĕr-kū-LŌ-sĭs): contagious infection caused by the *Mycobacterium tuberculosis* organism, primarily affecting the lungs but sometimes also spreading to and affecting other organ systems

puncture (PŬNGK-chŭr): hole or wound made by a sharp, pointed instrument

pustule (PŬS-tūl): small, pus-filled blister

pyelonephritis (pī-ĕ-lō-nĕ-FRĪ-tĭs): inflammation and infection caused by bacterial growth in the renal pelvis and kidney

R

Raynaud's disease (rĕ-NŌZ dĭ-ZĒZ): disorder that affects blood vessels in the fingers, toes, ears, and nose, marked by vessel constriction and reduced blood flow in response to triggers such as cold temperature

renal calculus (RĒ-năl KĂL-kū-lŭs): small stone, composed of mineral salts, that may obstruct portions of the kidneys or a ureter; also called *kidney stone*

renal colic (RĒ-năl KŎL-ĭk): severe, intermittent pain caused by spasms of the ureter

renal failure (RĒ-năl FĀL-yĕr): acute or chronic failure of the kidneys to effectively eliminate fluids or wastes from the body

retinal detachment (RĔT-ĭ-năl dĭ-TACH-mŭnt): separation of the inner sensory layer of the retina from the outer pigment layer, caused by a break in the inner layer that permits vitreous fluid to leak under the retina and lift off its innermost layer; may cause blindness

retinopathy (rĕt-ĭn-ŎP-ă-thē): disease of the retina, often caused by diabetes

Reye's syndrome (rīz SĬN-drŏm): serious disease associated with aspirin use by children with viral illnesses, which may result in permanent brain damage or even death

rheumatic heart disease (roo-MĂT-ĭk hărt dĭ-ZĒZ): complication of rheumatic fever in which inflammation and damage occur to parts of the heart, usually the valves

rheumatoid arthritis (RA) (ROO-mă-toyd ăr-THRĪ-tĭs): autoimmune arthritis that causes progressive joint pain and deformity and may affect organ systems

rhonchi (RŎNG-kī): coarse, gurgling sound heard in the lungs with a stethoscope, caused by secretions in the air passages

rosacea (rō-ZĀ-sē-ă): chronic condition that causes flushing and redness of the face, neck, and chest

rotator cuff tear (rō-TĀ-tŏr kŭf tār): traumatic rip of one or more of the muscles or tendons within the rotator cuff of the shoulder

S

salmonellosis (săl-mō-nĕ-LŌ-sĭs): intestinal infection caused by various types of salmonella organisms

scabies (SKĀ-bēz): contagious skin disease transmitted by the itch mite, with symptoms of itching, scaly papules, insect burrows, and secondary infected lesions most prevalent in skin folds at the wrists and elbows, between the fingers, under the arms, in the groin, and under the beltline

scales (skālz): area of skin that is excessively dry and flaky

sciatica (sī-ĂT-ĭ-kă): pain, numbness, weakness, or tingling that is felt from the lower back along the pathway of the sciatic nerve into the legs

scleroderma (sklĕr-ă-DĔR-mă): group of chronic autoimmune diseases that cause inflammatory and fibrotic changes to skin, muscles, joints, tendons, cartilage, and other connective tissues

scoliosis (sko-lē-Ō-sĭs): abnormal S-shaped lateral curvature of the vertebrae

sebaceous cyst (sē-BĀ-shŭs sĭst): small sac or pouch below the skin surface filled with a thick fluid or semisolid oily substance called *sebum*

seborrheic keratosis (sĕ-bō-RĒ-ĭk kĕr-ă-TŌ-sĭs): benign, flat, irregularly shaped skin growths of various colors with a warty, waxy, "stuck-on" appearance

shingles (SHĬNG-gulz): unilateral painful vesicles occurring on the upper body, caused by the herpes zoster virus

shock (shŏk): syndrome of inadequate perfusion (circulation of blood, nutrients, and oxygen through tissues and organs) as a result of hypotension

short bowel syndrome (shŏrt BOW-ĕl SĬN-drōm): malabsorption and malnutrition disorder created by the loss of a significant portion of functioning bowel

silicosis (sĭl-ĭ-KŌ-sĭs): respiratory disease caused by chronic or repetitive inhalation of silica (quartz) dust

sinusitis (sī-nŭs-Ī-tĭs): inflammation of the lining of the sinus cavities

Sjögren's syndrome (SS) (SHŌ-grĕnz SĬN-drōm): autoimmune disorder that causes dysfunction of salivary glands in the mouth and lacrimal glands in the eyes and affects other areas of the body

small bowel obstruction (SBO) (smăl BOW-ĕl ŏb-STRŬK-shŭn): blockage of normal passage of intestinal contents

spina bifida (SPĪ-nă BĪ-fĭd-ă): incomplete closure of the spinal canal, which may result in protrusion of the spinal cord and meninges at birth and may cause paralysis; also called *neural tube defect*

spinal cord injury (SCI) (SPĪ-năl kord IN-jă-rē): traumatic bruising, crushing, or tearing of the spinal cord

spinal stenosis (SPĪ-năl stĕ-NŌ-sĭs): narrowing of an area of the spine that puts pressure on the spinal cord and spinal nerve roots

sprain (sprān): complete or incomplete tear in the ligaments around a joint

squamous cell carcinoma (SKWĀ-mŭs sĕl kăr-sĭ-NŌ-mă): type of cancer that usually appears in the mouth, esophagus, bronchi, lungs, or cervix, marked by a firm, red nodule or a scaly appearance; may ulcerate

sterility (stĕr-ĬL-ĭ-tē): inability to produce offspring

strabismus (stră-BĬZ-mŭs): deviation or misalignment of eyes that may adversely affect depth perception; types include *exotropia* (eyes turned outward), *esotropia* (eyes turned inward), *hypertropia* (eyes turned upward), and *hypotropia* (eyes turned downward)

strain (strān): trauma to a muscle and sometimes a tendon due to violent contraction or excessive forcible stretching

stress incontinence (strĕs ĭn-KŎNT-ĭn-ĕns): involuntary urine leakage upon physical stress, such as a cough or sneeze

stridor (STRĪ-dŏr): high-pitched upper-airway sound heard without a stethoscope, indicating airway obstruction; a medical emergency

stroke (strōk): death of brain cells due to loss of blood supply; also known as *cerebrovascular accident (CVA)* and *brain attack*

subdural hematoma (sub-DUR-ul hē-mă-TŌ-mă): collection of blood between the dura and the arachnoid (middle or second layer of the meninges)

syphilis (SĬF-ĭ-lĭs): multistage STI caused by the spirochete *Treponema pallidum*, with key symptoms including skin lesions; eventually fatal unless treated

systemic lupus erythematosus (SLE) (sĭs-TĔM-ĭk LOO-pŭs ĕr-ĭ-thē-mă-TŌ-sŭs): chronic autoimmune disorder that causes inflammation and degeneration of various connective tissues in the body, such as the skin, lungs, heart, joints, kidneys, blood, or nervous system

T

tendinitis (tĕn-dĭn-Ī-tĭs): condition of inflammation of a tendon due to overuse

tension headache (TĔN-shŭn HED-āk): nonmigraine headache in which pain is felt in all or part of the head

testicular torsion (tĕs-TĬK-ū-lăr TŌR-shŭn): condition in which the testicles become twisted and the spermatic cord, blood vessels, nerves, and vas deferens become strangled

tetanus (TĔT-ă-nŭs): noncontagious illness marked by severe, prolonged spasm of skeletal muscle fibers; also known as *lockjaw*

thoracic outlet syndrome (TOS) (thō-RĂS-ĭk OWT-lĕt SĬN-drōm): group of painful disorders involving compression of the nerves or vessels in the neck and arms

thromboangiitis obliterans (TAO) (thrŏm-bō-ăn-jē-Ī-tĭs ŏb-LĬT-ĕr-ănz): type of vascular disease associated with tobacco use, marked by inflammation and clot formation within small vessels of the hands and feet, which may lead to gangrene and surgical amputation; sometimes called *Buerger's disease*

thrombophlebitis (thrŏm-bō flĕ-BĪ-tĭs): development of a blood clot in a deep vein, usually in the legs; also known as *deep vein thrombosis (DVT)*

thyrotoxicosis (thī-rō-tŏks-ĭ-KŌ-sĭs): severe episode of worsening symptoms of hyperthyroidism

tinea (TĬ-nē-ă): fungal skin disease occurring on various parts of the body, also called *dermatophytosis* or *ringworm*; forms include tinea capitis (scalp), tinea corporis (trunk), tinea cruris (genital area, also called *jock itch*), tinea nodosa (mustache and beard), tinea pedis (feet, also called *athlete's foot*), and tinea unguium (nails)

tinnitus (tĭn-Ī-tŭs): perception of ringing, buzzing, tinkling, or hissing sound in the ear

toxic shock syndrome (TSS) (TŎKS-ĭk shŏk SĬN-drōm): rare disorder caused by bacterial exotoxins; most commonly occurs in young women who use tampons

transfusion incompatibility reaction (trănz-FŪ-zhŭn ĭn-kŏm-păt-ĭ-BĬL-ĭ-tē rē-ĂK-shŭn): reaction of antibodies present in transfused blood to RBCs in the recipient's blood or of antibodies in the recipient's blood to RBCs in the transfused blood

transient global amnesia (TGA) (TRĂNZ-ē-ĭnt GLŌ-băl ăm-NĒ-zē-ă): rare disorder, not caused by a neurological event or injury, that causes sudden, temporary loss of recent memory

transient ischemic attack (TIA) (TRĂNZ-ē-ĭnt ĭs-KĒ-mĭk ă-TĂK): temporary strokelike symptoms caused by a brief interruption of blood supply to a part of the brain

transplant rejection (TRĂNZ-plănt rē-JĔK-shŭn): identification of transplanted tissue as foreign by the recipient's immune system, which responds by attacking the tissue

traumatic brain injury (traw-MĂT-ĭk brān IN-jă-rē): injury to the brain following a blow to the head commonly caused by a fall or motor vehicle accident

trichomoniasis (trĭk-ō-mō-NĪ-ă-sĭs): STI infestation with *Trichomonas vaginalis* parasites; key symptoms include vaginitis, urethritis, and cystitis

trigeminal neuralgia (TN) (trī-JĔM-ĭn-ăl nū-RĂL-jē-ă): neurological disorder that causes severe, episodic facial pain along the pathway of the fifth cranial (trigeminal) nerve; also called *tic douloureux*

tubular necrosis (TŪ-bū-lăr nĕ-KRŌ-sĭs): renal failure caused by acute injury to the renal tubules

U

ulcer (ŬL-sĕr): lesion of the skin or mucous membranes, marked by inflammation, necrosis, and sloughing of damaged tissues

ulcerative colitis (ŬL-sĕr-ă-tĭv kō-LĪ-tĭs): chronic inflammatory disease of the lining of the colon and rectum marked by up to 20 liquid, bloody stools per day

upper-respiratory infection (URI) (Ŭ-pĕr rĕs-PĪR-ă-tō-rē ĭn-FĔK-shŭn): infection and inflammation of upper-airway structures, usually caused by a virus; often called the *common cold*

uremia (ū-RĒ-mē-ă): increased level of urea or other wastes in the blood

urge incontinence (UR-j ĭn-KŎNT-ĭn-ĕns): involuntary urine leakage directly following the strong urge to urinate

urgency (UR-jĕn-sē): need to urinate immediately

urinary incontinence (UI) (Ū-rĭ-nār-ē ĭn-KŎNT-ĭn-ĕns): involuntary urine leakage upon physical stress, such as a cough or sneeze (stress incontinence), after failing to reach a toilet in time (functional incontinence), or directly following the strong urge to urinate (urge incontinence)

urinary retention (Ū-rĭ-nār-ē rĭ-TĔN-shŭn): inability to urinate

urinary tract infection (UTI) (Ū-rĭ-nār-ē trăkt ĭn-FĔK-shŭn): inflammation and infection caused by bacterial growth in the urinary tract, usually the bladder

uterine fibroids (Ū-tĕr-ĭn FĪ-broyds): benign, smooth tumors made of muscle and fat; also called *leiomyomas*

uterine prolapse (Ū-tĕr-ĭn PRŌ-lăps): downward protrusion of the uterus into the vaginal opening

uveitis (ū-vē-Ī-tĭs): nonspecific term for any intraocular inflammatory disorder, which may affect the iris, ciliary body, choroid, or other parts of the eye

V

varicocele (VĂR-ĭ-kō-sēl): enlargement and dilation of the veins of the spermatic cord that drain the testis

varicose veins (VĂR-ĭ-kōs vānz): bulging, distended veins due to incompetent valves, most commonly in the legs

vertigo (VĔR-tĭ-gō): a feeling of spinning or moving in space

vesicle (VĔS-ĭ-kul): clear, fluid-filled blister

vesicoureteral reflux (VUR) (VĔS-ĭ-kō-ū-RĒ-tĕr-ăl RĒ-fluks): abnormal flow of urine from the bladder back into the ureter

vitiligo (vĭt-ĭl-Ī-gō): chronic skin disease that results in patchy loss of skin pigment; may also affect hair color and cause white patches or streaks

volvulus (VŎL-vū-lŭs): twisting of the bowel upon itself, causing obstruction

W

wart (wŏrt): small, benign skin tumor caused by various strains of the human papillomavirus (HPV); appearance varies from tiny to moderate-sized bumps or cauliflower-shaped growths

wheal (hwēl): rounded, temporary elevation in the skin, white in the center with a red-pink periphery and accompanied by itching

wheeze (hwēz): somewhat musical sound heard in the lungs, usually with a stethoscope, caused by partial airway obstruction (such as with asthma)

Wilms' tumor (vĭlmz TŪ-mor): rapidly growing type of kidney cancer that most commonly affects children; also known as nephroblastoma

GLOSSARY OF DIAGNOSTIC TESTS AND PROCEDURES

#
24-hour urine specimen: total urine excreted over 24 hours, collected for analysis

A
angiography: diagnostic or therapeutic radiography (radiological imaging) of the heart and blood vessels

arterial blood gases (ABGs): measurement of O_2 and CO_2 levels and acid-base balance (pH balance) in arterial blood

antinuclear antibody (ANA): test to detect the presence of autoantibodies which may suggest an autoimmune disorder such as rheumatoid arthritis

arthrography: radiological examination of a joint after injection of a contrast fluid into the joint space

audiometry: detailed measurement of hearing with an audiometer

automated external defibrillator (AED): small computer-driven defibrillator that analyzes the patient's rhythm, selects the appropriate energy level, charges the machine, and delivers a shock to the patient

automatic implanted cardioverter defibrillator (AICD): very small defibrillator, surgically implanted in patients with a high risk for sudden cardiac death, that automatically detects and treats life-threatening arrhythmias

average blood glucose (eAG): reflection of the average blood glucose level over the past 2 to 3 months reported by the same units (mg/dl) seen on glucose meters; directly correlates to HbA1c results

B
barium enema: enema containing a substance that shows up clearly under x-ray and fluoroscopic examination

barium swallow: x-ray examination of the esophagus after the patient has swallowed a liquid that contains barium

biopsy: removal of a tissue sample for microscopic examination

bladder ultrasound (bladder scan): noninvasive use of a portable ultrasound device to measure the amount of retained urine

blood urea nitrogen (BUN): lab value used to measure kidney function, based on nitrogen levels in the blood

bone marrow aspiration: removal of a bone marrow specimen from the cortex of a flat bone for analysis

bone scan: use of a gamma camera to detect abnormalities in bone density after injection of radioactive material

BOTOX: injection of a small amount of botulinum toxin into selected muscles of the face; interferes with muscle contraction, thereby reducing the appearance of wrinkles

bronchoscopy: visual examination of the airways of the lungs

C
C-reactive protein (CRP): test to detect or monitor inflammatory conditions

cardiac catheterization: evaluation of the heart vessels and valves via the injection of dye that shows up under radiology

cardiopulmonary resuscitation (CPR): emergency procedure that provides manual external cardiac compression and sometimes artificial respiration

cardioversion: restoration of normal sinus rhythm (NSR) by chemical or electrical means

CD-4 lymphocyte count: measurement of the number of specialized WBCs sometimes called *helper T cells,* used to identify whether a person's HIV infection is worsening

cerebrospinal fluid (CSF) analysis: analysis of CSF for blood, bacteria, and other abnormalities

chemical peel: application of a chemical solution to the skin to improve appearance by removing blemishes, fine wrinkles, uneven pigmentation, scars, and tattoos

chest x-ray (CXR): radiological picture of the lungs

cochlear implant: surgical insertion into the cochlea of a device that receives sound and transmits signals to electrodes implanted within the cochlea, allowing hearing-impaired persons to perceive sound

color vision tests: use of multicolored charts to evaluate the patient's ability to recognize color

computed tomography (CT) scan: computerized collection and translation of multiple x-rays into a three-dimensional picture, creating a more-detailed and accurate image than traditional x-rays; study of the brain and spinal cord using radiology and computer analysis

corneal transplant (keratoplasty): surgical replacement of a diseased cornea with a healthy one from a donor

coronary artery bypass graft (CABG): surgical creation of an alternate route for blood flow around an area of coronary arterial obstruction

creatine kinase (CK): test to measure isoenzymes released by skeletal and cardiac muscles into the blood when they are damaged

cryosurgery: destruction of abnormal tissue by freezing

cryotherapy: application of cold, such as with ice compresses, to decrease inflammation and pain

culture and sensitivity (C&S): process of growing microorganisms, then exposing them to antimicrobial drugs to determine which ones kill them most effectively

cystoscopy: visual examination of the bladder lining with a cystoscope

D

defibrillation: delivery of an electric shock with the goal of ending ventricular fibrillation and restoring normal sinus rhythm

dermabrasion: removal of small scars, nevi (moles), tattoos, or fine wrinkles with a wire brush or burr impregnated with diamond particles, leaving a smoother surface

dermaplaning: removal of small scars, nevi (moles), tattoos, or fine wrinkles with a dermatome (a device resembling an electric razor), leaving a smoother surface

dilation and curettage (D&C): dilation of the cervix followed by scraping of the endometrial lining

dual-energy x-ray absorptiometry (DEXA): radiological evaluation of bone density to detect osteoporosis

E

echocardiography (ECHO): ultrasound procedure used to detect cardiovascular disorders that allows visualization of the size, shape, position, thickness, and movement of all parts of the heart, as well as characteristics of blood flow through the heart

electrocardiography (ECG, EKG): creation and study of graphic records (electrocardiograms) of electric currents originating in the heart

electroencephalography (EEG): record of electrical activity of the brain on graph paper; study of electrical activity of the brain

electromyogram (EMG): record of skeletal muscle electrical activity, used to diagnose neuromuscular disorders

endoscopic retrograde cholangiopancreatography (ERCP): radiographic examination of vessels that connect the liver, gallbladder, and pancreas to the duodenum after a radiopaque material has been injected through a fiberoptic endoscope

enucleation: surgical removal of the entire eyeball

enzyme immunosorbent assay (EIA): rapid enzyme immunochemical method for identifying the presence of antigens, antibodies, or other substances in the blood, used as a primary diagnostic test for many infectious diseases including syphilis and HIV; formerly called *enzyme-linked immunosorbent assay (ELISA)*

erythrocyte sedimentation rate (ESR, sed rate): test used in the diagnosis and monitoring of many diseases that cause acute or chronic inflammation; measures the rate at which red blood cells settle in plasma or saline located in a tube of unclotted blood; an elevated ESR indicates inflammation

event recorder: portable monitoring device that transmits heart rhythms by telephone to a central laboratory where dysrhythmias can be detected and analyzed

exercise stress test: noninvasive test that measures cardiac function during physical activity; also called *treadmill test* or *stress test*

extracorporeal shock wave lithotripsy: procedure in which shock waves or sound waves crush stones in the kidneys or urinary tract

F

fasting blood glucose (FBG): test of blood glucose levels after a fast of 8 to 12 hours, used to screen for diabetes; also called *fasting blood sugar (FBS)*

fecal occult blood test (Hemoccult): test of fecal specimen for presence of hidden blood

finger stick blood sugar (FSBS): test of blood glucose from a drop of capillary blood obtained by pricking the finger; also called *finger stick blood glucose (FSBG)*

G

gastroccult: test of gastric contents for pH level and presence of blood

glucose tolerance test (GTT): measurement of blood glucose levels at specified intervals after ingestion of glucose

glycosylated hemoglobin (HbA1c): reflection of the average blood glucose level over the past 3 to 4 months

H

***Helicobacter pylori* test:** test that detects the presence of antibodies to *Helicobacter pylori*, the most common cause of gastric ulcers

Hemoccult (stool guaiac test): small sample of feces tested for presence of blood

hemodialysis: filtration of wastes and fluid from blood as it passes through selectively permeable membranes; also called *dialysis*

Holter monitor: portable device worn by patient during normal activity that records heart rhythm for up to 24 hours

I

international normalized ratio (INR): standardized method of checking the prothrombin time (PT); prothrombin is a blood-clotting factor that is used to monitor warfarin (Coumadin) therapy, and warfarin (Coumadin) is an anticoagulant medication that slows the clotting time of blood

intravenous pyelogram (IVP): x-ray examination of the kidneys, ureters, and bladder after injection of a contrast medium

K

KUB: radiological imaging (x-ray) of the abdomen, specifically the kidneys, ureters, and bladder

L

laparoscopy: exploration of abdominal contents with a laparoscope

laser-assisted in-situ keratomileusis (LASIK): procedure in which a laser is used to alter the shape of the deep corneal layer after a top flap in the surface is opened

laser photocoagulation: destruction of areas of the retina with a laser beam

laser resurfacing: use of short pulses of light to remove fine lines and damaged skin and to minimize scars and even out areas of uneven pigmentation; sometimes called a *laser peel*

liver function tests (LFTs): tests, including aspartate aminotransferase (AST) and alanine aminotransferase (ALT), that determine the liver's ability to perform its many complex functions

lower endoscopy: visual examination of the GI tract from rectum to cecum; variations include the colonoscopy, sigmoidoscopy, and proctoscopy

lower GI x-ray: x-ray of the large intestine after rectal instillation of barium sulfate

lumbar puncture (LP): puncture of subarachnoid layer at the fourth intervertebral space to obtain CSF for analysis

M

magnetic resonance imaging (MRI): use of an electromagnetic field and radio waves to create visual images on a computer screen

Mantoux test: intradermal injection of tuberculin purified protein derivative (PPD) just beneath the surface of the skin to identify whether the patient has been exposed to tuberculosis

metered dose inhaler (MDI): handheld device used to deliver medication to the patient's lower airways

microdermabrasion: similar to dermabrasion but less invasive, involving multiple treatments of gentle abrasion; useful in reducing fine lines, nevi (moles), age spots, and acne scars

monospot (heterophile): quick test used to screen for the presence of the heterophile antibody that is common in individuals with Epstein-Barr virus infection

myelography: radiography of the spinal cord and associated nerves after intrathecal injection (into the spinal canal) of a contrast medium

N

nebulizer: device that produces a fine spray or mist to deliver medication to a patient's deep airways

needle biopsy: aspiration of tissue or fluid through a large-gauge needle for analysis

P

pacemaker: device that can trigger the mechanical contractions of the heart by emitting periodic electrical discharges

Papanicolaou smear: removal of tissue cells from the cervix for analysis

partial thromboplastin time (PTT): measure of blood-clotting time, used to monitor heparin therapy; heparin is an anticoagulant medication that slows the clotting time of blood

patch test: test in which paper or gauze saturated with an allergen is applied to the skin beneath an occlusive dressing while the response is noted

pelvic sonography: ultrasound imaging of the structures in the female pelvis

percutaneous transluminal coronary angioplasty (PTCA): method of treating a narrowed coronary artery via inflation and deflation of a balloon on a double-lumen catheter inserted through the right femoral artery

peritoneal dialysis: filtration of fluid and wastes from the blood using the lining of the patient's peritoneal cavity as a dialyzing membrane

phacoemulsification: removal of the lens with an ultrasonic device to treat cataracts

pleurodesis: infusion of a sterile, irritating substance into the pleural space, causing the pleural linings to fuse to one another by developing scar tissue

postural drainage: placement of the patient in various positions that facilitate drainage of secretions from the lungs, often done along with chest physiotherapy (CPT)

prostate-specific antigen (PSA): blood test used to screen for prostate cancer

prothrombin time (PT): procedure that measures the clotting time of blood; used to assess levels of anticoagulation in patients taking warfarin (Coumadin)

pulmonary angiography: radiographic examination of pulmonary circulation after injection of a contrast dye

pulmonary function tests (PFTs): group of tests that provide information regarding lung capacity; sometimes called *spirometry*

pulse oximetry: indirect measurement of arterial-blood O_2 saturation level, also known as the SpO_2; the normal level in a person with healthy lungs is 97% to 99%

R

radial keratotomy: incision into the outer portion of the cornea to flatten it and help correct nearsightedness

radioactive iodine uptake: nuclear medicine study that measures how rapidly radioactive iodine is taken up from the blood after oral or intravenous administration

refractive error test: evaluation of the eye's ability to focus an image

rheumatoid factor: blood test used to identify rheumatoid arthritis and other disorders

Rinne test: hearing test that compares bone conduction to air conduction, using a tuning fork

S

scleral buckling: placement of a band of silicone around the eyeball to stabilize a detached retina

scratch test: test in which an allergen is placed on a scratched area of the skin and the response is noted

serum creatinine: lab value used to measure kidney function that is more specific than BUN

slit-lamp microscopy: examination of the posterior surface of the cornea with a slit lamp

sputum analysis: examination of mucus or fluid coughed up from the lungs

stool culture: examination of a fecal specimen for abnormal bacteria and other microorganisms

stress test: treadmill test that can show if the blood supply is reduced in the arteries that supply the heart; also called *exercise stress test*

T

thoracentesis: surgical puncture of the chest wall to remove fluid from the interpleural space; also called *pleurocentesis*

thyroid function test: reflection of thyroid function by measuring levels of thyroid-stimulating hormone (TSH), triiodothyronine (T3), and thyroxine (T4)

thyroid scan: radiographic evaluation of the thyroid after a radioactive substance is injected; identifies thyroid size, shape, position, and function

thyroid-stimulating hormone (TSH): measure of the ability of the thyroid gland to concentrate and retain circulating iodine for synthesis of thyroid hormone

tonometry: measurement of intraocular pressure or tension to detect glaucoma

total hip replacement (THR): procedure to replace an arthritic hip with a prosthetic device to restore mobility and function; also referred to as *total hip arthroplasty*

transcutaneous electrical nerve stimulation (TENS): delivery of a mild electrical current to a painful area to disrupt transmission of pain signals between the body and brain

transesophageal echocardiography (TEE): study of the heart via a probe placed in the esophagus

transurethral resection of the prostate (TURP): removal of tissue from the prostate gland with an endoscope, via the urethra

troponin: protein released into the body by damaged heart muscle, considered the most accurate blood test to confirm the diagnosis of a myocardial infarction (MI)

tubal ligation: sterilization procedure in which fallopian tubes are cut and ligated

tympanometry: procedure for evaluation of the mobility and patency of the eardrum, detection of middle-ear disorders, and evaluation of the patency of the eustachian tube

tympanoplasty: reconstruction of a perforated tympanic membrane

U

ultrasound: test in which ultrahigh-frequency sound waves are used to outline the shapes of various body structures

upper endoscopy: visual examination of the GI tract, from esophagus to duodenum

upper GI x-ray (UGI): x-ray that involves the use of a contrast medium to help visualize abdominal organs, including the stomach and esophagus

urinalysis (UA): visual and microscopic analysis of a urine specimen

urinary catheterization: insertion of a tube into the bladder via the urethra to drain urine, obtain a urine specimen, or instill medication

uterine ablation: procedure that destroys the entire surface of the endometrium and superficial myometrium

V

vasectomy: sterilization procedure in which a small section of the vas deferens is removed

viral load: measurement of the number of copies of the human immunodeficiency virus in the blood, used to monitor progression of HIV infection and AIDS

visual acuity test: examination that identifies the smallest letters, numbers, or objects that can be correctly identified on a standardized Snellen's vision chart from 20 feet

vital capacity (VC): measurement of the volume of air that can be exhaled after maximum inspiration

voiding cystourethrography (VCUG): radiological examination of the bladder and urethra during urination

W

Weber test: hearing test that evaluates bone conduction using a tuning fork

DRUGS AND DRUG CLASSIFICATIONS

There are several systems of drug classification. One is based on the body system that is most affected (e.g., respiratory drugs, cardiac drugs); another is based on the therapeutic action (e.g., antihypertensive, antacid); and another is based on the chemical action of the drug (e.g., cholinergic, selective serotonin reuptake inhibitor). As the following table indicates, most drugs fall into several classes.

This table contains a list of the most commonly prescribed medications in the United States. The first column lists the drugs alphabetically according to generic names, followed by the common brand names in the second column. The third column lists the drugs' therapeutic classifications, and the fourth column lists the most common uses of the drugs.

Generic Name *A*	Brand Name	Therapeutic Classification	Common Use
acarbose	Precose	Alpha-glucosidase inhibitor	Slows digestion of complex carbohydrates
acebutolol	Sectral	Beta blocker/Beta-adrenergic blocking agent	Decreases heart rate and cardiac output
acetaminophen	Tylenol	Analgesic and antipyretic	Relieves minor aches and pains; reduces fever
acetazolamide	Diamox	Carbonic anhydrase inhibitor: topical, oral, or intravenous	Treats glaucoma; decreases fluid production
adalimumab	Humira	Immunosuppressant	Treats rheumatoid arthritis, psoriasis; blocks tumor necrosis factor (TNF)
albuterol	AccuNeb, Proventil, Ventolin	Short-acting bronchodilator	Dilates, or opens up, bronchi for quick relief of acute asthma symptoms
alemtuzumab	Campath	Immunotherapy	Stimulates the immune system to recognize and attack cancer cells
alendronate	Fosamax	Bisphosphonate	Treats osteoporosis; increases bone density
allopurinol	Zyloprim	Xanthine oxidase inhibitor	Treats gout; blocks the production of uric acid in the body
alphagan	Brimonidine Tartrate	Alpha agonist (ophthalmic)	Treats glaucoma; decreases fluid production and/or increases fluid drainage

Generic Name A—cont'd	Brand Name	Therapeutic Classification	Common Use
alprostadil	Caverject, Edex, Muse	Impotence agent	Causes vasodilation and increases blood flow to penis to cause an erection
alteplase	Activase	Thrombolytic	Dissolves a thrombus
alupent	Metaproterenol	Short-acting bronchodilator	Dilates, or opens up, bronchi for quick relief of acute asthma symptoms
amantadine	Symadine, Symmetrel	Anti-influenza agent, antiviral (not a vaccine)	Relieves symptoms and reduces the duration of certain types of influenza
amiloride	Midamor	Diuretic (water pill)	Removes excess fluids and sodium from the body; relieves the heart's workload
amlodipine	Norvasc, Lotrel	Calcium channel blocker	Interrupts movement of calcium into cells; decreases the heart's pumping strength and relaxes blood vessels
amoxicillin	Amoxil	Penicillin	Antibiotic; prevents bacterial cell wall formation
ampicillin	Omnipen, Principen	Penicillin	Antibiotic; prevents bacterial cell wall formation
anthralin	Drithocreme, Micanol, Psoriatec, Zithranol	Antipsoriatic	Slows down the growth of skin cells
apraclonidine	Lopidine	Alpha agonist (ophthalmic)	Treats glaucoma; decreases fluid production and/or increases fluid drainage
arsenic trioxide	Arsenox	Differentiating agent	Forces cancer cells to mature into normal cells
aspart	NovoLog	Insulin	Insulin replacement; helps glucose get into cells
aspirin	Bayer, Bufferin, Ecotrin	Nonsteroidal anti-inflammatory drug (NSAID)	Reduces inflammation, pain, and fever
	Ascriptin, St. Joseph 81 mg	Platelet aggregation inhibitor, salicylate	Prevents thrombus formation; reduces pain and inflammation
atazanavir	Reyataz	Antiretroviral; nucleoside reverse transcriptase inhibitor (NRTI)	Prevents the HIV virus from spreading
atenolol	Tenormin	Beta blocker/Beta-adrenergic blocking agent	Decreases heart rate and cardiac output
atorvastatin	Lipitor	Cholesterol-lowering agent	Lowers LDL (bad) cholesterol; raises HDL (good) cholesterol; lowers triglyceride levels

Continued

Generic Name A—cont'd	Brand Name	Therapeutic Classification	Common Use
atropine	Isopto Atropine	Cycloplegic mydriatic	Dilates the pupil and/or causes temporary paralysis of accommodation during eye exam or procedure
azathioprine	Imuran	Immunosuppressive	Prevents organ transplant rejection and prevents the immune system from attacking the body in autoimmune disorders
azithromycin	Zithromax	Macrolide	Antibiotic; inhibits protein synthesis
azithromycin	AzaSite	Antibiotic (ophthalmic)	Treats blepharitis, conjunctivitis, and keratitis; kills or inhibits spread of bacteria
B			
bacitracin	Bacticin	Antibiotic (ophthalmic)	Treats blepharitis, conjunctivitis, and keratitis; kills or inhibits spread of bacteria
baclofen	Lioresal	Skeletal muscle relaxant	Reduces tone in skeletal muscle; decreases muscle pain
benazepril	Lotensin	Angiotensin-converting enzyme (ACE) inhibitor	Lowers angiotensin II levels; expands blood vessels and decreases resistance
bendamustine	Treanda	Alkylating agent	Treats cancer; prevents cancer cells from multiplying by directly damaging the DNA in the cell
benzoyl peroxide	Benoxyl, Benzac, Desquam, Fostex, Triaz, Vanoxide, Zoderm	Anti-acne agent	Reduces amount of acne-causing bacteria
benztropine	Cogentin	Anticholinergic antiparkinson agent	Compensates for lack of dopamine in Parkinson's disease
bepridil	Vascor	Calcium channel blocker	Interrupts movement of calcium into cells; decreases the heart's pumping strength and relaxes blood vessels
besifloxacin	Besivance	Antibiotic (ophthalmic)	Treats blepharitis, conjunctivitis, and keratitis; kills or inhibits spread of bacteria
betaxolol	Kerlone	Beta blocker/Beta-adrenergic blocking agent	Decreases heart rate and cardiac output

Generic Name B—cont'd	Brand Name	Therapeutic Classification	Common Use
bexarotene	Targretin	Differentiating agent	Forces cancer cells to mature into normal cells
bimatoprost	Lumigan	Prostaglandin (ophthalmic)	Treats glaucoma; increases fluid drainage
biperiden	Akineton	Anticholinergic antiparkinson agent	Compensates for lack of dopamine in Parkinson's disease
bisoprolol	Zebeta	Beta blocker/Beta-adrenergic blocking agent	Decreases heart rate and cardiac output
bisoprolol/ hydrochlorothiazide	Ziac	Beta blocker/Beta-adrenergic blocking agent	Decreases heart rate and cardiac output
Bismuth subsalicylate	Pepto-Bismol	Antidiarrheal	Reduces diarrhea by slowing forward propulsion of intestinal contents
bleomycin	Blenoxane	Antitumor antibiotic	Treats cancer; interferes with enzymes involved in DNA replication
bortezomib	Velcade	Targeted therapy: antineoplastic agent, proteasome inhibitor	Attacks specific cancer cells
brinzolamide	Azopt	Carbonic anhydrase inhibitor: topical, oral, or intravenous	Treats glaucoma; decreases fluid production
bromfenac	Prolensa, Xibrom	NSAID (Ophthalmic)	Decreases inflammation and reduces pain
bromocriptine	Parlodel	Growth hormone antagonist	Decreases production of growth hormone
budesonide (steroid) and formoterol	Symbicort	Long-acting beta-adrenergic agonist bronchodilator	Dilates, or opens up, bronchi for long-term control of asthma symptoms
bumetanide	Bumex	Diuretic: loop, thiazide, or potassium sparing	Removes excess fluids and sodium from the body; relieves the heart's workload; increases urine flow
C			
cabergoline	Dostinex	Prolactin inhibitor	Decreases production of prolactin
candesartan	Atacand	Angiotensin II receptor blocker/inhibitor	Prevents effects of angiotensin II; keeps blood pressure from rising
captopril	Capoten	Angiotensin-converting enzyme (ACE) inhibitor	Lowers angiotensin II levels; expands blood vessels and decreases resistance

Continued

Generic Name C—cont'd	Brand Name	Therapeutic Classification	Common Use
capecitabine	Xeloda	Antimetabolite	Treats cancer; interferes with DNA and RNA through substitution of the building blocks
carbidopa/levodopa	Parcopa, Sinemet	Dopaminergic antiparkinson agent	Replaces or prevents degradation of dopamine in Parkinson's disease
carbimazole	None	Antithyroid agent	Decreases production of thyroid hormone
carboprost	Hemabate	Uterine stimulant	Stimulates uterine muscle contractions
carisoprodol	Soma	Skeletal muscle relaxant	Reduces tone in skeletal muscle; decreases muscle pain
carteolol	Cartrol	Beta blocker/Beta-adrenergic blocking agent	Decreases heart rate and cardiac output
celecoxib	Celebrex	Nonsteroidal anti-inflammatory drug (NSAID)	Reduces inflammation, pain, and fever
cephalexin	Biocef, Keflex	Cephalosporin	Antibiotic; prevents bacterial cell wall formation
cetirizine	Zyrtec	Antihistamine	Relieves allergy symptoms
chlorambucil	Leukeran	Alkylating agent	Treats cancer; prevents cancer cells from multiplying by directly damaging the DNA in the cell
chlorothiazide	Diuril	Diuretic (water pill)	Removes excess fluids and sodium from the body; relieves the heart's workload
chlorpropamide	Diabinese	Sulfonylurea	Increases insulin production by the pancreas
chlorthalidone	Hygroton	Diuretic (water pill)	Removes excess fluids and sodium from the body; relieves the heart's workload
chlorzoxazone	Parafon Forte	Skeletal muscle relaxant	Reduces tone in skeletal muscle; decreases muscle pain
cimetidine	Tagamet	Histamine-2 blocker	Blocks histamine to reduce stomach acidity
ciprofloxacin	Cipro, Ciloxan	Fluoroquinolone	Antibiotic; prevents growth of bacteria
cladribine	Leustatin	Antimetabolite	Treats cancer; interferes with DNA and RNA through substitution of the building blocks
clindamycin	Cleocin	Antibacterial	Kills bacteria or prevents its growth

Generic Name C—cont'd	Brand Name	Therapeutic Classification	Common Use
clofarabine	Clolar	Antimetabolite	Treats cancer; interferes with DNA and RNA through substitution of the building blocks
clomiphene citrate	Clomid, Serophene	Synthetic ovulation stimulant	Stimulates ovulation
clopidogrel	Plavix	Platelet aggregation inhibitor, salicylate	Prevents thrombus formation; reduces pain and inflammation
clotrimazole	Lotrimin	Antifungal agent	Interferes with the formation of the fungal cell membrane
codeine	None	Opioid/Narcotic analgesic	Relieves moderate to severe pain
cromolyn sodium, nedocromil sodium	None	Mast cell stabilizer, anti-inflammatory	Decreases inflammation; prevents asthma attacks
cyclobenzaprine	Flexeril	Skeletal muscle relaxant	Reduces tone in skeletal muscle; decreases muscle pain
cyclopentolate	Cyclogyl	Cycloplegic mydriatic	Dilates the pupil and/or causes temporary paralysis of accommodation during eye exam or procedure
cyclophosphamide	Cytoxan	Alkylating agent	Treats cancer; prevents cancer cells from multiplying by directly damaging the DNA in the cell
cyclophosphamide	Cytoxan	Disease-modifying antirheumatic drug (DMARD), immunosuppressive	Treats rheumatoid arthritis; Prevents organ transplant rejection
cyclosporine	Sandimmune, Neoral	Immunosuppressive	Prevents organ transplant rejection and prevents the immune system from attacking the body in autoimmune disorders
cytarabine	Cytosar	Antimetabolite	Treats cancer; interferes with DNA and RNA through substitution of the building blocks
D			
dalteparin	Fragmin	Anticoagulant	Decreases the clotting ability of the blood
danaparoid	Orgaran	Anticoagulant	Decreases the clotting ability of the blood
darunavir	Prezista	Antiretroviral; nucleoside reverse transcriptase inhibitor (NRTI)	Prevents the HIV virus from spreading

Continued

Generic Name D—cont'd	Brand Name	Therapeutic Classification	Common Use
daunorubicin	Cerubidine	Antitumor antibiotic	Treats cancer; interferes with enzymes involved in DNA replication
delavirdine	Rescriptor	Antiretroviral; non-nucleoside reverse transcriptase inhibitor (NNRTI)	Prevents the HIV virus from spreading
denosumab	Prolia	Bone resorption inhibitor	Treats osteoporosis; slows the formation and action of cells that break down bone
dexamethasone	Decadron	Corticosteroid	Reduces inflammation; suppresses the immune system
dextromethorphan	Delsym, PediaCare, Robitussin Cough, Sucrets, Triaminic, Vicks	Antitussive	Suppresses cough
diclofenac	Voltaren	Nonsteroidal anti-inflammatory drug (NSAID)	Reduces inflammation, pain, and fever
digitoxin	Crystodigin	Digitalis glycoside	Increases the force of the heart's contractions
diltiazem	Cardizem, Tiazac	Calcium channel blocker	Interrupts movement of calcium into cells; decreases the heart's pumping strength and relaxes blood vessels
dimenhydrinate	Dramamine	Antiemetic	Prevents or treats motion sickness, nausea, and vomiting
dinoprostone	Cervidil	Uterine stimulant	Stimulates uterine muscle contractions
diphenhydramine	Benadryl, Nytol, Sominex, Twilite, Unisom	Antihistamine, anticholinergic antiparkinson agent	Relieves allergy symptoms; compensates for lack of dopamine in Parkinson's disease
dipivefrin ophthalmic	Propine	Alpha agonist (ophthalmic)	Treats glaucoma; decreases fluid production and/or increases fluid drainage
dipyridamole	Persantine	Antiplatelet agent	Prevents blood clot formation
docetaxel	Taxotere	Mitotic inhibitor	Treats cancer; stops mitosis or inhibits enzymes from making proteins needed for cell reproduction
docusate	Colace	Osmotic-type laxative	Increases water in the intestinal tract to soften or increase number of bowel movements

Generic Name D—cont'd	Brand Name	Therapeutic Classification	Common Use
donepezil	Aricept	Cholinesterase	Treats dementia associated with Alzheimer's disease
dorzolamide	Trusopt	Carbonic anhydrase inhibitor: topical, oral, or intravenous	Treats glaucoma; decreases fluid production
doxorubicin	Adriamycin	Antitumor antibiotic	Treats cancer; interferes with enzymes involved in DNA replication
doxycycline	Microdox, Periostat, Vibramycin	Tetracycline	Antibiotic; inhibits protein synthesis
E			
efavirenz	Sustiva	Antiretroviral; non-nucleoside reverse transcriptase inhibitor (NNRTI)	Prevents the HIV virus from spreading
enalapril	Vasotec	Angiotensin-converting enzyme (ACE) inhibitor	Lowers angiotensin II levels; expands blood vessels and decreases resistance
enoxaparin	Lovenox	Anticoagulant	Decreases the clotting ability of the blood
epinephrine ophthalmic	Epifrin	Alpha agonist (ophthalmic)	Treats glaucoma; decreases fluid production and/or increases fluid drainage
epirubicin	Ellence	Antitumor antibiotic	Treats cancer; interferes with enzymes involved in DNA replication
eprosartan	Teveten	Angiotensin II receptor blocker/inhibitor	Prevents effects of angiotensin II; keeps blood pressure from rising
erythromycin	E-Mycin, Pediazole	Macrolide	Antibiotic; inhibits protein synthesis
erythromycin ophthalmic	Ilotycin, Romycin	Antibiotic (ophthalmic)	Treats blepharitis, conjunctivitis, and keratitis; kills or inhibits spread of bacteria
esomeprazole	Nexium	Proton pump inhibitor	Decreases amount of acid in the stomach
estramustine	Emcyt	Mitotic inhibitor	Treats cancer; stops mitosis or inhibits enzymes from making proteins needed for cell reproduction
etanercept	Enbrel	Immunosuppressant	Treats rheumatoid arthritis and psoriasis; blocks tumor necrosis factor (TNF)
ethinyl estradiol/ drospirenone	Beyaz, Yasmine, Yaz	Contraceptive	Prevents ovulation

Continued

Generic Name E—cont'd	Brand Name	Therapeutic Classification	Common Use
ethinyl estradiol/ levonorgestrel	Alesse, Aviane, Lutera, Seasonique	Contraceptive	Prevents ovulation
ethinyl estradiol/ norgestimate	Ortho Tri-Cyclen, Sprintec, TriNessa	Contraceptive	Prevents ovulation
etravirine	Intelence	Antiretroviral; non-nucleoside reverse transcriptase inhibitor (NNRTI)	Prevents the HIV virus from spreading
exenatide	Byetta	Incretin mimetic	Increases insulin release
F			
famotidine	Pepcid	Histamine-2 blocker	Blocks histamine to reduce stomach acidity
felodipine	Plendil	Calcium channel blocker	Interrupts movement of calcium into cells; decreases the heart's pumping strength and relaxes blood vessels
fentanyl	Actiq, Duragesic, Fentora	Opioid/Narcotic analgesic	Relieves moderate to severe pain
fesoterodine	Toviaz	Antispasmodic	Treats urinary incontinence; prevents uncontrollable bladder contractions
fexofenadine	Allegra	Antihistamine	Relieves allergy symptoms
flurbiprofen	Ocufen	NSAID (ophthalmic)	Decreases inflammation and reduces pain
fluconazole	Diflucan	Antifungal agent	Interferes with the formation of the fungal cell membrane
fludarabine	Fludara	Antimetabolite	Treats cancer; interferes with DNA and RNA through substitution of the building blocks
fluticasone	Flovent	Steroid	Prevents inflammation; prevents asthma attack
fluticasone (steroid) and salmeterol	Advair	Long-acting beta-adrenergic agonist bronchodilator	Dilates, or opens up, bronchi for long-term control of asthma symptoms
fluvastatin	Lescol	Cholesterol-lowering agent	Lowers LDL (bad) cholesterol; raises HDL (good) cholesterol; lowers triglyceride levels
formoterol	Foradil, Perforomist	Long-acting beta-adrenergic agonist bronchodilator	Dilates, or opens up, bronchi for long-term control of asthma symptoms
fosamprenavir	Lexiva	Antiretroviral; nucleoside reverse transcriptase inhibitor (NRTI)	Prevents the HIV virus from spreading

Generic Name F—cont'd	Brand Name	Therapeutic Classification	Common Use
fosinopril	Monopril	Angiotensin-converting enzyme (ACE) inhibitors	Lowers angiotensin II levels; expands blood vessels and decreases resistance
furosemide	Lasix	Diuretic: loop, thiazide, or potassium sparing	Removes excess fluids and sodium from the body; relieves the heart's workload; increases urine flow
G			
galantamine	Razadyne	Cholinesterase inhibitor	Treats dementia associated with Alzheimer's disease
gatifloxacin ophthalmic	Zymaxid	Antibiotic (ophthalmic)	Treats blepharitis, conjunctivitis, and keratitis; kills or inhibits spread of bacteria
gefitinib	Iressa	Targeted therapy; signal transduction inhibitor	Attacks specific cancer cells
gemcitabine	Gemzar	Antimetabolite	Treats cancer; interferes with DNA and RNA through substitution of the building blocks
glargine	Lantus	Insulin	Insulin replacement; helps glucose get into cells
glimepiride	Amaryl	Sulfonylurea	Increases insulin production by the pancreas
glipizide	Glucotrol	Sulfonylurea	Increases insulin production by the pancreas
glucagon	None	Hormone	Treats severe hypoglycemia; increases blood glucose
glyburide	DiaBeta, Glynase, Micronase	Sulfonylurea	Increases insulin production by the pancreas
guaifenesin	Guiatuss, Mucinex, Organidin, Robitussin	Expectorant	Relieves congestion by thinning and loosening mucus in the airways
H			
haloperidol	Haldol	Miscellaneous antipsychotic agent	Treats dementia
heparin	None	Anticoagulant	Decreases the clotting ability of the blood
homatropine	Isopto Homatropine	Cycloplegic mydriatic	Dilates the pupil and/or causes temporary paralysis of accommodation during eye exam or procedure
human chorionic gonadotropin (hCG)	Chorex, Novarel, Ovidrel, Profasi, Pregnyl	Gonadotropin	Stimulates ovulation

Continued

Generic Name H—cont'd	Brand Name	Therapeutic Classification	Common Use
humulin	None	Combination isophane/ Regular insulin	Insulin replacement; helps glucose get into cells
hydralazine	Apresoline	Vasodilator	Relaxes blood vessels and increases blood supply and oxygen to the heart; reduces the heart's workload
hydrochlorothiazide	Esidrix, Hydrodiuril, Microzide	Diuretic: loop, thiazide, or potassium sparing	Removes excess fluids and sodium from the body; relieves the heart's workload; increases urine flow
hydrocodone	Lorcet, Lortab, Norco, Vicodin	Opioid/Narcotic analgesic	Relieves moderate to severe pain
hydrocortisone	Cortaid, Preparation H	Corticosteroid	Reduces inflammation; suppresses the immune system
hydromorphone	Dilaudid, Exalgo	Opioid/Narcotic analgesic	Relieves moderate to severe pain
hydroxyurea	Hydrea	Antimetabolite	Treats cancer; interferes with DNA and RNA through substitution of the building blocks

I

Generic Name	Brand Name	Therapeutic Classification	Common Use
ibandronate	Boniva	Bisphosphonate	Treats osteoporosis; increases bone density
ibuprofen	Motrin	Nonsteroidal anti-inflammatory drug (NSAID)	Reduces inflammation, pain, and fever
idarubicin	Idamycin	Antitumor antibiotic	Treats cancer; interferes with enzymes involved in DNA replication
imatinib	Gleevec	Targeted therapy; tyrosine kinase inhibitor	Attacks specific cancer cells
indapamide	Lozol	Diuretic (water pill)	Removes excess fluids and sodium from the body; relieves the heart's workload
indinavir	Crixivan	Antiretroviral; nucleoside reverse transcriptase inhibitor (NRTI)	Prevents the HIV virus from spreading
indomethacin	Indocin	Nonsteroidal anti-inflammatory drug (NSAID)	Reduces inflammation, pain, and fever
interferon-alfa	Intron A, Roferon-A	Immunotherapy	Stimulates the immune system to recognize and attack cancer cells
interferon beta	Avonex, Betaseron, Extavia, Rebif	Manufactured protein	Slows the progression of multiple sclerosis

Generic Name *I—cont'd*	Brand Name	Therapeutic Classification	Common Use
ifosfamide	Ifex	Alkylating agent	Treats cancer; prevents cancer cells from multiplying by directly damaging the DNA in the cell
ipratropium	Atrovent	Anticholinergic bronchodilator	Relaxes the smooth muscle of the bronchi
irbesartan	Avapro	Angiotensin II receptor blocker/inhibitor	Prevents effects of angiotensin II; keeps blood pressure from rising
isoproterenol	Isuprel	Short-acting bronchodilator	Dilates, or opens up, bronchi for quick relief of acute asthma symptoms
isosorbide dinitrate	Isordil	Vasodilator	Relaxes blood vessels and increases blood supply and oxygen to the heart; reduces the heart's workload
ixabepilone	Ixempra	Mitotic inhibitor	Treats cancer; stops mitosis or inhibits enzymes from making proteins needed for cell reproduction
K			
kaolin and pectin	Kaopectate	Antidiarrheal	Reduces diarrhea by slowing forward propulsion of intestinal contents
ketoconazole	Nizoral	Antifungal agent	Kills fungus or prevents its growth
ketoprofen	Orudis	Nonsteroidal anti-inflammatory drug (NSAID)	Reduces inflammation, pain, and fever
ketorolac	Toradol	Nonsteroidal anti-inflammatory drug (NSAID)	Reduces inflammation, pain, and fever
ketorolac tromethamine	Acular	NSAID (ophthalmic)	Decreases inflammation and reduces pain
L			
lanoxin	None	Digitalis preparation	Increases the force of the heart's contractions
lanreotide	Somatuline	Growth hormone antagonist	Decreases production of growth hormone
lansoprazole	Prevacid	Proton pump inhibitor	Decreases amount of acid in the stomach
latanoprost	Xalatan	Prostaglandin (ophthalmic)	Treats glaucoma; increases fluid drainage
lenalidomide	Revlimid	Immunotherapy	Stimulates the immune system to recognize and attack cancer cells

Continued

Generic Name L—cont'd	Brand Name	Therapeutic Classification	Common Use
levalbuterol	Xopenex	Short-acting bronchodilator	Dilates, or opens up, bronchi for quick relief of acute asthma symptoms
levobunolol HCL ophthalmic	Betagan	Beta blocker (ophthalmic)	Treats glaucoma; decreases fluid production
levofloxacin	Levaquin	Fluoroquinolone	Antibiotic; prevents growth of bacteria
levofloxacin ophthalmic	Iquix, Quixin	Antibiotic (ophthalmic)	Treats blepharitis, conjunctivitis, and keratitis; kills or inhibits spread of bacteria
levothyroxine	Levothroid, Levoxyl, Synthroid, Unithroid	Synthetic hormone	Replaces or provides more thyroid hormone
lidocaine	Akten	Local anesthetic (ophthalmic)	Blocks pain signals in the eye before eye exam or surgical procedure
liothyronine	Cytomel	Synthetic hormone	Replaces or provides more thyroid hormone
liraglutide	Victoza	Incretin mimetic	Increases insulin release
lisinopril	Prinivil, Zestril	Angiotensin-converting enzyme (ACE) inhibitor	Lowers angiotensin II levels; expands blood vessels and decreases resistance
lispro	Humalog	Insulin	Insulin replacement; helps glucose get into cells
lomustine	CeeNU	Alkylating agent	Treats cancer; prevents cancer cells from multiplying by directly damaging the DNA in the cell
loperamide	Imodium	Antidiarrheal	Reduces diarrhea by slowing forward propulsion of intestinal contents
loratadine	Claritin	Antihistamine	Relieves allergy symptoms
losartan	Cozaar	Angiotensin II receptor blocker/inhibitor	Prevents effects of angiotensin II; keeps blood pressure from rising
lovastatin	Altoprev, Mevacor	Cholesterol-lowering agent	Lowers LDL (bad) cholesterol; raises HDL (good) cholesterol; lowers triglyceride levels
M			
magnesium sulfate	None	Uterine relaxant	Inhibits uterine muscle contractions
mechlorethamine	Mustargen	Alkylating agent	Treats cancer; prevents cancer cells from multiplying by directly damaging the DNA in the cell

Generic Name M—cont'd	Brand Name	Therapeutic Classification	Common Use
meclizine	Antivert	Antiemetic	Prevents or treats nausea and vomiting
medroxyprogesterone	Depo-Provera, Provera	Contraceptive	Prevents ovulation
melphalan	Alkeran	Alkylating agent	Treats cancer; prevents cancer cells from multiplying by directly damaging the DNA in the cell
memantine	Namenda	Miscellaneous CNS agent	Treats dementia associated with Alzheimer's disease
menotropins	Menopur, Repronex	Gonadotropin	Stimulates ovulation
meperidine	Demerol	Opioid/Narcotic analgesic	Relieves moderate to severe pain
metaxalone	Skelaxin	Skeletal muscle relaxant	Reduces tone in skeletal muscle; decreases muscle pain
metformin	Glucophage, Glumetza, Fortamet, Riomet	Biguanide	Controls (lowers) high blood sugar
methadone	Dolophine, Methadose	Opioid/Narcotic analgesic	Relieves moderate to severe pain
methazolamide	Neptazane	Carbonic anhydrase inhibitor: topical, oral, or intravenous	Treats glaucoma; decreases fluid production
methimazole	Tapazole	Antithyroid agent	Decreases production of thyroid hormone
methocarbamol	Robaxin	Skeletal muscle relaxant	Reduces tone in skeletal muscle; decreases muscle pain
methotrexate	Trexall	Antimetabolite	Treats cancer; interferes with DNA and RNA through substitution of the building blocks
			Psoriasis; interferes with the growth of skin cells
methotrexate	Rheumatrex, Trexall	Disease-modifying antirheumatic drug (DMARD), immunosuppressive	Treats rheumatoid arthritis; prevents organ transplant rejection
methylprednisolone	Medrol, Solu-Medrol	Corticosteroid	Reduces inflammation; suppresses the immune system
metipranolol	OptiPranolol	Beta blocker (ophthalmic)	Treats glaucoma; decreases fluid production
metoprolol	Lopressor, Toprol-XL	Beta blocker/Beta-adrenergic blocking agent	Decreases heart rate and cardiac output
miglitol	Glyset	Alpha-glucosidase inhibitor	Slows digestion of complex carbohydrates

Continued

Generic Name *M—cont'd*	Brand Name	Therapeutic Classification	Common Use
mitomycin-c	Mutamycin	Antitumor antibiotic	Treats cancer; interferes with enzymes involved in DNA replication
moexipril	Univasc	Angiotensin-converting enzyme (ACE) inhibitor	Lowers angiotensin II levels; expands blood vessels and decreases resistance
mometasone furoate monohydrate	Nasonex	Steroid	Relieves nasal allergy symptoms; reduces nasal polyps
montelukast	Singulair	Leukotriene inhibitor	Prevents asthma attacks
morphine	None	Opioid/Narcotic analgesic	Relieves moderate to severe pain
moxifloxacin hydrochloride ophthalmic	Moxeza, Vigamox	Antibiotic (ophthalmic)	Treats blepharitis, conjunctivitis, and keratitis; kills or inhibits spread of bacteria
mupirocin	Bactroban, Centany	Antibacterial	Kills bacteria or prevents its growth
N			
nabumetone	Relafen	Nonsteroidal anti-inflammatory drug (NSAID)	Reduces inflammation, pain, and fever
nadolol	Corgard	Beta blocker/Beta-adrenergic blocking agent	Decreases heart rate and cardiac output
naproxen	Aleve, Naprosyn	Nonsteroidal anti-inflammatory drug (NSAID)	Reduces inflammation, pain, and fever
nateglinide	Starlix	Meglitinide	Increases insulin production by the pancreas
nelfinavir	Viracept	Antiretroviral; nucleoside reverse transcriptase inhibitor (NRTI)	Prevents the HIV virus from spreading
neomycin	Neo-Fradin, Mycifradin	Aminoglycoside	Antibiotic; inhibits protein synthesis
nepafenac	Nevanac	NSAID (ophthalmic)	Decreases inflammation and reduces pain
nesiritide	Natrecor	Vasodilator	Relaxes blood vessels and increases blood supply and oxygen to the heart; reduces the heart's workload
nevirapine	Viramune	Antiretroviral; non-nucleoside reverse transcriptase inhibitor (NNRTI)	Prevents the HIV virus from spreading
nifedipine	Adalat, Procardia	Calcium channel blocker	Interrupts movement of calcium into cells; decreases the heart's pumping strength and relaxes blood vessels

Generic Name N—cont'd	Brand Name	Therapeutic Classification	Common Use
nimodipine	Nimotop, Nymalize	Calcium channel blocker	Treats subarachnoid hemorrhage; interrupts movement of calcium into cells; decreases the heart's pumping strength and relaxes blood vessels
nisoldipine	Sular	Calcium channel blocker	Interrupts movement of calcium into cells; decreases the heart's pumping strength and relaxes blood vessels
nitrate	None	Vasodilator	Relaxes blood vessels and increases blood supply and oxygen to the heart; reduces the heart's workload
nitroglycerin	None	Vasodilator	Relaxes blood vessels and increases blood supply and oxygen to the heart; reduces the heart's workload
novolin	None	Combination isophane/regular insulin	Insulin replacement; helps glucose get into cells

O

octreotide	Sandostatin	Growth hormone antagonist	Decreases production of growth hormone
omeprazole	Prilosec	Proton pump inhibitor	Decreases amount of acid in the stomach
orphenadrine	Norflex	Skeletal muscle relaxant	Reduces tone in skeletal muscle; decreases muscle pain
oseltamivir phosphate	Tamiflu	Anti-influenza agent, antiviral (not a vaccine)	Relieves symptoms and reduces the duration of certain types of influenza
oxaprozin	Daypro	Nonsteroidal anti-inflammatory drug (NSAID)	Reduces inflammation, pain, and fever
oxybutynin	Ditropan, Oxytrol	Antispasmodic	Treats urinary incontinence; prevents uncontrollable bladder contractions
oxycodone	Oxycontin, Oxyfast, Percocet, Roxicodone	Opioid/Narcotic analgesic	Relieves moderate to severe pain
oxymorphone	Opana	Opioid/Narcotic analgesic	Relieves moderate to severe pain
oxytocin	Pitocin, Syntocinon	Uterine stimulant	Stimulates uterine muscle contractions

Continued

Generic Name P	Brand Name	Therapeutic Classification	Common Use
paclitaxel	Taxol	Mitotic inhibitor	Treats cancer; stops mitosis or inhibits enzymes from making proteins needed for cell reproduction
pemetrexed	Alimta	Antimetabolite	Treats cancer; interferes with DNA and RNA through substitution of the building blocks
pentostatin	Nipent	Antimetabolite	Treats cancer; interferes with DNA and RNA through substitution of the building blocks
perindopril	Aceon	Angiotensin-converting enzyme (ACE) inhibitor	Lowers angiotensin II levels; expands blood vessels and decreases resistance
phenylephrine	Mydfrin	Cycloplegic mydriatic	Dilates the pupil and/or causes temporary paralysis of accommodation during eye exam or procedure
phosphorated carbohydrate solution	Emetrol	Antiemetic	Prevents or treats nausea and vomiting
pilocarpine	Isopto Carpine, Pilocar, Pilopine	Cholinergic	Treats glaucoma; increases fluid drainage
pioglitazone	Actos	Thiazolidinedione	Lowers insulin resistance; reduces glucose
pirbuterol	Maxair	Short-acting bronchodilator	Dilates, or opens up, bronchi for quick relief of acute asthma symptoms
piroxicam	Feldene	Nonsteroidal anti-inflammatory drug (NSAID)	Reduces inflammation, pain, and fever
pitavastatin	Livalo	Cholesterol-lowering agent	Lowers LDL (bad) cholesterol; raises HDL (good) cholesterol; lowers triglyceride levels
polyethylene glycol	Miralax	Osmotic-type laxative	Increases water in the intestinal tract to soften or increase number of bowel movements
potassium chloride	Klor-Con, Micro-K	Mineral supplement	Prevents low potassium levels
pramipexole	Mirapex	Dopaminergic antiparkinson agent	Replaces or prevents degradation of dopamine in Parkinson's disease
pravastatin	Pravachol	Cholesterol-lowering agent	Lowers LDL (bad) cholesterol; raises HDL (good) cholesterol; lowers triglyceride levels

Generic Name P—cont'd	Brand Name	Therapeutic Classification	Common Use
prednisolone	Prelone	Corticosteroid	Reduces inflammation; suppresses the immune system
prednisone	Deltasone	Corticosteroid	Reduces inflammation; suppresses the immune system
probenecid	Probalan	Uricosuric agent	Treats gout; lowers uric acid level in the body
procyclidine	Kemadrin	Anticholinergic antiparkinson agent	Compensates for lack of dopamine in Parkinson's disease
promethazine	Phenergan, Promethegan	Antiemetic	Prevents or treats motion sickness, nausea, and vomiting
proparacaine	Alcaine, Ocu-Caine, Ophthetic, Parcaine	Local anesthetic (ophthalmic)	Blocks pain signals in the eye before eye exam or surgical procedure
propranolol	Inderal	Beta blocker/Beta-adrenergic blocking agent	Decreases heart rate and cardiac output
propylthiouracil	None	Antithyroid agent	Decreases production of thyroid hormone
pseudoephedrine	Contac Cold, Drixoral, Neo-Synephrine, Sudafed	Decongestant	Reduces swelling and drainage in the nasal passage
psyllium	Metamucil	Osmotic-type laxative	Increases water in the intestinal tract to soften or increase number of bowel movements
Q			
quinapril	Accupril	Angiotensin-converting enzyme (ACE) inhibitor	Lowers angiotensin II levels; expands blood vessels and decreases resistance
R			
rabeprazole	Aciphex	Proton pump inhibitor	Decreases amount of acid in the stomach
raloxifene	Evista	Selective estrogen receptor modulator	Treats osteoporosis; decreases bone breakdown that occurs after menopause
ramipril	Altace	Angiotensin-converting enzyme (ACE) inhibitor	Lowers angiotensin II levels; expands blood vessels and decreases resistance
repaglinide	Prandin	Meglitinide	Increases insulin production by the pancreas
ranitidine	Zantac	Histamine-2 blocker	Blocks histamine to reduce stomach acidity

Continued

Generic Name	Brand Name	Therapeutic Classification	Common Use
R—cont'd			
rilpivirine	Edurant	Antiretroviral; non-nucleoside reverse transcriptase inhibitor (NNRTI)	Prevents the HIV virus from spreading
rimantadine	Flumadine	Anti-influenza agent, antiviral (not a vaccine)	Relieves symptoms and reduces the duration of certain types of influenza
risedronate	Actonel	Bisphosphonate	Treats osteoporosis; increases bone density
ritonavir	Norvir	Antiretroviral; nucleoside reverse transcriptase inhibitor (NRTI)	Prevents the HIV virus from spreading
rituximab	Rituxan	Immunotherapy	Stimulates the immune system to recognize and attack cancer cells
rivastigmine	Exelon	Cholinesterase inhibitor	Treats dementia associated with Alzheimer's disease
ropinirole	Requip	Dopaminergic antiparkinson agent	Replaces or prevents degradation of dopamine in Parkinson's disease
rosiglitazone	Avandia	Thiazolidinedione	Lowers insulin resistance; reduces glucose
rosuvastatin	Crestor	Cholesterol-lowering agent	Lowers LDL (bad) cholesterol; raises HDL (good) cholesterol; lowers triglyceride levels
S			
salicylic acid	Duofilm, Virasil	Keratolytic	Treats acne, warts; dissolves the substance that causes skin cells to stick together
salmeterol	Serevent	Long-acting beta-adrenergic agonist bronchodilator	Dilates, or opens up, bronchi for long-term control of asthma symptoms
saquinavir	Invirase	Antiretroviral; nucleoside reverse transcriptase inhibitor (NRTI)	Prevents the HIV virus from spreading
scopolamine	Transderm	Antivertigo agent	Treats motion sickness; reduces nausea and vomiting
sildenafil	Viagra	Impotence agent	Causes vasodilation and increases blood flow to penis to cause an erection
simvastatin	Zocor	Cholesterol-lowering agent	Lowers LDL (bad) cholesterol; raises HDL (good) cholesterol; lowers triglyceride levels

Generic Name S—cont'd	Brand Name	Therapeutic Classification	Common Use
simvastatin and ezetimibe	Vytorin	Cholesterol-lowering agent	Lowers LDL (bad) cholesterol; raises HDL (good) cholesterol; lowers triglyceride levels
solifenacin	Vesicare	Antispasmodic	Treats urinary incontinence; prevents uncontrollable bladder contractions
somatropin	Genotropin, Humatrope, Norditropin, Nutropin, Serostim, Zorbtive	Growth hormone	Treats growth failure; increases production of growth hormone
sotalol	Betapace	Beta blocker/Beta-adrenergic blocking agent	Decreases heart rate and cardiac output
spironolactone	Aldactone	Diuretic: loop, thiazide, or potassium sparing	Removes excess fluids and sodium from the body; relieves the heart's workload; increases urine flow
streptomycin	None	Aminoglycoside	Antibiotic; inhibits protein synthesis
streptozotocin	Zanosar	Alkylating agent	Treats cancer; prevents cancer cells from multiplying by directly damaging the DNA in the cell
sulfacetamide sodium ophthalmic	AK-Sulf, Bleph-10, Ocusulf, Sturzsulf, Sulster	Antibiotic (ophthalmic)	Treats blepharitis, conjunctivitis, and keratitis; kills or inhibits spread of bacteria
sulindac	Clinoril	Nonsteroidal anti-inflammatory drug (NSAID)	Reduces inflammation, pain, and fever
sunitinib	Sutent	Targeted therapy	Attacks specific cancer cells
T			
tacrine	Cognex	Cholinesterase inhibitor	Treats dementia associated with Alzheimer's disease
tadalafil	Cialis	Impotence agent	Causes vasodilation and increases blood flow to penis to cause an erection
tafluprost	Zioptan	Prostaglandin (ophthalmic)	Treats glaucoma; increases fluid drainage
tazarotene	Tazorac	Retinoid	Treats acne; decreases inflammation and other skin changes
telmisartan	Micardis	Angiotensin II receptor blocker/inhibitor	Prevents effects of angiotensin II; keeps blood pressure from rising

Continued

Generic Name T—cont'd	Brand Name	Therapeutic Classification	Common Use
terbinafine	Lamisil	Antifungal agent	Kills fungus or prevents its growth
terbutaline	Brethine	Uterine relaxant	Inhibits uterine muscle contractions
teriparatide	Forteo	Parathyroid hormone and analog	Treats osteoporosis; stimulates bone growth and slows bone loss
tetracaine	Altacaine, Opticaine, TetraVisc	Local anesthetic (ophthalmic)	Blocks pain signals in the eye before eye exam or surgical procedure
tetracycline	Panmycin, Sumycin	Tetracycline	Antibiotic; inhibits protein synthesis
thalidomide	Thalomid	Immunotherapy	Stimulates the immune system to recognize and attack cancer cells
thyrocalcitonin	Calcimar, Miacalcin	Calcitonin	Treats osteoporosis; regulates calcium levels
ticlopidine	Ticlid	Platelet aggregation inhibitor	Prevents thrombus formation
timolol	Biocadren	Beta blocker/Beta-adrenergic blocking agent	Decreases heart rate and cardiac output
timolol hemihydrate	Betimol	Beta blocker (ophthalmic)	Treats glaucoma; decreases fluid production
timololmaleate ophthalmic	Timoptic-XE	Beta blocker (ophthalmic)	Treats glaucoma; decreases fluid production
tinzaparin	Innohep	Anticoagulant	Decreases the clotting ability of the blood
tiotropium	Spiriva	Anticholinergic bronchodilator	Relaxes the smooth muscle of the bronchi
tipranavir	Aptivus	Antiretroviral; nucleoside reverse transcriptase inhibitor (NRTI)	Prevents the HIV virus from spreading
tizanidine	Zanaflex	Skeletal muscle relaxant	Reduces tone in skeletal muscle; decreases muscle pain
tobramycin	Nebcin	Aminoglycoside	Antibiotic; inhibits protein synthesis
tobramycin ophthalmic	AKTob, Tobradex	Antibiotic (ophthalmic)	Treats blepharitis, conjunctivitis, and keratitis; kills or inhibits spread of bacteria
tolazamide	None	Sulfonylurea	Increases insulin production by the pancreas
tolbutamide	None	Sulfonylurea	Increases insulin production by the pancreas

Generic Name T—cont'd	Brand Name	Therapeutic Classification	Common Use
tolterodine	Detrol	Antispasmodic	Treats urinary incontinence; prevents uncontrollable bladder contractions
trandolapril	Mavik	Angiotensin-converting enzyme (ACE) inhibitor	Lowers angiotensin II levels; expands blood vessels and decreases resistance
travoprost	Travatan Z	Prostaglandin (ophthalmic)	Treats glaucoma; increases fluid drainage
tretinoin	Atralin, Renova, Retin-A	Differentiating agent, retinoid	Forces cancer cells to mature into normal cells; treats acne; keeps skin pores clear; treats sun damage
trihexyphenidyl	Artane	Anticholinergic antiparkinson agent	Compensates for lack of dopamine in Parkinson's disease
tropicamide	Mydriacyl	Cycloplegic mydriatic	Dilates the pupil and/or causes temporary paralysis of accommodation during eye exam or procedure
U			
urofollitropin	Bravelle, Fertinex, Metrodin	Gonadotropin	Stimulates ovulation
ustekinumab	Stelara	Immunosuppressant	Treats rheumatoid arthritis and psoriasis; blocks tumor necrosis factor (TNF)
V			
valsartan	Diovan	Angiotensin II receptor blocker/inhibitor	Prevents effects of angiotensin II; keeps blood pressure from rising
vardenafil	Levitra	Impotence agent	Causes vasodilation and increases blood flow to penis to cause an erection
verapamil	Calan, Isoptin, Verelan	Calcium channel blocker	Interrupts movement of calcium into cells; decreases the heart's pumping strength and relaxes blood vessels
vinblastine	Velban	Mitotic inhibitor	Treats cancer; stops mitosis or inhibits enzymes from making proteins needed for cell reproduction
vincristine	Oncovin	Mitotic inhibitor	Treats cancer; stops mitosis or inhibits enzymes from making proteins needed for cell reproduction

Continued

Generic Name *V—cont'd*	Brand Name	Therapeutic Classification	Common Use
vinorelbine	Navelbine	Mitotic inhibitor	Treats cancer; stops mitosis or inhibits enzymes from making proteins needed for cell reproduction
W			
warfarin	Coumadin, Jantoven	Coumarin and indandione, anticoagulant	Treats thromboembolic stroke prophylaxis; decreases the clotting ability of the blood
Z			
zanamivir	Relenza	Anti-influenza agent, antiviral (not a vaccine)	Relieves symptoms and reduces the duration of certain types of influenza
zoledronic acid	Reclast	Bisphosphonate	Treats osteoporosis; increases bone density

ABBREVIATIONS

APPENDIX

F

SYMBOLS

~ or ≈	approximately
Δ	change
↓	down, downward, decreased, diminished
♀	female
♂	male
Ø	no, none
#	number (#5) or pounds (5# wt.)
×	number of times (×5, 5×) or minutes (×5 min)
/	per
1°	primary
2°	secondary, secondary to
↔	to and from
→	to, progressing toward, approaching
↑	up, upward, increased
ā	before
c̄	with
p̄	after
s̄	without

A

A&O	alert and oriented
AAROM	active assistive range of motion
AB	antibody, abortion
abd	abdomen, abduction
ABGs	arterial blood gases
AC	axillary crutches
a.c.	before meals
ACL	anterior cruciate ligament
add	adduction
ad lib.	as desired, at discretion
ADH	antidiuretic hormone
ADHD	attention-deficit hyperactivity disorder

ADLs	activities of daily living
AE	above the elbow
AED	automated external defibrillator
AF, A-fib	atrial fibrillation
AFB	acid-fast bacillus
AG, Ag	antigen
AGN	acute glomerulonephritis
AICD	automatic implanted cardioverter defibrillator
AIDS	acquired immune deficiency syndrome
AK	above the knee
AKA	above-the-knee amputation
ALS	amyotrophic lateral sclerosis (Lou Gehrig's disease)
a.m.a.	against medical advice
ANS	autonomic nervous system
ant	anterior
AOM	acute otitis media
AP	anteroposterior
ARDS	acute respiratory distress syndrome
ARF	acute renal failure
AROM	active range of motion
AS	ankylosing spondylitis, astigmatism
ASHD	arteriosclerotic heart disease
ATN	acute tubular necrosis
AV, A-V	atrioventricular

B

BCC	basal cell carcinoma
BE	below the elbow
BG, BS	blood glucose, blood sugar
bid, b.i.d.	twice a day
BK	below the knee
BKA	below-the-knee amputation

BM	bowel movement
BMD	bone mineral density
BMI	body mass index
BMR	basal metabolic rate
BNO	bladder neck obstruction
BOTOX	botulinum toxin
BP	blood pressure
BPH	benign prostatic hypertrophy (benign prostatic hyperplasia)
bpm	beats per minute
BRP	bathroom privileges
B/S	bedside
BSE	breast self-examination
BUN	blood urea nitrogen
Bx, bx	biopsy

C

C&S	culture and sensitivity
C1–C7	first cervical vertebra, second cervical vertebra, etc.
Ca	calcium
CA	cancer, carcinoma
CABG	coronary artery bypass graft
CAD	coronary artery disease
CAT	cataract
cath	catheterization, catheter
CC or c/c	chief complaint
CCU	coronary care unit
CF	cystic fibrosis
CFS	chronic fatigue syndrome
CHF	congestive heart failure
CIRC	circumcision
CK	creatine kinase
CMC	chronic mucocutaneous candidiasis
CNS	central nervous system
c/o	complain (ed/ing/s/t) of
CO^2	carbon dioxide
cont.	continue
COPD	chronic obstructive pulmonary disease
CP	cerebral palsy, chest pain
CPAP	continuous positive airway pressure

CPR	cardiopulmonary resuscitation
CPT	chest physiotherapy
CRF	chronic renal failure
C-section	cesarean section
CSF	cerebrospinal fluid
CT	computed tomography
CTS	carpal tunnel syndrome
CV	cardiovascular
CVA	cerebrovascular accident
CWP	coal worker's pneumoconiosis
CXR	chest x-ray
cysto	cystoscopy

D

D&C	dilation and curettage
D/C or d/c	discharge, discontinue
decub	decubitus ulcer
derm	dermatology
DEXA	dual-energy x-ray absorptiometry
DI	diabetes insipidus
DIC	disseminated intravascular coagulation
DJD	degenerative joint disease (osteoarthritis)
DKA	diabetic ketoacidosis
DM	diabetes mellitus
DME	durable medical equipment
DNR	do not resuscitate
DOB	date of birth
DOE	dyspnea on exertion
DRE	digital rectal examination
DTR	deep tendon reflex
DVT	deep vein thrombosis
Dx	diagnosis

E

EBV	Epstein-Barr virus
ECG, EKG	electrocardiogram
ECHO	echocardiogram
ED	erectile dysfunction
EDC	estimated date of confinement (due date)
EENT	eyes, ears, nose, and throat

EEG	electroencephalography
EGD	esophagogastroduodenoscopy
EIA	enzyme immunosorbent assay
ELOS	estimated length of stay
EM, em	emmetropia
EMG	electromyogram, electromyography
ENT	ears, nose, and throat
EOB	edge of bed
EOM	extraocular movement
ERCP	endoscopic retrograde cholangiopancreatography
ERT, HRT	estrogen replacement therapy, hormone replacement therapy
ESR	erythrocyte sedimentation rate (sed rate)
ESRD	end-stage renal disease
eval.	evaluate, evaluation
ext	extension

F

FBG, FBS	fasting blood glucose, fasting blood sugar
FH	family history
FHR	fetal heart rate
flex	flexion
FSBS	finger stick blood sugar
FWB	full weight bearing
FWW	front wheel walker
Fx	fracture

G

G, glc	glaucoma
GBS	Guillain-Barré syndrome
GC	gonorrheal
GERD	gastroesophageal reflux disease
GH	growth hormone
GI	gastrointestinal
GTT	glucose tolerance test
GU	genitourinary
GVHD	graft-versus-host disease
GYN	gynecology

H

H&P	history and physical
h, hr	hour
H_2O	water
HbA1c	glycosylated hemoglobin
HD	hemodialysis
HF	heart failure
HIV	human immunodeficiency virus
HNP	herniated nucleus pulposus
h/o	history of
HOB	head of bed
HPV	human papilloma virus
HR	heart rate
HRT	hormone replacement therapy
ht.	height
HTN	hypertension (high blood pressure)
HW	hemi walker
Hx, hx	history

I

I&D	incision and drainage
I&O	intake and output
IBD	inflammatory bowel disease
IBS	irritable bowel syndrome
ICP	intracranial pressure
ICU	intensive care unit
ID	intradermal (injection)
IDDM	insulin-dependent diabetes mellitus (type 1 diabetes)
Ig	immunoglobulin
IM	intramuscular
INR	international normalized ratio
IP	ice pack
ITP	idiopathic thrombocytopenic purpura
IUD	intrauterine device
IV	intravenous
IVF	in vitro fertilization
IVP	intravenous pyelogram

J

JRA	juvenile rheumatoid arthritis

K

K	potassium
KS	Kaposi's sarcoma
KUB	kidney, ureter, and bladder

L

L	left
L&D	labor and delivery
L1–L5	first lumbar vertebra, second lumbar vertebra, etc.
LA	left atrium
LASIK	laser-assisted in-situ keratomileusis
lat	lateral
LBQC	large base quad cane
LE	lower extremity
LFT	liver function test
LLE	left lower extremity
LLQ	left lower quadrant
lmp	last menstrual period
LOC	level of consciousness, loss of consciousness
LOS	length of stay
LP	lumbar puncture
LTG	long-term goal
LUE	left upper extremity
LUQ	left upper quadrant
LV	left ventricle

M

MD	macular degeneration, muscular dystrophy
MDI	metered-dose inhaler
med	medial
meds	medications
MET, met	metastasis, metastasize
MHP	moist hot pack
MI	myocardial infarction
MM	malignant melanoma
MMT	manual muscle test
MR	mitral regurgitation
MRI	magnetic resonance imaging
MS	multiple sclerosis, mitral stenosis
MVA	motor vehicle accident
MVP	mitral valve prolapse

N

N&V	nausea and vomiting
Na	sodium
NG, ng	nasogastric
NIDDM	non–insulin-dependent diabetes mellitus (type 2 diabetes)
Noc, noct.	night, at night, in the night
NPO	nothing by mouth
NSAID	nonsteroidal anti-inflammatory drug
NWB	non–weight bearing

O

O^2	oxygen
OA	osteoarthritis
OB-GYN	obstetrics and gynecology
OC	oral contraceptive
OCD	obsessive-compulsive disorder
OOB	out of bed
ORIF	open reduction internal fixation
ortho	orthopedic, straight
OSA	obstructive sleep apnea
OT	occupational therapy
OTC	over-the-counter

P

P	pulse
Pa, P-A	posteroanterior
PAC	premature atrial contraction
PAD	peripheral artery disease
Pap	Papanicolaou smear
pc	after meals
PCP	*Pneumocystis carinii* pneumonia
PE	physical examination, pulmonary embolism
per	through or by
PERRLA	pupils are equal, round, reactive to light and accommodation
PFT	pulmonary function test
pH	potential of hydrogen (measure of acidity or alkalinity)
PID	pelvic inflammatory disease
PKD	polycystic kidney disease
PLOF	prior level of function
PM	polymyositis, afternoon/evening

PMS	premenstrual syndrome
PND	paroxysmal nocturnal dyspnea
PNS	peripheral nervous system
PO, p.o.	orally, by mouth
post.	posterior
post-op	after surgery (operation)
PPD	purified protein derivative (TB test)
PR	per (through the) rectum
pre-op	before surgery (operation)
prn, p.r.n.	as needed
PROM	passive range of motion
PSA	prostate-specific antigen
Pt. or pt.	patient
PT	prothrombin time, physical therapy, physical therapist
PTA	prior to admission, physical therapist assistant
PTCA	percutaneous transluminal coronary angioplasty
PTH	parathyroid hormone
PTT	partial thromboplastin time
PUD	peptic ulcer disease
PUW	pick up walker
PVC	premature ventricular contraction
PWB	partial weight bearing

Q

q	every
q2h	every 2 hours
qam	every morning
qd, q.d.	every day, once daily
qh, q.h.	every hour
qhs, q.h.s.	each evening (hour of sleep)
qid, q.i.d.	four times a day
qod, q.o.d.	every other day

R

R	respiration, right
RA	rheumatoid arthritis, right atrium, room air
RBC	red blood cell, red blood count
RD	retinal detachment
re:	regarding, concerning
RK	radial keratotomy

RLE	right lower extremity
RLQ	right lower quadrant
R/O or r/o	rule out
ROM	range of motion
ROS	review of systems
RP	retrograde pyelogram
RUE	right upper extremity
RUQ	right upper quadrant
RV	right ventricle
Rx	prescription, intervention plan

S

S1–S5	first sacral vertebra, second sacral vertebra, etc.
SBO	small bowel obstruction
SBQC	small base quad cane
SCC	squamous cell carcinoma
SCI	spinal cord injury
SG, sp. gr.	specific gravity
SIDS	sudden infant death syndrome
Sig.	directions for use, give as follows, let it be labeled, write on label
SLE	systemic lupus erythematosus
SOAP	subjective, objective, assessment, plan
SOB	shortness of breath
S/P	status post, no change after
SPC	single point cane
SS	Sjögren's syndrome
stat.	immediately
STD, STI	sexually transmitted disease, sexually transmitted infection
STG	short-term goal
STM	soft tissue mobilization; massage
SubQ	subcutaneous
Sx	symptom(s)

T

T&A	tonsillectomy and adenoidectomy
T1–T12	first thoracic vertebra, second thoracic vertebra, etc.
T3, T4	triiodothyronine, thyroxine (thyroid hormones)
TAH	total abdominal hysterectomy

TAH-BSO	total abdominal hysterectomy, bilateral salpingo-oophorectomy
TAO	thromboangiitis obliterans
TB	tuberculosis
TBI	traumatic brain injury
TEE	transesophageal echocardiography
TENS	transcutaneous electrical nerve stimulation
TGA	transient global amnesia
THA, THR	total hip arthroplasty, total hip replacement
TIA	transient ischemic attack
tid, t.i.d.	three times a day
tiw, t.i.w.	three times a week
TKA, TKR	total knee arthroplasty, total knee replacement
TM	tympanic membrane
TN	trigeminal neuralgia
TO or t.o.	telephone order
tol	tolerate, tolerated, tolerance
TOS	thoracic outlet syndrome
Trich	trichomoniasis
TSE	testicular self-examination
TSH	thyroid-stimulating hormone
TSS	toxic shock syndrome
TTWB	toe touch weight bearing
TURP	transurethral resection of the prostate
TV	tidal volume
Tx	treatment, traction

U

UA	urinalysis
UC	urine culture

UE	upper extremity
UGI	upper GI x-ray
ung.	ointment
URI	upper respiratory infection
UTI	urinary tract infection

V

VA	visual acuity
VC	vital capacity
VCUG	voiding cystourethrography
VD	venereal disease; sexually transmitted disease
V-fib	ventricular fibrillation
VO or v.o.	verbal order
VS	vital signs
V^T	tidal volume
VT, V-tach	ventricular tachycardia
VTE	venous thromboembolism
VUR	vesicoureteral reflux

W

WBAT	weight bearing as tolerated
WBC	white blood cell, white blood count
WC	wheelchair
wt.	weight

Y

y/o	years old

DISCONTINUED ABBREVIATIONS

The following abbreviations may be found in current medical records. However, the use of these terms is strongly discouraged because of the high rate of errors in transcription or interpretation.

Discontinued Abbreviation	Rationale	Replacement
AD: right ear	Mistaken for: AS, AU, OD, OS, OU	Write: right ear
AS: left ear	Mistaken for: AD, AU, OD, OS, OU	Write: left ear
AU: both ears	Mistaken for: U (units) when poorly written	Write: both ears
cc: cubic centimeter	Mistaken for: U (units) when poorly written	Write: mL
dc, DC, D/C: discharge or discontinue	Mistaken for: each other	Write: discharge or discontinue
IU: international unit	Mistaken for: IV	Write: international unit
$MgSO_4$: magnesium sulfate	Mistaken for: MSO_4	Write: magnesium sulfate
MS, MSO_4: morphine	Mistaken for: $MgSO_4$	Write: morphine sulfate
OD: right eye	Mistaken for: AD, AS, AU, OS, OU	Write: right eye
OS: left eye	Mistaken for: AD, AS, AU, OD, OU	Write: left eye
OU: both eyes	Mistaken for: AD, AS, AU, OD, OS	Write: both eyes
qd.: every day	Mistaken for: q.o.d.	Write: daily
qod.: every other day	Mistaken for: q.d. or q.i.d.	Write: every other day
SC, SQ: subcutaneous	Mistaken for: SL (sublingual) or 5 every	Write: subcut. or subcutaneous, SubQ or Sub-Q
ss: sliding scale	Mistaken for: 55	Write: sliding scale
u: unit	Mistaken for: 0, 4, or cc	Write: unit
µg: microgram	Mistaken for: mg	Write: mcg
<,>: less than, greater than	Mistaken for: each other	Write: less than or greater than
trailing zero (4.0 mg)	Decimal point may be missed, resulting in an overdose of 10 times the prescribed amount	Never write an unnecessary zero after a decimal point.
lack of leading zero (.4 mg)	Decimal point may be missed, resulting in an overdose of 10 times prescribed amount	Always use a zero before a decimal point to indicate its presence (0.4 mg).

MEDICAL TERMINOLOGY FAQS

Question: *How do I decide which word part to use when there is more than one choice?*

Answer: *It is often helpful to think of selecting the word part that is the most "user-friendly" to pronounce and that sounds best to the ear.*

Example: Create a term that means "pertaining to the neck."

Choosing a combining form is easy because there is only one, cervic/o, which means "neck." However, there are 12 suffixes that mean "pertaining to." These are listed below with the selected combining form. Try pronouncing each version of the new term listed below. The first one, cervical, is the easiest to pronounce and sounds best to the ear.

> cervical
> cervicac
> cervicar
> cervicary
> cerviceal
> cervicial
> cervicic
> cervicical
> cervicory
> cervicous
> cervicotic
> cervicotous

Question: *What if two options seem equally correct and desirable?*

Answer: *Use the term preferred by your colleagues or facility.*

Example: Create a term that means "pain of the neck."

There are two possible options: cervicalgia and cervicodynia. Either one is technically correct. There is no harm in asking a colleague which term should be used. As you converse with and listen to your fellow medical professionals, you will quickly learn the preferred terminology.

Question: *When a term includes more than one combining form, how do I know what order to put them in?*

Answer: *If the term refers to a procedure, place the word parts in the order that corresponds with the procedure. If the term pertains to anatomy, move from most proximal to most distal.*

Example: Create a term that means "visual examination of the esophagus, stomach, and duodenum."

As this procedure is performed, the scope first enters the esophagus, then the stomach, and then the duodenum. So when you create the medical term, put the word parts in the same order (with the suffix last): esophag/o, gastr/o, duoden/o,-scopy.

Question: *I hear some terms pronounced in more than one way. How do I know which pronunciation is correct?*

Answer: *First, refer to the pronunciation guide in this book. It should guide you in most cases. Second, in some cases, more than one pronunciation may be considered acceptable. Third, remember that the most common mistake people make is to emphasize the wrong syllable. When word parts are linked with a combining vowel (usually o), the emphasis is usually on the syllable with the combining vowel.*

Example: The tendency is to pronounce colonoscopy as kō-lŏn-ō-SKŌ-pē. But the correct pronunciation is kō-lŏn-ŎS-kō-pē.

SUFFIX AND PREFIX MASTER LIST

SUFFIXES THAT INDICATE MEDICAL SPECIALTY

Suffix	Pronunciation	Meaning
-iatrics,-iatry	ī-ă-trĭks, ī-ă-trē	field of medicine
-iatrist,-ician,-ist	ī-ă-trĭst, ĭ-shŭn, ĭst	specialist
-logist,-ologist	lō-jĭst, ŏl-ō-jĭst	specialist in the study of
-logy,-ology	lō-jē, ŏl-ō-jē	study of

SUFFIXES THAT INDICATE SURGERIES, PROCEDURES, OR TREATMENTS

Suffix	Pronunciation	Meaning
-centesis	sĕn-tē-sĭs	surgical puncture
-cidal,-cide	sī-dăl, sīd	destroying, killing
-desis	dē-sĭs	surgical fixation of bone or joint, binding, tying together
-dilation	dī-lā-shŭn	widening, stretching, expanding
-ectomy	ĕk-tō-mē	excision, surgical removal
-graphy	gră-fē	process of recording
-metry	mĕ-trē	measurement
-pexy	pĕk-sē	surgical fixation
-plasty	plăs-tē	surgical repair
-rrhaphy	ră-fē	suture, suturing
-scopy	skō-pē	visual examination
-therapy	thĕr-ă-pē	treatment
-tomy	tō-mē	cutting into, incision
-tripsy	trĭp-sē	crushing

SUFFIXES THAT INDICATE SENSORY EXPERIENCE, SENSATION, OR SUBJECTIVE FEELING

Suffix	Pronunciation	Meaning
-acusia,-acusis,-cusis	ă-koo-zē-ă, ă-koo-sĭs, koo-sĭs	hearing
-algesia,-algesic,-algia,-dynia	ăl-jē-zē-ă, ăl-jē-zĭk, ăl-jē-ă, dĭ-nē-ă	pain
-dipsia	dĭp-sē-ă	thirst
-esthesia	ĕs-thē-zē-ă	sensation
-opia,-opsia,-opsis,-opsy	ō-pē-ă, ōp-sē-ă, ŏp-sĭs, ŏp-sē	vision, view of
-osmia	ŏz-mē-ă	smell, odor
-phobia	fō-bē-ă	fear
-phoria	fō-rē-ă	feeling

SUFFIXES THAT INDICATE ACTION OR MOVEMENT

Suffix	Pronunciation	Meaning
-clasis,-clast	klăs-ĭs, klăst	to break
-ectasis	ĕk-tă-sĭs	dilation, expansion
-emesis	ĕm-ĕ-sĭs	vomiting
-gen, -genesis, -genic, -genous	jĕn, jĕn-ĕ-sĭs, jĕn-ĭk, jĕn-ŭs	creating, producing
-kinesia, -kinesis	kĭ-nē-zē-ă, kĭ-nē-sĭs	movement
-lysis	lĭ-sĭs	destruction
-pause, -stasis	pawz, stă-sĭs	cessation, stopping
-phage, -phagia	fāj, fā-jē-ă	eating, swallowing
-phasia	fā-zē-ă	speech
-rrhage, -rrhagia	rĭj, ră-jē-ă	bursting forth
-rrhea	rē-ă	flow, discharge
-rrhexis	rĕk-sĭs	rupture
-spasm	spă-zŭm	sudden involuntary contraction
-uresis	ū-rē-sĭs	urination

SUFFIXES THAT INDICATE DISEASES, DISORDERS, OR CONDITIONS

Suffix	Pronunciation	Meaning
-cele	sēl	hernia
-constriction	kŏn-strĭk-shŭn	narrowing
-cytosis	sī-tō-sĭs	a condition of cells
-derma	dĕr-mă	skin
-edema	ĕ-dē-mă	swelling
-emia	ē-mē-ă	a condition of the blood
-gravida	gră-vĭ-dă	pregnant woman
-ia,-ism	ē-ă, ĭz-ŭm	condition
-iasis	ī-ă-sĭs	pathological condition or state
-it is	ī-tĭs	inflammation
-lepsy,-leptic	lĕp-sē, lĕp-tĭk	seizure
-lith	lĭth	stone
-malacia	mă-lā-sē-ă	softening
-megaly	mĕg-ă-lē	enlargement
-necrosis	nĕ-krō-sĭs	tissue death
-oid	oyd	resembling
-oma	ō-mă	tumor
-osis	ō-sĭs	abnormal condition
-oxia	ŏk-sē-ă	oxygen
-paresis	pă-rē-sĭs	slight or partial paralysis
-partum,-tocia	părt-ŭm, tō-sē-ă	childbirth, labor
-pathy	pă-thē	disease
-penia	pē-nē-ă	deficiency
-pepsia	pĕp-sē-ă	digestion
-phonia	fō-nē-ă	voice
-plasia,-plasm	plā-zē-ă, plăz-ŭm	formation, growth
-plastic	plăs-tĭk	pertaining to formation or growth
-plegia	plē-jē-ă	paralysis
-plegic	plē-jĭk	pertaining to paralysis
-pnea	nē-ă	breathing
-pneic	nē-ĭk	pertaining to breathing
-ptosis	tō-sĭs	drooping, prolapse
-salpinx	săl-pĭnks	uterine (fallopian) tube
-sclerosis	sklĕ-rō-sĭs	hardening
-static	stă-tĭk	not in motion, at rest
-stenosis	stĕ-nō-sĭs	narrowing, stricture
-thorax	thōr-ăks	chest
-trophy	trō-fē	nourishment, growth
-uria	ū-rē-ă	urine

SUFFIXES THAT INDICATE INSTRUMENTS

Suffix	Pronunciation	Meaning
-graph	grăf	recording instrument
-meter	mĕ-tĕr	measuring instrument
-scope	skōp	viewing instrument
-tome	tōm	cutting instrument

SUFFIXES THAT MEAN "PERTAINING TO"

Suffix	Pronunciation	Meaning
-ac,-al,-ar, -eal	ăk, ăl, ăr, ăr-ē, ē-ăl, ē-ăl	pertaining to
-ial,-ic,-ical, -ory,-ous	ĭk, ĭ-kăl, ō-rē, ŭs, tĭk, tŭs	
-tic*,-tous*		

*-tic, a variation of-ic, is sometimes used; -tous, a variation of-ous, is sometimes used.

OTHER SUFFIXES

Suffix	Pronunciation Guide	Meaning
-cyte,-cytic	sīt, sīt-ĭk	cell
-gram	grăm	record
-ole,-ule	ōl, ūl	small
-prandial	prăn-dē-ăl	meal
-stomy	stō-mē	mouthlike opening

PREFIXES THAT INDICATE SIZE, QUANTITY, OR NUMBER

Prefix	Pronunciation	Meaning
a-, an-, in-	ā, ăn, ĭn	without, not, absence of
ambi-	ăm-bē	both, both sides, around, about
bi-	bī	two
di-	dī	twice, two, double
hemi-, semi-	hĕm-ē, sĕm-ē	half
iso-	ī-sō	same, equal
macro-	mă-krō	large
micro-	mī-krō	small
mono-, uni-	mŏ-nō, ū-nĭ	one, single
multi-	mŭl-tē	many
poly-	pŏ-lē	much
oligo-	ō-lĭ-gō	deficiency
pan-	păn	all
quadri-, tetra-	kwŏ-drĭ, tĕ-tră	four
tri-	trī	three

PREFIXES THAT INDICATE LOCATION, DIRECTION, OR TIMING

Prefix	Pronunciation	Meaning
ab-	āb	away from
ad-	ād	toward
anti-	ăn-tē	against
brady-	bră-dē	slow
con-	kŏn	together, with
contra-	kŏn-tră	against, opposite
circum-	sĕr-kŭm	around
dia-, trans-	dī-ă, trănz	through, across
ec-, ecto-	ĕk, ĕk-tō	out, outside
en-, end-, endo-, in-, intra-	ĕn, ĕnd, ĕn-dō, ĭn, ĭn-tră	in, within, inner
epi-	ĕ-pĭ	above, upon
eso-	ĕs-ō	inward
ex-, exo-, extra-	ĕks, ĕk-sō, ĕk-stră	away from, outside, external
hyper-, super-, supra-	hī-pĕr, soo-pĕr, soo-pră	excessive, above
hypo-, infra-, sub-	hī-pō, ĭn-fră, sŭb	below, beneath
inter-	ĭn-tĕr	between
para-, peri-	pă-ră, pĕr-ĭ	beside, near
post-	pōst	after, following
pre-	prē	before
pro-	prō	before, forward
re-, retro-	rē, rĕ-trō	behind, back
tachy-	tăk-ē	rapid
ultra-	ŭl-tră	beyond

OTHER PREFIXES

Prefix	Pronunciation	Meaning
auto-	aw-tō	self
dys-	dĭs	bad, painful, difficult
eu-	ū	good, normal
mal-	măl	bad, inadequate
neo-	nē-ō	new
tox-	tŏks	poison, toxin

INDEX

Page numbers followed by "f" indicate figures; those followed by "t" indicate tables.

epi-
ĕp-ĭ

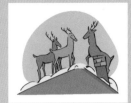

post-
pōst

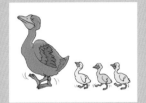

anti- **contra-**
ăn-tē kŏn-tră

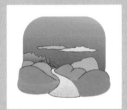

circum-
sĕr-kŭm

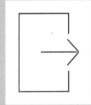

ab-
ăb

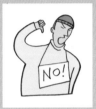

ex- **exo-** **extra-**
ĕks ĕks-ō ĕks-tră

mal-
măl

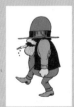

dys-
dĭs

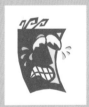

pre-
prē

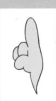

pro-
prō

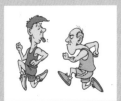

after, following

above, upon

around

against, opposite

away from, outside, external

away from

bad, painful, difficult

bad, inadequate

before, forward

before

re- **retro-**
rē rĕt-rō

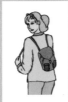

hypo- **sub-** **infra-**
hī-pō sŭb ĭn-fră

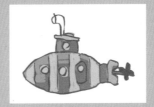

para- **peri-**
păr-ă pĕr-ĭ

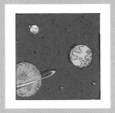

inter-
ĭn-tĕr

ultra-
ŭl-tră

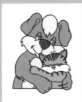

ambi-
ăm-bē

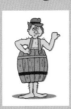

oligo-
ōl-ĭ-gō

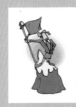

hyper- **super-** **supra-**
hī-pĕr soo-pĕr soo-pră

quadri- **tetra-**
kwŏd-rĭ tĕ-tră

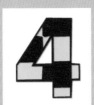

eu-
ū

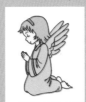

below, beneath	behind, back
between	beside, near
both, both sides, around, about	beyond
excessive, above	deficiency
good, normal	four

hemi- **semi-**
hĕm-ē sĕm-ē

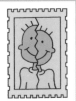

en- **end-** **endo-** **in-** **intra-**
ĕn ĕnd ĕn-dō ĭn ĭn-tră

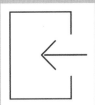

eso-
ĕs-ō

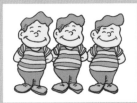

macro-
măk-rō

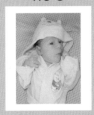

multi- **poly-**
mŭl-tē pŏl-ē

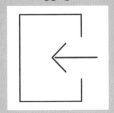

neo-
nē-ō

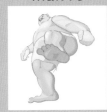

uni- **mono-**
ū-nĭ mŏ-nō

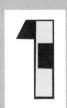

ec- **ecto-**
ĕk ĕk-tō

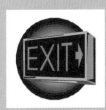

tox-
tŏks

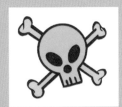

tachy-
tăk-ē

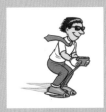

in, within, inner	half
large	inward
new	many, much
out, outside	one, single
rapid	poison, toxin

iso-
ī-sō

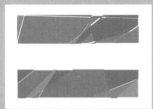

auto-
aw-tō

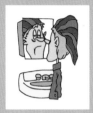

brady-
brăd-ē

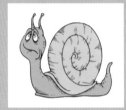

micro-
mī-krō

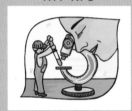

tri-
trī

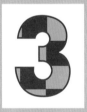

dia-   trans-
dī-ă   trănz

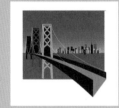

ad-
ăd

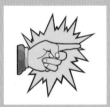

bi-   di-
bī   dī

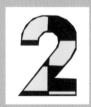

a-   an-   in-
ā   ăn   ĭn

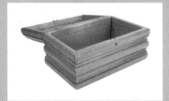

-algesia   -algesic   -algia   -dynia
ăl-jē-zē-ă   ăl-jē-sĭk   ăl-jē-ă   dĭn-ē-ă

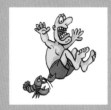

self	same, equal
small	slow
through, across	three
two	toward
pain	without, not, absence of

-cele
sēl

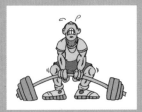

-centesis
sĕn-tē-sĭs

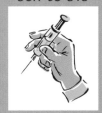

-cidal   **-cide**
sĭ-dăl   sīd

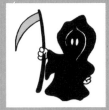

-clasis   **-clast**
klă-sĭs   klăst

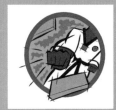

-cyte   **-cytic**
sīt   sīt-ĭk

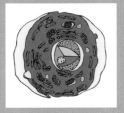

-derma
dĕr-mă

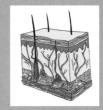

-dipsia
dĭp-sē-ă

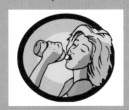

-ectasis
ĕk-tă-sĭs

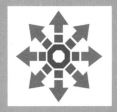

-ectomy
ĕk-tō-mē

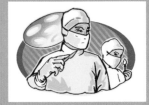

-edema
ĕ-dē-mă

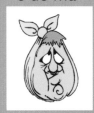

surgical puncture	hernia
to break	destroying, killing
skin	cell
dilation, expansion	thirst
swelling	excision, surgical removal

-emia
ē-mē-ă

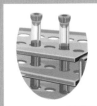

-emesis
ĕm-ĕ-sĭs

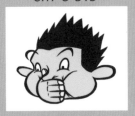

-esthesia
ĕs-thē-zē-ă

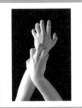

-gen   **-genesis**   **-genic**   **-genous**
jĕn   jĕn-ĕ-sĭs   jĕn-ĭk   jĕn-ŭs

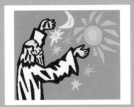

-gram
grăm

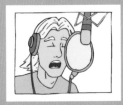

-graph
grăf

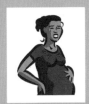

-graphy
gră-fē

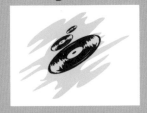

-gravida
grăv-ĭ-dă

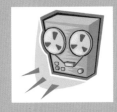

-ia   **-ism**
ē-ă   ĭ-zum

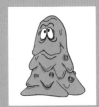

-iasis
ī-ă-sĭs

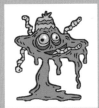

vomiting

a condition of the blood

creating, producing

sensation

recording instrument

record

pregnant woman

process of recording

pathological condition or state

condition

-iatrist **-ician** **-ist** **-logist** **-ologist**
ī-ă-trĭst ĭ-shŭn ĭst lō-jist ŏl-ō-jist

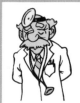

-itis
ī-tĭs

-kinesia **-kinesis**
kĭ-nē-zē-ă kĭ-nē-sĭs

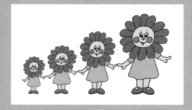

-lith
lĭth

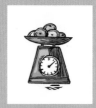

-megaly
mĕg-ă-lē

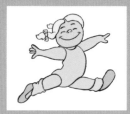

-meter
mĕ-tĕr

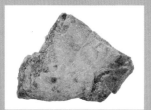

-lysis
lĭ-sĭs

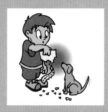

-malacia
mă-lā-sē-ă

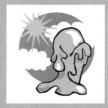

-ole **-ule**
ōl ūl

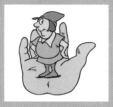

-oma
ō-mă

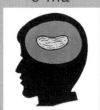

inflammation	specialist, specialist in the study of
stone	movement
measuring instrument	enlargement
softening	destruction
tumor	small

-metry
mĕ-trē

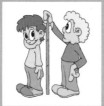

-oid
oyd

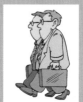

-oxia
ŏk-sē-ă

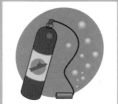

-paresis
păr-ē-sĭs

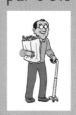

-opia   -opsia   -opsis   -opsy
ō-pē-ă   ōp-sē-ă   ōp-sis   ōp-sē

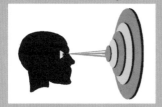

-osis
ō-sĭs

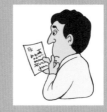

-penia
pē-nē-ă

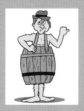

-pepsia
pĕp-sē-ă

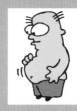

-pathy
pă-thē

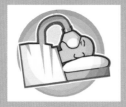

-pause   -stasis
pawz   stă-sĭs

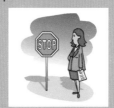

resembling	measurement
slight or partial paralysis	oxygen
abnormal condition	vision, view of
digestion	deficiency
cessation, stopping	disease

-phasia
fā-zē-ă

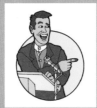

-phobia
fō-bē-ă

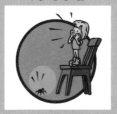

-pexy
pĕk-sē

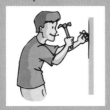

-phage   -phagia
fāj   fā-jē-ă

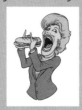

-plasty
plăs-tē

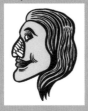

-plegia
plē-jē-ă

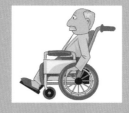

-phoria
fō-rē-ă

-plasia   -plasm
plā-zē-ă   plă-zum

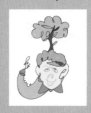

-rrhage   -rrhagia
rĭj   ră-jē-ă

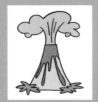

-rrhaphy
ră-fē

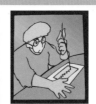

fear

speech

eating, swallowing

surgical fixation

paralysis

surgical repair

formation, growth

feeling

suture, suturing

bursting forth

-pnea
nē-ă

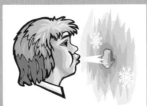

-ptosis
tō-sĭs

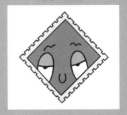

-scope
skōp

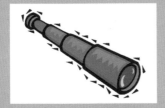

-scopy
skō-pē

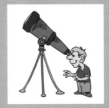

-rrhea
rē-ă

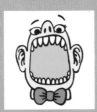

-rrhexis
rĕk-sĭs

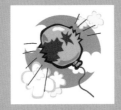

-stomy
stō-mē

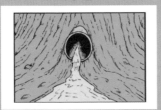

-therapy
thĕr-ă-pē

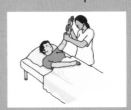

-stenosis
stĕ-nō-sĭs

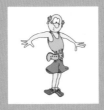

-tripsy
trĭp-sē

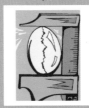

drooping, prolapse

breathing

visual examination

viewing instrument

rupture

flow, discharge

treatment

mouthlike opening

crushing

narrowing, stricture

-trophy
trō-fē

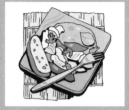

-tome
tōm

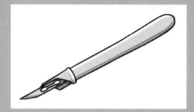

-tomy
tō-mē

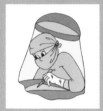

-acusia **-acusis** **-cusis**
ă-koo-zē-ă ă-koo-sĭs koo-sĭs

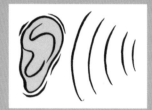

-osmia
ŏz-mē-ă

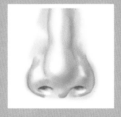

-uria
ū-rē-ă

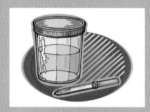

-static
stă-tik

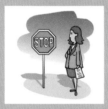

-salpinx
săl-pĭnks

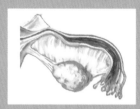

-thorax
thōr-ăks

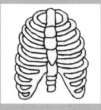

-lepsy **-leptic**
lĕp-sē lĕp-tĭk

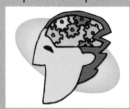

cutting instrument	nourishment, growth
hearing	cutting into, incision
urine	smell, odor
uterine (fallopian tube)	not in motion, at rest
seizure	chest

-phonia
fō-nē-ă

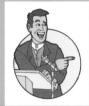

-partum   -tocia
părt-ŭm   tō-sē-ă

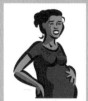

-ac	-al	-ar	-ary	-eal	-ial
ăk	ăl	ăr	ār-ē	ē-ăl	ē-ăl
-ic	**-ical**	**-ory**	**-ous**	**-tic**	**-tous**
ĭk	ĭ-kăl	ō-rē	ŭs	tĭk	tŭs

-iatrics   -iatry
ī-ă-trĭks   ī-ă-trē

-logy   -ology
lō-jē   ŏ-ō-jē

-desis
dē-sĭs

-dilation
dī-lā-shŭn

-spasm
spă-zŭm

-uresis
ū-rē-sĭs

-constriction
kŏn-strĭk-shŭn

childbirth, labor	voice
field of medicine	pertaining to
surgical fixation of bone or joint, binding, tying together	study of
sudden involuntary contraction	widening, stretching, expanding
narrowing	urination

-cytosis
sī-tō-sĭs

-necrosis
nĕ-krō-sĭs

-plastic
plăs-tĭk

-plegic
plē-jĭk

-pneic
nē-ĭk

-sclerosis
sklĕ-rō-sĭs

-prandial
prăn-dē-ăl

abduction

adduction

anterior
anter/o

tissue death

a condition of cells

pertaining to paralysis

pertaining to formation or growth

hardening

pertaining to breathing

movement toward the side, away from the body

meal

toward or near the front; ventral

movement toward the side, toward the body

posterior
poster/o

base

apex

bilateral

unilateral

contralateral

ipsilateral

deep

superficial

horizontal adduction

the lower or supporting part of any structure

toward or near the back; dorsal

both sides

the pointed tip of a conical structure

the opposite side

one side

further into the body

the same side

movement of the arm toward the midline, or anterior, when at shoulder level

nearer to the surface of the body

horizontal abduction	medial medi/o
lateral later/o	eversion
inversion	flexion
extension	medial rotation
lateral rotation	pronation

toward the midline; nearer to the middle

movement of the arm away from midline, or posterior, when at shoulder level

movement of the ankle causing the bottom of the foot to face toward the side or laterally

away from the midline; toward the side

movement toward the front or anterior (exception at the knee joint)

movement of the ankle causing the bottom of the foot to face toward the midline or medially

movement of the shoulder or hip toward the midline; internal rotation

movement toward the back or posterior (exception at the knee joint)

rotation movement of the forearm to palm down; palm facing posterior

rotation movement of the shoulder or hip away from the midline; external

supination

protraction

retraction

proximal
proxim/o

distal
dist/o

radial deviation

ulnar deviation

superior
super/o

inferior
infer/o

supine

movement of the scapula away from the spinal column; scapular abduction

rotation movement of the forearm to palm up; palm facing anterior

nearer to the axial body

movement of the scapula toward the spinal column; scapular adduction

movement of the wrist toward the radius or away from the body; wrist abduction

further from the axial body

toward or nearer to the head; cranial

movement of the wrist toward the ulna or toward the body; wrist adduction

lying horizontally facing upward

toward or nearer to the feet: caudal

prone

ventral

dorsal

corne/o   **kerat/o**
kōr-nē-ō   kĕr-ăt-ōo

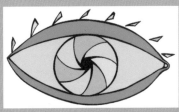

adip/o   **lip/o**   **steat/o**
ăd-ĭ-pō   lĭ-pō   stē-ă-tō

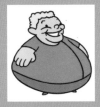

cutane/o   **derm/o**   **dermat/o**
kū-tā-nē-ō   dĕr-mō   dĕr-mă-tō

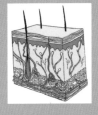

onych/o
ŏn-ĭ-kō

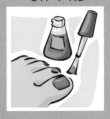

scler/o
sklĕ-rō

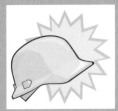

myc/o
mī-kō

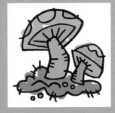

necr/o
nĕ-crō

front; anterior	lying horizontally facing downward
keratinized tissue, cornea	back; posterior
skin	fat
hardening, sclera	nail
dead	fungus

pil/o   trich/o
pī-lō   trĭ-kō

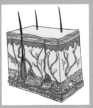

cyan/o
sī-ă-nō

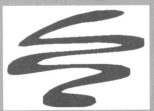

xer/o
zē-rō

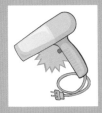

albin/o   leuk/o
ăl-bĭ-nō   loo-kō

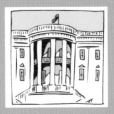

melan/o
mĕl-ă-nō

cirrh/o   xanth/o
sĭ-rō   zăn-thō

hydr/o
hī-drō

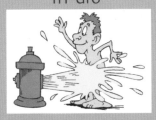

cyt/o
sī-tō

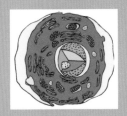

eti/o
ē-tē-ŏ

hidr/o
hī-drō

blue

hair

white

dry

yellow

black

posterior
(toward or near the back; dorsal)

water

sweat

cause

idi/o
ĭd-ē-ō

morph/o
mōr-fŏ

path/o
pă-thŏ

rhytid/o
rĭt-ĭ-dō

seb/o
sĕ-bō

son/o
sŏ-nō

chromat/o
krō-mă-tō

erythem/o   **erythr/o**
ĕr-ĭ-thēm-ō   ĕ-rĭth-rō

shape	unknown, peculiar
wrinkle	disease
sound	sebum
red	color